INNOVATIONS IN

HEALTHCARE DESIGN

INNOVATIONS IN
HEALTHCARE DESIGN

Selected Presentations from the First Five

Symposia on Healthcare Design

◆

◆

◆

◆

◆ Edited by SARA O. MARBERRY

Postscript by Wayne Ruga, AIA, IIDA, Allied Member ASID

JOHN WILEY & SONS, INC.

New York   Chichester   Weinheim   Brisbane   Singapore   Toronto

Cover design: *Jon Herder*

This publication is designed to provide accurate and authoritative
information in regard to the subject matter covered. It is sold with the
understanding that the publisher is not engaged in rendering professional
services. If professional advice or other expert assistance is required,
the services of a competent professional person should be sought.

Library of Congress Cataloging-in-Publication Data:
Symposium on Healthcare Design.
    Innovations in healthcare design : establishing a new paradigm :
selected presentations from the first five Symposia on Healthcare
Design / edited by Sara O. Marberry ; postscript by Wayne Ruga.
        p.   cm.
    Includes bibliographical references and index.
    ISBN 0-471-28637-0
    1. Health facilities—Design and construction—Congresses.
    2. Health facilities—Decoration—Congresses.   I. Marberry, Sara
O., 1959– .   II. Title.
725'.5—dc20   94-45677

Printed in the United States of America

10 9 8 7 6 5 4 3

CONTENTS

ACKNOWLEDGMENTS

I would like to thank the following individuals for allowing me to use their Symposium presentations in this book and supplying accompanying illustrations:

Edward Carter
Russell C. Coile, Jr.
Sue Baier
Margaret P. Calkins
Felicia Cleper-Borkovi, AIA
Martin H. Cohen, AIA
James Diaz, FAIA
Millicent Gappel, IFDA
Barbara Geddis, AIA
Richard Gerber, M.D.
Wanda J. Jones, M.P.H.
Mozhan Khadem
Neil Kellman, M.D. M. Arch.
Diana Kissil, AIA
Patrick E. Linton
Jain Malkin
Susan Mazer

Robin Nicholson, MA, MSc, RIBA
David Noferi
Anita Rui Olds
Helen G. Orem
Robin Orr, M.P.H.
Iqbal Paroo
Derek Parker, FAIA, RIBA
Thomas Payette, FAIA, RIBA
George Pressler, AIA
Annette Ridenour
Blair Salder
Dallas Smith
David Swain, AIA
Antonio Torrice/Ro Logrippo
Roger S. Ulrich, Ph.D.
Margaret Williams, R.N.

In addition, I would like to acknowledge the following individuals for their special support and encouragement:

Anne Fallucchi, editor emeritus of *Facilities Design & Management,* for giving my proposal her personal "thumbs up."

Dianne Davis, founder, Hospitality Healthcare Designs, for also giving my proposal a "thumbs up."

Wendy Lochner, senior editor at VNR, for getting the book approved and under way quickly.

Richard Marberry, my husband, for his legal advice and ongoing love.

Wayne Ruga, president and CEO, The Center for Health Design, for his vision and friendship, and for graciously giving me the rights to use this material.

My association with the National Symposium on Healthcare Design began in 1987 when I was a senior editor with *Contract* magazine (now called *Contract Design*). While at a reception at the San Francisco Merchandise Mart, I was approached by a small, soft-spoken man who introduced himself as Wayne Ruga. He began to tell me about a symposium he was planning for the following April on healthcare design, which would bring together design professionals, healthcare executives, and product manufacturers to talk about how the design of the physical environment could positively affect health and well-being.

I listened intently and told him what every editor tells people who approach them with information, "Send me something on it when you have more specifics."

Little did I know that this (to quote the final line from the movie *Casablanca*) would be the "beginning of a beautiful friendship" that would prove to be professionally, as well as personally, rewarding. Not only did Wayne send me something, but he also enlisted my support by inviting me to become a member of the Symposium's Advisory Council. Subsequently he asked me to be the "emcee" of the First Symposium in April 1988 at the La Costa Hotel and Spa in Carlsbad, California.

Since then, I have emceed five more Symposia; been named to The Center for Health Design's (which produces the Symposium) Board of Directors and Executive Committee; served as its communications consultant; and edited the Symposium's quarterly newsletter, *Æsclepius*, as well as four volumes of the *Journal of Healthcare Design* (the taped proceedings from each Symposia).

I have watched Wayne plant the seeds, as he did with me at our first meeting, with many others, enlisting their support to help "grow" his dream and share in his conviction that the design of the physical environment can positively affect the quality of healthcare. His biggest reward from all of this, I believe, has been his ability to empower others to explore new avenues for professional achievement and growth.

Such is the case with me. My involvement with The Center and Symposium has profoundly changed my life and influenced the direction of my work. It has given me a deeper understanding of design as an integral part of human life—an essential component of our physical, mental, and spiritual needs. Its importance in the healthcare environment, in which those needs are intensified, cannot be underestimated, and should not be under-utilized.

So, this book is a collection of 24 presentations by various professionals who share those same beliefs and have translated them into their work. Ninety-one other presentations from past Symposia are documented in the *Journal of Healthcare Design, Volumes I-V,* from which these 24 were selected. Unfortunately, there are many fine presentations that I could not include in this book.

Unlike the *Journals*, however, this book offers illustrations and is intended to provide an overview of the issues central to healthcare design today. In addition, it offers many fine models and examples (hence, the title *New Paradigms*) that can, and are, being put into place.

Most of the presentations in this book were edited from transcribed audio tapes; a few are papers that were written specifically for publication. It has been my experience that readers find the translation from the spoken word to the written word acceptable, even though the presenters often complain!

The idea for this book, of course, came from Wayne, who I asked to write a Postscript to outline the next steps to achieve a desired future for healthcare design. His insightful views come at the end of what I hope will prove to be one of the most enriching and rewarding reading experiences of healthcare design currently in publication.

Sara O. Marberry

◆

◆

◆

◆

◆ Chapter

ONE

N E W   P O S S I B I L I T I E S

THE OUTLOOK FOR HEALTHCARE DESIGN IN THE ERA OF REFORM

Russell C. Coile, Jr.

Editor's Note: Mr. Coile's presentation titled "New Possibilities" at the Fourth Symposium on Healthcare Design in Boston, 1991, was updated in December 1993 for this book.

Sweeping reforms in American public policy and the healthcare marketplace will restructure America's hospitals and medical care settings between now and the 21st century. The social goal of universal coverage for health insurance is likely to be enacted, enabling some 30 to 40 million Americans to have full access to physician and hospital services. But the additional costs, estimated at more than $300 million in the first five years, could place major new restrictions and payment controls on the U.S. health industry.

What will be the impact of these trends for health facility construction, one of the economy's most recession-resistant sectors of the design–build field? And will financial pressures retard a promising trend toward the design of "healing environments" in hospitals and health facilities? There are no certain answers, but early trends signal the directions the future may take for healthcare and design.

Trend #1: Health Reform Enactment

The Health Security Act is the most sweeping new venture in social policy in half a century. President Bill Clinton and Hillary Rodham Clinton personally delivered the 1336-page proposal to Congressional leaders on October 27, 1993, providing long-awaited details for a fundamental restructuring of America's $900 billion healthcare industry (Devroy and Priest, 1993). Now the real health debate begins, with dozens of Congressional hearings, competing proposals, and partisanship. At stake is the future of American healthcare, the nation's 5500 community hospitals and 600,000 physicians. What will be decided is whether the U.S. can afford to extend basic health insurance to the 37 million Americans who lack coverage, despite the fact that we are already spending 14 percent of the gross domestic product on healthcare.

Whatever passes will be a patchwork quilt of compromises that may bear little resemblance to the recommendations of the 500-member White House task force headed by Mrs. Clinton. Five weeks after the President's initial launch of the health reform proposal, the revised plan to overhaul America's $900 billion health industry has already undergone significant revisions:

- "Capped entitlements" will limit government subsidies to small businesses and early retirees.
- More small businesses will qualify for subsidies as the definition of a "small business" was raised in size from 50 to 75 employees.
- Regulatory powers of state-run purchasing alliances have been scaled back.
- States can more easily choose a "single-payor" system to satisfy Congressional Democrats who prefer the Canadian model.
- Financing of the plan has been clarified and the amount of deficit reduction cut to $58 billion.

The prediction? There will be health reform but perhaps not universal coverage. Lawmakers may exempt the smallest employers and phase-in coverage for others over three to five years. Congress will ease Medicare cuts by adding other revenue sources, such as taxes on insurance premiums or provider revenues. Some of the expensive "goodies" Mr. Clinton promised may be cut back, including the early retirees subsidy as well as new drug and long-term benefits for the elderly (Wartzman and Stout, 1993). Details will be left to the states.

Implications for Healthcare Design: Industry observers are trying to calculate the "winners" and "losers" under health reform. General acute hospitals face a financial threat and will be losers, assuming that substantial Medicare cuts are part of reform's financing package. Medicare reimbursement for capital has already been restricted and could be eliminated. Psychiatric hospitals may feel the pinch, too, if the 30-day limit on psychiatric stays is enacted. But ambulatory care should grow and be a winner under health reform. The Clintons give strong emphasis to primary care. Long-term care may be another reform beneficiary with incremental expansion under the Clinton health plan.

Trend #2: The "Hillary Effect"

Hillary Rodham Clinton's health reform plan is already making an impact on the nation's $900 billion health industry—lower inflation, empty hospital beds, and declining use rates for healthcare services. Medical care prices are falling and demand is slipping across the nation. The earliest evidence of the Hillary Effect is reflected in the mid-1993 rate of medical care inflation as measured by the Consumer Price Index. The slowdown in health inflation has yielded the lowest provider price increases in more than a decade, less than twice the overall CPI.

Thanks to Hillary Clinton, employer health costs are dropping fast. The average employer's health benefits costs rose only eight percent in 1993, the smallest increase in six years (Memmott, 1993). Health insurance benefits costs rose 11 percent in 1992, according to KMPG Peat Marwick's survey of 1000 employers with more than 200 workers. Health insurance prices are moderating as insurers try to avoid being the symbolic targets of reformers. Mrs. Clinton publicly lashed out at insurers in November over an antireform television campaign sponsored by the Health Insurance Association of America (HIAA). The President joined the counterattack on the insurers, promising that the Clinton reform plan would "limit the extent to which you can be gouged in a system over which you have no control" (Jehl, 1993). The Clinton attack puts the spotlight on health insurers, which should hold down premium increases in 1994.

Implications for Healthcare Design: Uncertainty surrounding health reform is already having a "chilling" impact on decisions about new health facilities projects. Although healthcare construction spending held level at $11.3 billion in 1992, only projects in the pipeline are sustaining capital investment now. Designers and architects report that many clients have placed major projects on hold, awaiting clearer signals from Washington about health reform.

Trend #3: Networks

Tomorrow's regional healthcare delivery system will be a "network" of hospitals, physicians, and insurance partners who provide comprehensive health services to thousands of enrollees on a capitated basis. Networks are the next step toward fully integrated regional delivery systems. Business arrangements—not asset-based mergers—will link network participants in a "seamless" web of care (Kenkel, 1993a).

Employers like networks because they retain employee choice. Point-of-service (POS) plans incorporate broader choice of providers. Although only 11 percent of employers offer POS plans today, compared with 61 percent of companies with HMO plans, the number of POS options is growing rapidly (Mandelker, 1993). The University of Vermont introduced an HMO in 1987, but signed up only 100 employees, the rest staying with the college's generous indemnity plan. Costs rose 14 to 15 percent per year. So the University eliminated its indemnity plan in July 1993 and switched to POS, estimating a cost savings of 25 percent.

Cost saving performance like this will be the test of networks. Can these loosely structured arrangements deliver high-quality, low-cost services? More important, can network participants equitably share a limited capitation payment without fighting or self-interested behaviors? Their problems will include:

- Limited experience in managing patients under capitation.
- Attempts to keep hospital beds full with network patients.
- Motivating physicians to practice collegially in groups.
- Lack of shared vision and common management control.
- Inadequate information systems and clinical guidelines.

Implications for Healthcare Design: Healthcare designers' newest customers may be networks. These new organizations will need to quickly find and furnish corporate offices, but that is only the beginning. Networks will oversee the development of regional primary care networks, located in new ambulatory care centers, outpatient surgery centers, and medical office buildings. Networks will also drive the consolidation of hospitals and high-tech facilities into fewer, strategically located sites. Networks are likely to identify one hospital as their regional hub and concentrate tertiary services in a single location—eg., open-heart procedures, cancer care, and hand surgery.

Trend #4: Payor/Provider Integration

An emerging trend in payor/provider integration will bring America's healthcare provider into a new, closer relationship with HMOs and insurers. Payors are switching tactics from strong-arm contracting to joint ventures, acquisitions, and mergers. The largest payor/provider merger was the announcement of a deal between California Blue Shield and Burbank-based UniHealth in mid-1993, although technical issues ultimately frustrated the unification effort.

In managed care hotbed Minneapolis–St. Paul, Minnesota, Blue Cross and Blue Shield are developing a partnership with the Aspen Medical Group, a 120-doctor primary care organization. An agreement with Aspen would service Blue Cross/Shield enrollees out of Aspen's eight locations in the St. Paul/East Metro market (*Health Care Competition Week,* 1993). More payor/provider deals are likely in the Twin Cities, as providers and insurers gear up for implementation of "Minnesota Care," the state's health reform initiative scheduled to go into effect in July 1994. In another Twin Cities transaction, Health Partners of Minneapolis, a large staff-model HMO, announced merger plans with Ramsey HealthCare, the one-time county hospital, which operates a hospital and clinics in St. Paul (Sardinha, 1993).

Implications for Healthcare Design: Integrated payor/provider networks will grow quickly in the 1990s. Much of this growth will be in ambulatory care. To attract and serve thousands of enrolled consumers, network-building will focus on the strategic deployment of ambulatory care clinics and medical offices, which will house dozens to hundreds of employed physicians across a region or state.

Trend #5: Capitation

The Clinton health reform plan will plunge hospitals and physicians into the world of capitation. Most providers are unprepared for the risks of capitation. This prepaid reimbursement strategy pays providers a preset fee to provide all covered health services. It sounds simple. If providers cannot accurately estimate their costs, or control them, the providers lose money. Keep costs and utilization down, and make money.

Capitation is more complex than fee-for-service payment. This means managing the delivery of patient care in a way that produces cost-effective clinical outcomes. States like California and Minnesota are way ahead in organizing for capitation. The most important asset is a large medical group practice that practices conservatively. That occurs when more than one-third of a medical group's revenues come from capitation, according to James Hillman, CEO of the Unified Medical Group Practice Association, a California-based trade association for physician groups that deal only with prepaid healthcare (de LaFuente, 1993). Successful group practices have found that capitated managed care requires specialized management and information systems, practice guidelines, incentives, and a strong medical director.

Managing capitated patients is risky business. Successful capitation captures huge cash-flow streams and tightly manages hospital and medical expenses. Organizations such as the Mullikin Medical Centers of Artesia, California, channeled $274 million in revenues in 1992 to its 400 doctors and hospitals. Mullikin operates its own hospital, 94-bed Pioneer Hospital, and has recently created a strategic affiliation with the Daughters of Charity Health System in southern California. Other providers are following Mullikin's lead. In Chicago, the Lutheran General Health Plan, a 483-doctor Independent Practice Association has achieved hospital use rates in the low 200s per 1000 covered lives, well below the area average of 300–350 per 1000 enrollees (Droste, 1993).

Implications for Healthcare Design: Taking capitation contracts places physicians and hospitals together in risk-sharing ventures. Successful organizations like Mullikin operate dozens of small ambulatory care clinics, with four to ten physicians per site. These medical offices are built for group practice. Hospital use is strongly controlled. Mullikin owns a small hospital, and its inpatient utilization rates are among the lowest in the nation. Under capitation, some hospitals will close, while others will downsize. Hospital and health system clients may ask their architects and builders to share capitation arrangements, as clients demand that new or remodeled facilities be efficient.

Trend #6: Primary Care Networks

The success of healthcare reform may depend upon whether primary care networks can be organized to provide routine health services and manage referrals to costly specialists. Today's medical schools will produce only 6100 family practice residents in the next five years. The American Medical Association predicts that one in four physicians will practice in primary care by the year 2000—only half what managed care experts predict will be needed (Kenkel, 1993b).

Hospitals and health systems are rushing to acquire medical group practices in preparation for health reform and managed care. This is not just a California trend. In Tupelo, Mississippi, the state's largest hospital and rural referral center has signed an affiliation with the state's second largest multispeciality group practice (Greene, 1993). A new foundation will be created by 685-bed North Mississippi Medical Center and Internal Medical Associates, a 22-doctor group practice.

Primary care networks will succeed only if they boost pay for family practitioners. Even in HMOs, primary care doctors averaging $100,000 per year make one-third less than cardiologists and half the salary of orthopedists. HMOs, group practices, and hospitals are increasing compensation to attract primary care doctors. In some HMOs, primary care physicians may receive bonuses of up to 40 percent, depending upon how well they control costs (Kenkel, 1993b). California-based Capp Care is introducing a new physician payment program based on Medicare's RBRVS (Resource-Based Relative Value System), which gives greater financial rewards to primary care doctors over specialists.

Implications for Healthcare Design: The development of primary care networks is another confirmation of the shift to ambulatory care. For healthcare designers and builders, the message is that the restructuring of American medicine is going to require the construction of thousands of new medical office buildings, built for high-volume primary care and multispeciality group practices.

Trend #7: Physician-Hospital Organizations

To participate in managed care and health reform, hospitals and physicians must integrate their services and finances. Without shared market clout, doctors and hospitals will be vendors at the mercy of more powerful HMOs, insurers, and government purchasers. A majority of hospitals and their physicians understand the need for integration; 57 percent of the 249 hospitals surveyed by TriBrook have initiated PHO developments (Melville, 1993).

In Maryland, CEO Robert Pezzoli of Baltimore's St. Agnes is designing an alliance of physicians, hospitals, and healthcare companies capable of serving an enrolled population of two million (Meisol, 1993). Pezzoli convinced 225 St. Agnes physicians to organize for capitation and bid for patients in package deals with insurers. This is an all-new market: "It's the Wild West of

Medicine," says J.D. Kleinke, a principal with HICA, a Baltimore-based analyst of Medicare cost data. He means Baltimore is becoming like California—an intensely competitive managed care market. St. Agnes bought a free-standing ambulatory surgery center and is offering surgery at prices from 11 to 29 percent below market rates. The hospital and doctors group closed five deals with HMOs and insurers in October. Baltimore analysts predict that 100 percent of Maryland physicians will be involved in similar managed care arrangements in five years, up from 25 percent today.

When PHOs take on capitation contracts, hospitals need to understand how the PHO will make money—by reducing hospitalization. Under capitation, hospital care is a cost, not a revenue. The PHO wants to see hospital beds empty, not full. One of the new rules of the game is that "hospitalization must be looked at as a failure of the system," according to John McDonald, chief executive of Mullikin Medical Centers, one of the most cost-effective medical groups in the United States (Kenkel, 1993). McDonald states: "If the hospital is paid on a per diem or a case rate basis, the incentives aren't aligned with the medical providers who are working like crazy (under capitation) to try to keep the patients out of the hospital."

Implications for Healthcare Design: As hospitals and physicians move into vertically organized healthcare networks, the hospital campus will be a focal point for development. New medical offices will be needed, because from 35 to 50 percent of a hospital's physicians may practice on campus. Satellite ambulatory campuses will feature ambulatory surgical centers and high-volume, group-practice medical offices.

Trend #8: Clinical Efficiency

How will hospitals and physicians possibly "do more for less" under health reform and managed care? The answer is clinical efficiency. Managing the pattern of medical care will be the most important strategy for cost containment in the 1990s. Clinical efficiency is essential under capitation. Once provider payments are capped by capitation, there is no way to "game the system" by unbundling services, upcoding discharges to increase revenues, or providing marginally necessary tests or procedures.

ScrippsHealth's "CareTrac" program closely monitors patient care using a set of preestablished clinical guidelines (Buser, 1993). Since CareTrac was implemented by the San Diego-based health system in 1992, overall hospital charges have been reduced by 21 percent. This care management system is very efficient. Length of stay has been cut 19 percent and intensive care unit patients average less than one-day stays in the expensive critical care units.

Scripps physicians put patients on predetermined regimes. Nurses monitor patient progress using a preestablished charting system. Patients and families are involved, too, reviewing completed medical "tasks" on their own. Everyone is enthusiastic about the new approach. Nurse charting time has been reduced by 50 percent. Physicians believe their patients receive more predictable care. Patients and families are better informed and less anxious, because expectations about the care process and outcomes are clarified.

Implications for Healthcare Design: The search for clinical efficiency is driving a new wave of hospital remodeling, as health facilities are redesigned to make care processes more efficient and low cost. Experiments with "patient-focused care" in dozens of hospitals show promise. With the decentralization of many ancillary services, for example, costs are reduced when routine diagnostic tests and X-rays can be run in minifacilities on the patient floor. Putting a pharmacist in the surgical suite and on patient units has generated more savings, as well as improving quality. These experiments will result in new configurations for inpatient and ambulatory facilities, both new construction and remodeling.

Trend #9: Managed Care Dominance

The solutions to the nation's healthcare crisis are already evident—managed care plans. If the Clinton health plan is successful, it will "hitch Hillary's wagon" to managed care. The shift to managed care is now a certainty. HMO and PPO enrollment nears 100 million covered lives (Table 1–1). National enrollment in HMOs reached 43.7 million at the end of 1992 and is expected to reach 52 million by the end of 1994, as HMOs grow eight percent per year (Henderson, 1993). According to the SMG Marketing Group of Chicago, another 58 million people are eligible for Preferred Provider Organizations. PPOs and Point of Service (POS) Plans grew 24 percent in 1991 and 34 percent in 1992. This is a national trend. In 19 states, more than 15 percent of the population are enrolled in an HMO (InterStudy, 1993).

SMG's John Henderson predicts a consolidation among types of managed care plans. The biggest health plans will dominate the managed care market.

◆ **TABLE 1–1** National enrollment in HMOs is expected to reach 55 million by the end of 1995. (*Chart design:* Glenn Ruga.)

FORECAST OF MANAGED CARE ENROLLMENT
(IN MILLIONS)

PAYOR TYPE	1990	1992	1995
HMO (Traditional)	36	39	47
HMO-POS	2	5	8
PPO	19	26	33
Indeminity (managed)	80	70	59
Indeminity (traditional)	22	17	6
Medicare (non-HMO)	32	33	33
Medicare (HMO)	1	3	7
Medicaid	21	22	25
Medical Uninsured	34	37	25
National Health Reform?	0	0	15
TOTAL	**247**	**252**	**258**

Source: SMG Marketing Group, *SMG Marketing Letter,* August 1993.

By the end of 1992, the ten largest HMOs had a total enrollment of 28 million, covering two out of three HMO members. National health reform will be an HMO. Multistate HMOs and PPOs will evolve into national, integrated health plans (IHPs) covering as much as 65 percent of the non-Medicare population by the year 2000.

Implications for Healthcare Design: If healthcare designers want to see the future under managed care, look at California's Kaiser health plan. The nation's largest HMO operates in more than a dozen states, serving more than seven million enrollees. Kaiser is a "staff" (salaried physicians) model. Its doctors are organized and housed in large multispeciality clinics. Kaiser is expanding its ambulatory care facilities. Most Kaiser clinics house at least 10–15 physicians. Larger medical clinics are staffed by hundreds of doctors, with high-volume adult and pediatric walk-in clinics that provide most of the urgent care in the system, instead of emergency rooms. Kaiser is building four new "gateway" hospitals in California that will be low-tech facilities in new markets where there are not enough enrollees to justify a full-service hospital of 200–300 beds.

Trend #10: Demand Reduction

Managed care will shift from cost/utilization management to demand reduction strategies as capitation becomes the new form of reimbursement. "Demand reduction" programs encourage healthier enrollees who don't require as many services or expensive treatments. Hospital interest is resurging in health promotion and wellness. In October 1993, a conference sponsored by the Riverside Health System drew over 300 participants to Williamsburg, Virginia, to see the latest models in hospital-sponsored wellness programs.

In California, the HealthTrac program is a joint venture with California Blue Shield. The program provides customized health education and counseling to enrollees. Evaluation of pilot efforts with the Bank of America show promising results in lowering the overall costs of care through health promotion. HealthTrac is marketing nationally to partner with insurers and self-insured employers. The trend in corporate wellness programs is toward more comprehensive efforts (Haughie, 1993).

Implications for Healthcare Design: Is the hospital of the future a health club? No, but most hospitals will have rehabilitation and fitness facilities. So will comprehensive ambulatory care centers. But the emphasis on health promotion and demand reduction is only part of a wider trend toward redesigning health facilities as healing environments that promote quality of life. The challenge for healthcare designers is to build spaces that actively promote a sense of well-being and security for patients. (Conclusion: It's hard to believe that hospitals are still building hospitals!)

Despite the arrival of national health reform and managed care, a majority (58.6 percent) of the nation's hospitals are planning expansions or renovations now (Melville, 1994). (See Table 1–2.) They don't get it. Managed care is driving hospital use down. Patient days may drop by 25 percent in the next five to seven years. Wall Street healthcare analyst Ken Abramowitz predicts that hospital occupancy will fall from 62 percent today to from 57 to 60 percent in the next five years (Abramowitz, 1993).

Why are they doing this when the future demand for hospital beds is likely to decline? "For the very reason they fear they will be worse off, they are

◆ **TABLE 1–2** Despite the arrival of national health reform and managed care, a majority of the nation's hospitals were planning expansions or renovations in 1993. (*Chart design: Glenn Ruga.*)

MOST HOSPITALS ARE PLANNING/CONSTRUCTING FACILITIES

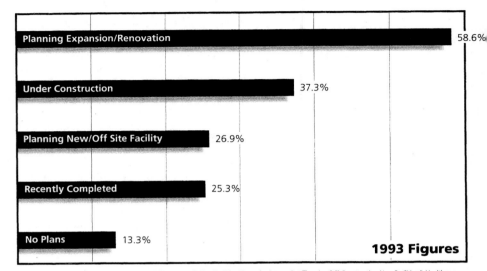

Planning Expansion/Renovation — 58.6%
Under Construction — 37.3%
Planning New/Off Site Facility — 26.9%
Recently Completed — 25.3%
No Plans — 13.3%

1993 Figures

Source: TriBrook Group, 1993, cited in Beth Melville, "Hospitals May Be Grim About the Future, But They Are Still Constructing New Facilities." *Healthcare Competition Week*, September 17, 1993.

moving forward with plans for the marketplace as they envision it a couple of months or years from now," says consultant Douglas Rich of TriBrook Group of Westmont, Illinois. Concerns about the future are causing many hospitals to accelerate making facilities investments, according to a survey of hospital executives (Melville, 1993). Although half of the hospitals are building new facilities, fewer than one in four (24.9 percent) have accelerated their strategic planning, while uncertainty has slowed planning in 21.2 percent of the facilities.

America's hospitals already have a glut of excess capacity. Nearly 40 percent of the nation's hospital beds are empty every day. Additional debt is the last thing hospitals need as they seek managed care contracts. Managed care buyers are looking for low-cost providers. Taking on heavy debt service in this market makes little sense.

Hospitals should be making strategic investments today in these critical areas:

- Building a primary care network
- Information systems
- Equity stake in HMOs
- Purchasing physician practices
- Expanding ambulatory care capacity
- Multihospital regional network

The TriBrook survey found a pall of pessimism in the outlooks of America's healthcare executives. More than one-third of the CEOs were not hopeful about the future of the hospital industry. So they are speeding up capital investments, hoping to get projects completed "under the wire" when health reform and managed care may close the door on hospital borrowing. The failure to plan is the most serious deficiency found in the TriBrook study. Today is exactly when hospitals should be planning for tomorrow. Shortsighted facilities are building facilities. Wrong! They should be preparing for capitation, organizing doctors, and building high-volume ambulatory care facilities.

Sources/Readings

Abramowitz, Kenneth S. 1993. Data Point to Problems, Opportunities for Hospitals over Next Five Years. *Strategies for Healthcare Excellence* 6(10): 10–11.

Buser, Martin. 1993. Pre-Established Care Guides Patients to Recovery. *California Hospitals* 7(4): 10–12. July-August.

de LaFuente, Donna. 1993. Considering the Risks of Change. *Modern Healthcare.* 23(40): 53–59. Oct. 4.

Devroy, Ann, and Priest, Dana. 1993. Clinton Health Bill Opens Hill Debate. *Washington Post,* Oct. 28: A1, A19.

Droste, Therese M. 1993. Midwest Maverick Is Ahead of the Integration Game. *Medical Staff Strategy Report* 2(10): 1–5.

Findlay, Steven. 1993. Eleven Steps to Health Reform. *Business & Health.* 11(11): 26–32. Mid-September.

Greene, Jay. 1993. Two Large Mississippi Providers to Affiliate. *Modern Healthcare* 23(37): 28. Sept. 13.

Harwood, John. 1993. Rival Plans Gain Strength But None Claims Majority. *Wall Street Journal,* Oct. 28: A18.

Haughie, Glenn E. 1993. Corporate Wellness Programs: Are They a Cost-Effective Benefit? *Pension World,* July.

Health Care Competition Week. 1993. Minnesota Blue Cross and Medical Group Forming Integrated Delivery Network, 10(18): 10. Sept. 17.

Henderson, John A. 1993. Not Waiting for Reform: Managed Care Takes Charge. *SMG Market Letter,* 7(7): 1–5. August.

InterStudy. 1993. The InterStudy Competitive Edge, Aug.; cited in *Medical Benefits,* 10(17): 2–3. Sept. 15.

Jehl, Douglas. 1993. Clinton Joins Counterattack on Insurers' TV Ads. *New York Times,* Nov. 4: A13.

Kenkel, Paul J. 1993a. Filling Up Beds Is No Longer the Name of the System Game. *Modern Healthcare* 23(37): 39–48. Sept. 13.

———. 1993b. Primary Doctors Vital to Reform, Health Plans. *Modern Healthcare* 23(37): 42. Sept. 13.

Mandelker, Jeannie. 1993. Employers Shun HMOs to Retain Employee Choice. *Business & Health,* 11(11): 20–24. Mid-September.

Meisol, Patricia. 1993. St. Agnes: Fighting Back. *Baltimore Sun,* Oct. 24: 1D, 6D.

Melville, Beth. 1993. Hospitals May Be Grim About the Future, But They're Still Constructing New Facilities. *Health Care Competition Week,* 10(18): 4–5. Sept. 17.

Memmott, Mark. 1993. Health Inflation Slows, But Still Above Inflation. *USA Today,* Oct. 25: B1.

Sardinha, Carol. 1993a. MCO Merger Madness, Spurred by Reform, Shows No Signs of Abating. *Managed Care Outlook,* 6(18): 1–3. Sept. 24.

———. 1993b. Tighter UR, New Doc Practice Patterns Boost HMO Profits. *Managed Care Outlook* 6(18): 3–4. Sept. 24.

Stout, Hilary, and Wartzman, Rick. 1993. Clinton Submits Health Bill to

Congress; and Handicapping Begins on What Will Be Scrapped First. *Wall Street Journal*. Oct. 28: A18.

Wolf, Richard, and Hasson, Judi. 1993. Congress Readies for Surgery. *USA Today*, Oct. 27: 3A.

Futurist Russell C. Coile, Jr., is the president of the Health Forecasting Group of Santa Clarita, California. His latest books are Revolution *(Whittle Books/Grand Rounds Press, 1993) on the future of medicine, and* The New Governance *(Health Administration Press, 1994) on strategies and models for hospital trustees.*

◆ ◆ ◆

ACUTE CARE DESIGN: EMERGING TRENDS

Fifth Symposium on Healthcare Design, San Diego, 1992

Wanda J. Jones, M.P.H.

To understand emerging trends in healthcare facilities, one should explore the sociology, economics, philosophy, psychology, anthropology, and humor of hospital development and design.

Many healthcare professionals went through graduate school learning how to deal with physician psychology, what kind of nursing schools to support, and how Medicare reimbursement worked. Then, as soon as managers began working, an administrator would say, "You're in charge of the building program." With no preparation, managers learned about contracts, about what sewers do to site planning when they run right under a hospital, and many other things managers were never trained to know.

Managers, also, in many states, were captured by a "Certificate of Need (CON) psychology." A CON mindset involves a very short mental time span in which hospital administrators look three years back, and only three years forward, as well as strive to "game" the regulatory system as best they can. Executives concentrated on licensed beds as the rich asset to control and develop; complying with norms is a means to that end. The result of CON psychology is that new hospitals tend to look like older ones.

Managers in acute care share a cultural mindset that includes an idea of what a hospital is supposed to look like. As difficult as it may be, current managers should set aside preconceptions of what a hospital is and decide to think anew, plan anew, and decide anew. As the Fifth Symposium's keynote speaker, Jeff Goldsmith, stated, "The future healthcare paradigm is vastly different from the one we know now." It is easy to forget that hospitals last a long time. Most managers plan them to solve today's space needs. While accomplishing that goal, many hospital designs also "freeze-in" today's organizational patterns. Hospital administrators and their staffs share a medical culture bias toward consensus-building that is expressed through asking teams of people at the operating level to deal with day-to-day or month-to-month issues and annual budgets. Every seven to 15 years, however, a similar team will be asked to plan for a facility that may last 40 or more years and cause the generation of many millions of dollars of operating expenses. Such planning calls for perspective—a willingness to make a grand change worthy of the future value of the project and to take risks that are normally "bred out" of daily hospital life.

It is worth the task of putting the vast sweep of historical changes in hospital design in perspective to appreciate the dimensions of the changes to which current projects should adapt.

A *Historical Perspective*

Healthcare had no separate structure for thousands of years before the Middle Ages; the temple and the home were the principal places of healing.

The Crusades from the 11th through the 13th centuries saw the advent of professional nursing. At first, women who were the caregivers for children went on the Children's Crusade. When they returned from the Crusades, these women, if they survived, became nuns and fulfilled their nursing role in convents associated with cathedrals. So there is a long history of nurses associated with a physical place with a religious sponsorship, caring both for local residents and traveling pilgrims.

After the plagues of the 14th century that inaugurated the first national public health efforts and quarantines, the next big turning point for healthcare was the Crimean War. In Crimea, Florence Nightingale gained fame for her nursing skills. At the end of the war Nightingale became committed to designing hospitals, because up until that time hospitals often had been converted from homes, public buildings, or sometimes even stables. Some hospitals were asylums that were nothing more than jails for people considered public health risks. Nightingale devised a series of concepts that had to do with light, air, and cleanliness. Her basic design for an open patient care pavilion with windows is still the model today, even as the number of patients per room has gradually declined.

At the turn of the 20th century, X-rays, antiseptics, and anesthesia brought a totally new capability to hospitals—that of technically assisted diagnosis and treatment. Prior to this, hospitals were for infectious diseases, childbirth, and for crude, unsupported surgery, such as amputations without anesthesia. There have been "built-to-suit" hospitals in America since Ben Franklin built one in Philadelphia, but they were generally only places in which the care and comfort of the patient was seen to by nurses associated with the building. Physicians had offices in their homes and treated most people in the patients' own homes; they did give volunteer time to patients in the hospital. The separation between the surgeon and the nurse associated with the cathedral, home, or special place of asylum has remained with us in the form of the separate organizational structure of the hospital medical staff.

In many ways, the two-branched hospital organization has been dysfunctional; fortunately we are beginning to move away from it. Recently, El Camino Hospital in Mountain View, California, voted to create a corporate structure that put a portion of the medical and hospital staff together in a single risk-sharing corporation, a trend now well underway in the United States.

The space age that flowered in the 1960s was another turning point in hospital design. Electronic devices developed for NASA included CRTs (cathode ray tubes) for monitors and imaging devices. Spaces were added in the lower floors of hospitals for those devices, in newly organized departments.

Today, the weight of economics, social values, and futurist ideas necessitates a reassessment of this series of "gifts" of history. Some of these gifts

◆ **FIGURE 1–1** Attempts to reform healthcare delivery are working against a strong pull from the past, a stronger pull than a desired future.

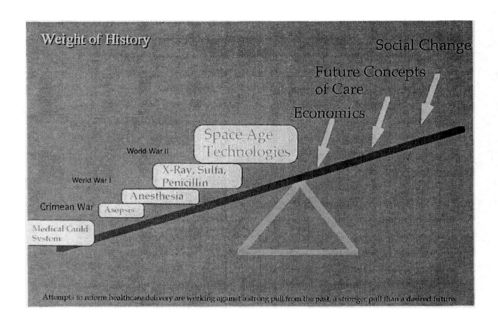

have become liabilities. The reasons for original design are important; if they are understood, it will be easier to decide whether the reasons apply today. If not, new designs should be created (Figure 1–1).

The Old Forms

Old hospital forms were "opportunistic" spaces, or essentially anything available. Such hospitals offered only shelter, food, and maybe some cleanliness.

Florence Nightingale-inspired wards were long, low pavilions connected by corridors, with open bays and windows on both sides. Wards were often designated not by specialty or disease, but by the attending physicians, or by the sex of the patient (Figure 1–2).

The so-called modern hospital can be said to have begun with the invention of the elevator. In some hospital projects, the size of the elevator core was the central design issue. One example is a hospital with a pristine, 30-acre campus that had a 200-bed facility centered on the site. An addition was being planned by the architect to proceed perpendicularly from the front door. When asked why he chose to disturb the entrance to the hospital rather than locate this addition to the side, he said, "Well, if we just bridge over to the hospital we can keep the same elevator core." He would, of course, have created chaos within the whole structure for several years and eventually crammed too much traffic through that elevator core.

Elevators allowed the stacking of the Nightingale pavilion (Figure 1–3). The central elevator core determined the size of nursing units, influencing travel distances for nurses. In early elevator-influenced hospital design, there was no base block, only a bed tower. New equipment and/or diagnostic services were placed within the vertical envelope by "cannibalizing" space.

By the late 1950s and early 1960s, a vertical tower with no base block was too restrictive. There were too many special purpose services to be housed. So, the base block began to grow horizontally, then from one story, to two,

◆ **FIGURE 1–2** Florence
Nightingale-inspired wards were
long, low pavilions connected by
corridors, with open bays and
windows on both sides.

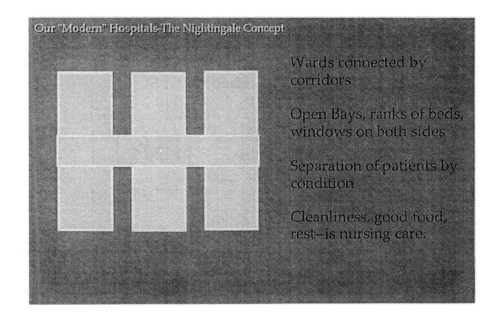

three, or four, plus one or two basement levels. In the 1970s and 1980s, the
tower began to be uncoupled from the base block, either to the side, or on
ground level in two or more segments. But the separation of base block activities and nursing floors persisted, causing patients to traverse ever longer
distances during each stay. In the 1990s, it is apparent that the ability to extend the base block to accommodate everything that hospitals use for diagnosis and treatment is exceeding hospitals' ability to handle patient travel logistics.

When patients are admitted to a modern hospital, they are brought to a

◆ **FIGURE 1–3** Elevators allowed
the stacking of the Nightingale
pavilion.

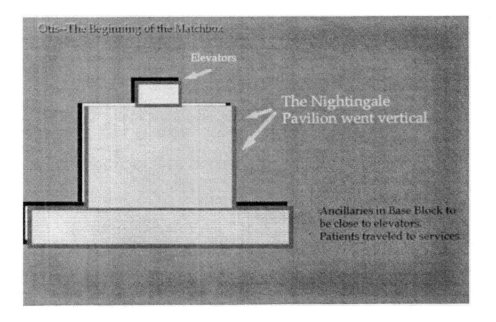

patient room, then almost immediately brought down to the base block for service, then taken back up to their room; back down to the base block, up to the room, down to the base block, etc. The average patient changes his or her room assignment four times in a typical admission. An estimated 40 percent of nursing hours are used to manage patient logistics, labor is overly subdivided.

U.S. hospitals are poised for a new cycle of construction related to earlier "waves" of new construction with the subsequent aging of hospitals.

During the World Wars, the United States tended not to build any new structures. Civilian investment was deferred, because investments were made in military hardware. So immediately after each war, hospital construction accelerated. The Hill-Burton Program that started in 1946 and remained in operation into the early 1970s was responsible for much of the building in the suburbs, to support the housing constructed for returning veterans. If we consider hospitals to have a 40-year life, we can anticipate that the 1990s will be a period of major replacement of hospitals built immediately after World War II. Because hospital demand is declining, ambulatory care is increasing, and medical care is very different from 40 years ago, new hospitals should be totally re-thought.

Doing Things Differently

What would a 1990s hospital administration do differently? First of all, the operating system (how patient care is organized) should be redesigned in basic ways. In a future-oriented operating system, routine services are brought to the bed cluster so that patient travel is reduced, the number of separate people associated with patient care is reduced, and the idea of departments is replaced with the concept of professional function and support functions.

Ancillary departments are artifacts of history. Much of the reason why we have excessive departmentalism is that there is physician specialization around a single service or procedure. Nuclear medicine is nuclear medicine. It is not general X-ray. When that service is added, an office for the physician and space to perform the service is added. The physician is in charge of his budget, his staff, his space, and so on. Department space planning is controlled by the department head; no one in the old hospital planning process considered how the total collection of departments functioned from the standpoint of patients.

Departmentalism is choking us to death. There are hospitals with 50 or more department heads. Why? This number is not needed for span of control or management. Managers think they have separate departments because of the narrowness of knowledge specialization. The era of increasing narrowness has become too expensive to sustain; the reverse trend is toward more cross-training within a few general categories. As with general industry, middle managers are experiencing layer of labor that can be reduced with little consequence.

The United States is evolving a total delivery system in which the acute hospital plays a relatively small part. The total system will encompass home, pharmacy, primary care, specialty care, hospital, and postacute care, then work back to the home. One of the reasons hospital design will be tricky during this transition period is that hospital services are still migrating to the ambulatory setting, so that it is hard to tell what the residual programs will be. Keynoter Goldsmith said about 85 percent of all surgeries in the future will be outpatient, compared with about 50 percent now. Even with the strong outpatient surgery trend, the management team, physicians, and nurses—everyone—will have a tendency to plan as if the surgery service will be about the same in the future as it is now. The team will plan the usual eight or 12 ORs, all in one central location, with central supply in the basement. Moreover, the hospital will be planned first, not the outpatient services.

To loosen our image of the traditional OR, it is helpful to see other arrangements for surgery. In Scandinavia, surgery can take place in the patient room using a plastic bubble with sleeves in it. In Japan, high-volume eye surgery takes place in a room with a set of surgeons acting in sequence for each patient. To simply decentralize specialized ORs to a few, large patient floors as one concept is not a big jump.

Basis for Redesign

Generally, an architect can expect that if an organization has not yet developed a strategic plan and a total community service/delivery plan, it will probably overdesign its building. The architectural team should be prepared to plan for all the settings that patients will use in order to determine what the hospital structure itself should be. In addition to aiding with the size and placement decisions, architects should help clients consider the through-put efficiency, or "flow" of the patient through the core process.

One of the multifold theories in futurism that applies to every business in the United States is that there is a huge trend toward providing services on an "any time" basis from the standpoint of the buyer, or user. This means that the user's time is considered an asset. Consumers have been trained in the fast-food world to expect a meal in a minute or less, or seven minutes for those who are really patient. The idea of sitting down to a seven-course meal that takes 45 minutes to prepare is foreign to many people. Banking is no longer done by standing in line for a bank clerk for 15 minutes; the automatic teller takes only 30 seconds.

Yet providers ask patients to go from the physician's office to the hospital to have a test, come back to the physician's office to learn the result of the test, be retested, be referred to yet another building where a specialist resides, have the specialist then return them to the hospital for more tests, then be scheduled at another time for a procedure. This is very time-expensive for patients. This pattern is designed to satisfy the time efficiency requirements of the professional.

To straighten this situation out, it will be tempting to rely on committee work, voluntary compliance, and professionals doing things cooperatively to gradually improve patient flow. A more effective approach would be to design a good patient flow in a totally new building and then invite practitioners to come in, be trained in that way of working, and proceed. It is extremely hard to correct old problems in place in old structures.

For example, Group Health of Puget Sound for most of its history used the staff model of full-time paid physicians to deliver care to subscribers. But as it moved into areas in which it had to serve new subscribers, it tended to offer contract opportunities to local group practices. Management and medical leaders attempted to communicate the Group Health mentality of prevention, wellness, education, continuity, and follow-up. This was on top of the episodic model that most civilian, non-HMO physicians follow.

After a few years, Group Health executives began to understand that this method was simply not working. It had two models of care offered side-by-side within this HMO. Company executives said, "We've really got to plan for whatever community we go into to work a very short time with a local group, but to know that we must put capital, management, and people into that site or it will never be a Group Health site."

Past and Future Systems

How does a healthcare team and its architect arrive at better hospital design? For a future facility to actually fit the future patient and not rehouse past methods, the team should trace the pathway of main patient types, access all steps, then redesign the pathway for simplicity.

This redesign is not only a task leading to a new configuration of space, but it is a major organizational development effort. It brings people from different departments together to look at how the system works from the patient's point of view. Lab and nursing staff, physicians, and staff from admitting and security will all deal with the total patient care process rather than departmental space planning.

At a higher level of abstraction, large providers and buyers have the problem of redeploying dollars for the greatest benefit. The largest amount of money is now spent on the terminal phase of acute illnesses and the acute phase of chronic illnesses. Funds should move to the earliest stages where a little intervention can produce a great deal of benefit. Inevitably, hospitals will assume a quasi-public health role—and managers will have to become conversant with the clinical side of hospital work so they can make good judgments about the most appropriate setting for each type of patient.

Managers tend to define themselves as being in a supporting role with regard to physicians, as not having their own mission or professional concept of what they want to accomplish. They have left clinical planning to physicians.

With the advent of managed care, they must understand what the clinical product of their organization is and the need for them to mold it and guide it. If managers do not understand the relative value of their clinical product lines, they will not be able to judge the new technologies that Goldsmith outlined, particularly genetics technologies in which very few physicians have been trained. Providers will be able to absorb this technology only if the CEO understands its meaning and becomes at least conversant with the language and the delivery implications, then sees to it that the medical and hospital staff are trained.

If genetics technologies were fully absorbed, hospitals would be handling people in family units and groups. This is not done now. Hospital design assumes care for one patient at a time—one procedure or activity at a time. Just to overcome the singularity of our actions—and move to group action in which a family unit or a risk group is associated with a team of people responsible for the primary prevention—will take a concerted reeducation of those managers and physicians who came into the profession in the past two or three decades. And it will lead to new space design.

Technically, it is possible even now for educated patients to go to an admitting desk in a neighborhood health center or hospital, pull out a computer keyboard, open up their own records, enter their current symptoms, and call up the schedule of their care team, or any diagnostic service. Patients could go directly to the testing area, have those tests, have them electronically communicated to the physician, be in his office as he calls up the test results, negotiate with him on what treatment plan is best, and obtain a video to take home to do a guided decision process. If they elect to have a procedure, patients could call up the surgery schedule on their own computer, schedule the procedure, and present themselves on the duly appointed day.

Next to the excluded poor, the proactive patient is the most ill served by our present system. We can educate patients and family members to be proactive. In fact, the whole family, as a group, can be educated to a greater degree than is common practice. Mature HMOs such as Group Health Minneapolis, HIP in New York, and Harvard Community Health Plan have what amounts to a "junior college" for their memberships. Group Health in Puget Sound offers more than 200 different classes per month in every kind of medical problem.

Regional healthcare systems will be the "brain trust" for designing the future patient core patterns and setting; they should become adept at population-based planning, and total delivery system design.

A single hospital project, in this view, is not isolated but fits into a larger delivery framework. Is it a centerpiece hospital? If so, what are its satellites? Is it a satellite? If so, what are the edges between it and the centerpiece hospital?

In addition to a wider view of a hospital's place in the total system, planners should factor in modern social views of the role of healthcare services in a community. There are two trends at work simultaneously: to create large medical campuses and contrarily, to decentralize services. The traditional health campus idea is now being understood as excessively isolating healthcare from the community it is supposed to serve. The most egregious example of this is Los Angeles County's plan to replace County Medical Center at a cost of billions of dollars. This plan, in effect, requires the residents of the county to travel from their homes to this site (the largest of five county hospitals in California) for not only hospital care, but for outpatient care, simple diagnostics, wellness, maternity services, etc. That travel cost is extremely high. The campus is isolated from the county and its neediest communities. The reason for the central replacement is one word: teaching. The faculty—in this case, the USC faculty—controls where teaching takes place and believes that it is more efficient to have its residents seeing faculty members and patients together in one high-tech, capable place. Perhaps the economic problems in Los Angeles will prompt a redesign for several smaller hospitals, built in sequence.

When designing the care for a total delivery system, caregivers have to start with care at the home or office level and ask, "What will we be providing in those locations next, and what will that then cause us to do on our central campus?" The central campus may have a building that is largely devoted to management, that handles the entire patient core case management system for the organization.

As with central campuses, central diagnostic and treatment departments are giving way to separate inpatient and outpatient departments, as has been done with outpatient surgery. Services are also moving to the patient floor and to the bedside.

A Kodak process (Ektachrome) allows nonlab staff to perform lab tests using a dry film slide one inch in diameter. In seven minutes, a patient's test can be completed, as opposed to the usual turnaround time of one to two hours. These machines are the size of an electric typewriter or small computer and are fiber optically read. This kind of processing can be in each ICU, the emergency room, and every special care unit.

This decentralization and downsizing trend should be followed to its furthest expression. A planning team should ask, "How small can this get? How decentralized can this get?" There are technologies abroad that are extremely portable and inexpensive. These smaller technologies can be added incrementally; whereas large equipment, central departments, and large campuses all require huge, lumpy investments of capital. There will be fewer such large, lumpy investments of capital under managed care.

Death to Departments

Finally, planning a new hospital is a chance to break the bonds created by the present department-based organizational structure (Figure 1–4). The planning structure for a project should reflect not the current, but the future hospital. Planning teams should reflect program and system, not be composed of representatives from each department. Planning teams should be coached by management so they know that only functions, not departmental boundaries, are to be built into the future design. (Example: not a central lab, but lab services.)

Finally, hospitals should be designed for easy adaptability, since it is not possible to predict with certainty such things as the right proportion of critical care beds, new computer uses, and new treatments. Since a building

◆ **FIGURE 1–4** Planning a new hospital is a chance to break the bonds created by the present department-based organizational structure.

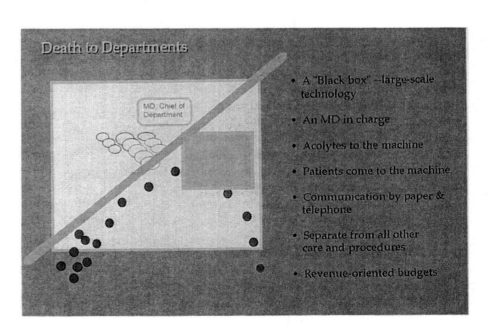

erected today will last past the third decade of the next century, the "teachable moment" of the planning period for new facilities is the best time to be as aggressive as the culture will bear. Flexibility as a key goal leads to larger patient rooms, in separable suites; large free-span spaces for professional and support services; and sufficient extra space to support periodic remodeling. Future hospitals will be long, low, and fat, as the base-and-tower model does not support patient-focused care to its fullest.

Coordinated Planning

A hospital design effort actually starts much earlier than the building. It starts with defining the market and the "risk groups" within the market. Risk groups are people predisposed to a specific medical condition. The medical condition has a "disease life cycle" of predisposition, early symptoms, acute symptoms, a postacute period, and then a continuing maintenance period. That disease life cycle picture becomes a template for planning a set of services, locations where services may take place, linking among the services, and the physical plant that will house each service. All of these elements are influenced by contracts, demographics, technology, manpower, and other factors, so that good planning support will include modeling of a total delivery system.

The "end" of a planning project is not the building—it is the improvement in health brought about by services that the building helps support.

Wanda J. Jones is president of New Century Healthcare Institute, a San Francisco, California, research, development, and educational organization concerned with population-based planning of regional healthcare systems. As an interpreter of future delivery trends, Jones has led planning projects for sites, hospital campuses, medical office buildings, community health centers, primary care networks, and tertiary institutes. Her interests include program management, clinical information system planning, community and target group-based planning, and patient-focused care.

◆ ◆ ◆

AMBULATORY CARE DESIGN: THE NEW GENERATION

Fifth Symposium on Healthcare Design, San Diego, 1992

George Pressler, AIA

The intent of my presentation is to examine briefly the past and current movement toward ambulatory care and to focus on what the future may hold for the next generation. Finally, I will examine what providers, planners, and designers should do in preparation.

It is important to look briefly at the past in order to build a more logical foundation from which to address the next generation of healthcare delivery. The following was reported in the American Hospital Association's (AHA) "Hospital Statistics."

- In 1970, there were 5859 hospitals providing 848,000 beds (Table 1–3). Occupancy was 80.3 percent with 181 million outpatient visits. The first free-standing surgical center was opened in Phoenix, Arizona, by Drs.

◆ **TABLE 1–3** As the number of hospitals, beds, and occupancy rates declines, outpatient visits have continued to increase.

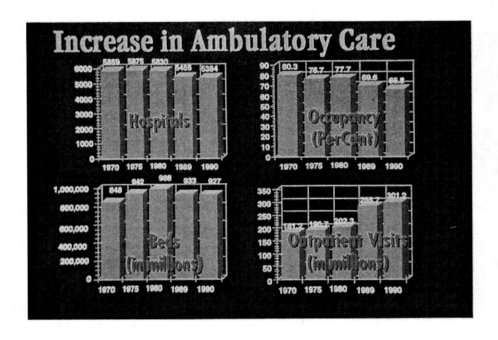

Wallace Reed and John Ford. Actually the first outpatient surgery departments within a hospital were at George Washington University in Washington, D.C., and at the University of California, Los Angeles (UCLA) Medical Center in the late 1960s.

• In 1971, the American Medical Association (AMA) endorsed the utilization of surgery centers. Outpatient surgical procedures were then and are now usually limited to patients who are under 65 years old, who are healthy, and who do not have a history of chronic disease or show any signs that would lead to complications during surgery.

• In 1975, occupancy dropped to 76.7 percent, and outpatient visits rose to 190,672 million. In the mid-1970s, the American College of Surgeons finally approved the use of free-standing surgery centers, which resulted in the number of facilities within the United States doubling within a year.

• In 1980, the occupancy rate rose slightly to 77.7 percent, but outpatient visits increased to 202.3 million. The number of hospitals had decreased to 5830, with the number of beds actually increasing to 988,000.

• In 1983, Congress passed legislation to establish the diagnostic related groups (DRG) prospective pricing system.

• The year 1986 marked the shift, with outpatient visits surpassing inpatient days for the first time.

• By 1989, there were 5455 hospitals with 933,000 beds. Occupancy had decreased substantially to 69.6 percent, with outpatient visits increasing to 285,712 million. Surgical centers now numbered 1227. Also, since 1987, the number of outpatient surgeries had increased by more than 35 percent to almost 2 million.

The majority of these free-standing facilities were owned and operated by physicians looking for strategies to increase or replace lost income. The SMG

Marketing Group reminds us of the 1930s and 1940s when physicians established hospitals for the same economic reasons.

According to the California Association of Hospitals and Health Systems, in 1990, the number of hospitals had dropped to 5384, and beds had decreased to 927,360, with the number of outpatient visits numbering 301.3 million. During the past eight years, outpatient visits per hospital have been 18 to 30 percent higher in California than the United States average. I will discuss the reasons for this trend a little later. For the first time ever, in 1990, the number of outpatient surgeries performed in the United States exceeded the number of inpatient procedures.

Outpatient specialty surgical procedures now include: ophthalmology, OB-Gyn, ENT, orthopedic, general, plastic, podiatry, urology, gastroenterology, dental, pain block, and neurology. Medicare and Medicaid acceptance and reimbursement, of course, is a primary factor in the development of these facilities, as is the importance of Medicare and state certifications of facilities. More than 800 surgical procedures can now be conducted on an outpatient basis, without requiring an overnight stay. It is estimated that over 60 percent of all procedures will be outpatient by 1995. Outpatient surgery has been more evident historically in countries outside the Unites States, such as Great Britain, Switzerland, and Germany. However, in the United States, as outpatient DRGs are enacted, we can expect further major increases in the number and types of outpatient procedures.

In his book, published in 1976, *The Post-Physician Era: Medicine in the 21st Century*, Jerrold Maxmen predicted that doctors would be replaced by computers and a new type of healthcare professional. He believed that with computers assuming the technical, functional responsibilities, nonphysicians will be accepted by patients to administer medical care. He stated then that "interpersonal talents will replace scientific sophistication." As we continue to look into the next generation as part of this presentation, I will include more of Maxmen's predictions from nearly two-thirds of a generation ago.

Current Trends

Leland Kaiser has referred to the past five years of healthcare planning and design as the "white water" period, in which survival was the primary objective. This resulted in severe competition, discounting, capitation, acquisition, merger, divestiture, and diversification. He predicts the next 15 years of healthcare will be revolutionized by technology, with an even higher percentage of United States GNP (gross national product) dedicated to healthcare.

My objective for this presentation is to discuss the new generation, which by definition is the time between the birth of the parents and that of their offspring—approximately 30 years. So, the targeted year for this discussion is about 2022. As those of us in the facility planning and design field well understand, the commencement of the process of programming, planning, financing, constructing, and equipping a major healthcare facility that would be operational at about that time could actually start within the next 10 years.

As a result, the primary message of the remainder of this presentation will be focused on that time frame. I will review many of today's current trends and those that are predicted for the near future, but I will limit this discussion to how they may affect the next generation of planning—culminating in the year 2022.

As Leland Kaiser predicts, that time period will be dominated by molecular biology and bioelectronics. He believes that life spans can, and will, be prolonged. As positive as that is, the impact on our nation's healthcare delivery system is rather incredible. It will continue to be incredible unless preparations begin today. As the elderly population consumes more resources, Kaiser affirms that it will become the largest sector of our healthcare market. He predicts that by 2007, healthcare costs will consume 22 percent of the GNP.

Roy Amara, president of the Institute of the Future, believes that the physician surplus will continue through our target year of 2022 (but keep in mind the 1976 prediction of the need for doctors). In support of this theory, a nationwide survey conducted by the National Research Corporation stated that 66 percent of those polled saw the need for increased options for homecare. As healthcare moves into the home environment, individuals are now seeking a much more thorough understanding of health treatment implications. The *Physician's Desk Reference* has now become one of the best-selling nonfiction books. Our population now demands access to information and requires access to education from healthcare providers.

In his attack on the U.S. healthcare system, Dr. C. Everett Koop, at this past year's AHA convention in Denver, confirmed the need to train a new kind of physician for the next century. These would act more like family physicians, regardless of their specialty. His closing remarks stated that "we need to place emphasis on healthCARE and not CURE. Curing costs billions, but caring comes from the soul."

Futurists have predicted that in the year 2000, ambulatory care will be just as important to hospitals as acute care, that more than 50 percent of the average hospital's revenues will come from ambulatory care services.

As medical diagnostic and treatment technology continues to advance, the cost of purchasing and providing this technology will far exceed potential financial resources. As a result, a difficult question must be answered, a question that puts economics head-to-head with ethical issues. With our limited access to dollars, will we be forced to choose technology that reduces operational costs, or technology that positively impacts medical outcomes? An argument can be made for both points of view, but the answer to this question will have a tremendous impact on healthcare delivery and the facilities and environments that planners and designers will create to support the system. I believe we each understand the impact of this decision from our own vantage points; and, interestingly, if we had to choose a direction here this afternoon, most likely we would make a nearly unanimous choice.

The AHA Society of Ambulatory Care Professionals' Board of Directors and the Strategic Planning Committee developed a five-year strategic plan. The results of this 1992–1993 ambitious work effort yielded: a comprehensive listing of 41 "megatrend" issues affecting ambulatory care (Figure 1–5); and a listing of forecasts for ambulatory care in the year 2000.

Some of the issues this task force identified were:

- Payment reform
- Hospital and medical group network development
- Cost effectiveness of ambulatory care

Ambulatory Care Megatrend Issues

- Payment Reform
- Hospital & Medical Group Network
- Cost Effectiveness
- Immigration
- High Tech Explosion
- Government Regulation
- Physician & Hospital Cooperation
- Information Systems

- Aging
- Rising Acuity
- Case Management
- Utilization review
- Convenience
- Health Promotion
- Education
- Home Care

- Immigration into the United States
- High-tech explosion
- Increase in governmental regulation
- Hospital-based physician and hospital cooperation
- Information systems
- Aging
- Rising acuity
- Case management
- Utilization review
- Convenience
- Health promotion/prevention
- Education of population
- Home care

I will explore in detail many of these megatrends as they affect our target year 2022. Likewise, many of the projected characteristics for the year 2000 will continue with even greater momentum beyond the turn of the century and will serve as the planning parameters for our "new generation" of ambulatory care. Selectively, from this AHA Society's more extensive list, I believe the constraints and opportunities that will remain or further develop in defining ambulatory care in 2022 include the following:

- Computer network practices
- Convenience and consumer-driven delivery
- Continuum of care
- Emphasis on prevention
- Service oriented/operational efficiency
- Hospital in the home
- Patient/family teaching
- More bureaucracy
- Quality of life focus
- Self-care
- Higher acuity

- Controlled healthcare/fewer choices
- Technology

As a result of The Healthcare Forum Foundation Leadership Center and The Institute for Alternative Futures' study, "Bridging the Leadership Gap in Healthcare," the predict-and-manage paradigm emerged. "Advances in our understanding of aging, disease, and genetics will allow us to predict normal declines and the course of illness. Better behavioral change techniques and a host of advanced therapies and preventive approaches will allow us to 'manage' health, leading to lower morbidity."

The Hospital Council of Southern California Center of Health Resources developed a 1991–1995 "View of the Future" in which it predicted that 66 percent of the active acute care beds will be controlled by multihospital systems. As a result, even with the assumed growth and aging of the population, fewer beds will be required because of a more efficiently controlled managed care delivery system, as well as the influx of more alternatives to traditional inpatient care.

Aging

In the next six seconds, 24 people will be added to the world population. Within the next hour, 11,000, and by the end of today, 260,000. And in three days, the growth will be equal to the population of San Francisco. The world's five-and-a-half billion population was reached in four million years. By our target year of 2022, only 30 years from now, we will have added yet another billion. And by 2050, our world's population may approach 11 billion people. Unfortunately, the majority of these people will reside in undeveloped third world countries.

The impact of the increase in population on our U.S. healthcare delivery

◆ **TABLE 1–4** By the year 2000, the number of people over the age of 75 in the United States will have grown by 35 percent.

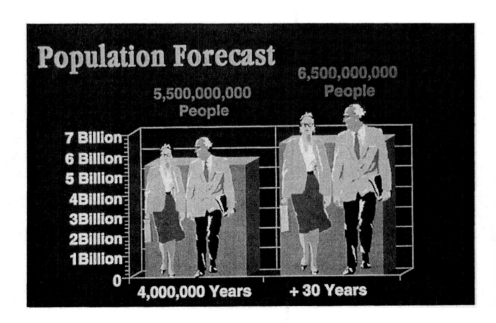

system becomes magnified when we realize that by the year 2000, the number of people over the age of 75 will have grown by 35 percent (Table 1–4). In 1980, the population over 65 was 25 million or 11.3 percent of the population. In 2000, it will be 35 million, or 13.1 percent. In our year 2022, the number of Americans younger than 50 will rise by only one percent, compared with the total of those individuals 50 and older, which will rise by 74 percent. In 2050, 67 million or 21.7 percent of the population will be over the age of 65. Analysis has shown that 25 to 55 percent of Medicare's annual expenditures are consumed by only five to six percent of total enrollees in their last year of life.

Now we all have heard advocates of rationing medical care to individuals over the age of 70 and, as in the state of Oregon's plan, of making decisions based on lifesaving potential and degree of improvement in the quality of life as a result of costly treatments. I posed an ethical question as to the application of new technologies based on operation cost savings versus medical outcomes earlier in this presentation. An additional ethical question is raised by the fact that high-tech treatments not covered by insurance are, and most likely will continue to be, available to those who have the ability to pay.

Other statistics forecast that by 2022, men can be expected to live an additional 19 years and women an additional 23. As a result, longer life expectancies means that spouses will be living together longer after retirement.

Genetics

All that we have heard over the past few years regarding the tremendous impact and burden that our aging American population will have on our future healthcare delivery system will be positively affected by yet another event. The results of this next revolution, Jeff Goldsmith wrote in a June 1992 article for *The Healthcare Forum Journal*, will "demolish what remains of the acute care paradigm and force our health insurance system and society to confront the increased predictability of disease risk." This revolution will originate in the clinical laboratory and pharmacy.

In more recent years, significant advances in diagnostic and therapeutic technologies have permitted more patients to be seen on an ambulatory basis. Management of many illnesses and diseases associated with the aging process are now addressed without admitting patients to the hospital.

The next revolution I am referring to regards genetic engineering, which has revealed the greatest potential to affect positively the quality of life. The Human Genome project currently in progress will map and sequence the estimated 100,000 genes in the human body. The "genome" is the complete set of instructions for making an organism. It contains the master blueprint for all cellular structures and activities for the lifetime of the cell or organism. Within the nucleus of each of a person's trillions of cells (except for red blood cells which do not have a nucleus), the human genome consists of tightly coiled threads of DNA. Each DNA molecule contains many genes, which are the basic physical and functional units of heredity.

As I just stated, there are an estimated 100,000 genes within the human genome. The ultimate goal of genome research is to develop tools for using this information in the study of human biology and medicine. The completed DNA sequencing map, which describes the gene order, will help medical researchers unravel the mechanisms of all inherited diseases.

According to Mark Guyer, of the National Center for Human Genome Research, this project—currently underway and expected to be completed within the next ten years—will enable the "new medical practitioner" or genetic screening technician (or our new health practitioner as forecast earlier in this presentation) to predict the risk of certain inherited diseases.

Russ Coile stated in the *Hospital Strategy Report* newsletter in January 1989: "Genetic probes will enhance diagnosis; genetic markers will guide clinicians to the disease; genetically coded drugs will go directly to the affected cells; genetic engineering may block and eliminate the 2000 to 4000 plus birth defects; and genetic therapy may repair existing genetic damage, aiding self-healing and regeneration."

As an aside, males are at higher risk for genetic disorders. The long-term results of genetic counseling and screening, as it is applied as early as conception, will have an unforeseen impact on our future aging population's quality and longevity of life. The potential impact of managing and/or delaying certain diseases until ten years later in one's life will affect not only our healthcare delivery system and its associated costs, but also the types of services and facilities that will be required to support this technology.

Genetic screening will affect the following: Duchenne's muscular dystrophy, diabetes, cardiovascular disease, inherited cancers, Down's syndrome, sickle-cell anemia, Alzheimer's disease, Tay-Sachs disease, hemophilia, hypertension, Lou Gehrig's disease, fragile X syndrome, and cystic fibrosis. Of interest pertaining to cystic fibrosis is the fact that one in 25 Caucasian Americans carries the gene, and 25,000 persons a year are diagnosed with this disease.

The Genome Database, which is the repository for compiling the efforts of this multi-billion dollar research from all over the world, is located at Johns Hopkins University in Baltimore, Maryland.

As I mentioned earlier when we forecast ambulatory care for the next generation, there are both opportunities and, unfortunately, continuing obstacles. These hurdles must be knocked down, moved, crawled under, or jumped over. They must be surpassed, because too much is at stake with regard to the availability and quality of life for the next generations. These barriers, which have existed since the beginning of time, are those associated with advances in technology, politics, sociology—and the two that are always in conflict—ethics and economics.

Considering the predicted reduced demand for institutional care, ambulatory and home care become the focus for less acute health intervention. The ambulatory setting will become more capable and receptive to the diagnosis and treatment of our aging citizens than is possible now. Refer to my earlier statement that today the majority of individuals over 65 requiring most forms of surgery are now admitted as inpatients.

As positive as the outlook is to improve the quality and quantity of life, the aging process will continue. Aging, as defined by the American Institute of Architect's (AIA) Task Force on Design for Aging, "is a dynamic process that begins at birth and continues unabated until death." As a result, facilities will continue to be required to accommodate persons with decreased muscle mass and mental awareness. The most positive side of this forecast for the next generation of healthcare is that fewer of an individual's remaining years will be affected by illness. It is predicted that the probability of being well will extend 20 years beyond our experience today. Prediction, modification, and management of chronic diseases will occur at a much younger age than we have seen in the past, when diagnosis was made after symptoms emerged, then followed by treatment. Now we see the actual possibility of a proactive, preventive approach.

Pharmaceutical Research

Along with the potential impact of genetic research on healthcare delivery, credit must be given to America's pharmaceutical industry, which invests nearly $11 billion a year on drug research and development. This is equivalent to the amount spent by the U.S. government on medical research. Ninety-five percent of the top-100-selling patented drugs were developed by private industry; only three percent by universities and governments; and two percent by individuals. According to the Pharmaceutical Manufacturers Association, half of all medical progress between now and our targeted year of 2022 is likely to come from drug research and development.

With regard to cancer, which accounts for 22 percent of all deaths in the United States, the Batelle Memorial Institute predicts that pharmaceutical advances over the next 25 years will reduce: leukemia deaths by 83,000 or 17 percent; cardiovascular deaths by 4.4 million; deaths due to colorectal cancer by 12 percent; and lung cancer deaths by almost half a million.

The leading cause of death by disease is heart disease. This, combined with the third most prevalent cause of death, stroke, affects the lives of 68 million Americans, and causes 982,000 deaths a year. The annual economic impact exceeds $100 billion. As Americans continue to improve their lifestyles and biomedical research continues to develop new treatments, experts estimate that heart disease and related deaths can be cut by over two-thirds by our new generation in 2022.

More than four million Americans suffer from Alzheimer's disease, and of these 100,000 die each year. The cost to the U.S. healthcare system and the economy is a staggering $88 billion per year. Cognitive enhancers, or drugs to improve the memory, are the focus of current research, as are drugs that increase brain activity and a nerve growth factor that encourages neurons to regrow. The National Institute on Aging estimates that an Alzheimer's disease treatment that could keep just ten percent of patients out of nursing homes for one year could save nearly $9 billion per year.

Three AIDS medicines were introduced in 1991; five more are waiting approval from the FDA; and 88 more are in development. Since the first medicine was approved in 1987, 13 more have entered the market. Seven vaccines are currently in clinical trials.

Attention was given during the Presidential debates to the fact that it now takes an average of 12 years to bring a new drug to market, with an accompanying price tag averaging $231 million.

For just seven uncured diseases—cancer, cardiovascular diseases, Alzeimer's, arthritis, depression, diabetes, and osteoporosis—the cost to society amounts to an estimated $379 billion annually. Genetics and molecular biology are bringing us much closer to understanding the causes of disease. This understanding will lead to pharmaceuticals that are targeted more exactly to the disease or diseased area.

Self-Health

Since everyone at this Symposium has been sitting for a few days, I thought I'd like to do a stand-up/sit-down exercise before moving to the next section of this presentation:

- If you had breakfast this morning, stand up.
- If you had eggs, bacon, or pancakes with butter and syrup, sit down.
- If you jogged or did any type of exercise this morning, last night, or sometime during your stay in San Diego, stand up.
- If you exercise on a regular basis, such as several times a week, stand up.
- If you have even remotely thought about joining a health club, stand up.
- If you smoke, sit down.
- If you have set a goal to stop smoking this year or in the next three years, you may stand.
- If you have not had a vacation of at least a week in the past year, sit down.
- If you use illegal drugs, sit down.
- If you use illegal drugs but do not inhale, you may stand. Oh, I see one person in the back of the room just stood up.
- If you have worked every weekend for the past two months, sit down.
- If you have had a least one fun outing with family or friends in the last month, stand up.
- If you have a hobby and/or a pet, stand up.
- If you have not had a cholesterol test, blood pressure taken, or a physical exam in the past year, sit down.
- If you have had a dental exam or cleaning in the past six months, stand up.
- If you plan on living until the age of 95, stand up.
- If you plan on being healthy until you are 94.999 years old, stand up.

Welcome to the next generation of ambulatory care. You may all sit down now.

Running parallel with the positive impact of genetic engineering on improving and extending the quality of life, particularly for the increasing numbers of our population over the age of 65, another phenomenon is occurring. At this time, since I have not yet learned any new jargon to increase our healthcare vocabulary, I am going to assume that responsibility.

In the 5th century B.C., Hippocrates stated, "The best way to avoid disease is to lead a wholesome life." I want to share a passage from a book I recently found:

While infectious disease is being brought under control, mental illness and emotional disturbance continue to increase in this complex Space Age. Heart disease has become the leading cause of death today; cancer has become our second most dangerous killer. The number of instances of both mental illness and heart disease can be reduced, to a great extent, by the simple measure of learning to live properly. The weapons which have proved effective against cancer offer little hope to a person who has neglected early symptoms and warnings. These are only a few of the challenges modern health education faces today.

This passage was quoted from a grade school textbook, *Modern Health*, published in 1955, over a generation ago.

And now I offer a new phrase to be added to our ever-increasing health-care vocabulary: *Self-health.*

The 1948 charter of the World Health Organization includes the following worthy goal: "To raise the physical and mental health level of all people, going far beyond the old concept of health as a mere absence of illness." This statement is much like the challenge of Dr. Koop that I quoted earlier, about focusing on "healthCARE" rather than "CURE."

A majority of all the professional health organizations today share a similar goal of looking at the community to integrate health/care, education, and prevention. The Healthcare Forum, in its continued dedicated emphasis on the global community, and AHA's Healthy People 2000 initiative both support the theory that this approach may be the optimum solution to avoid many of the negatively oriented forecasts for the new generation.

At its spring annual meeting in 1993, The Healthcare Forum will be focusing on the creation of healthier communities. It is currently reviewing communities located all over the world that may serve as models of collaboration and leadership, stressing improvement in the health status of community residents.

Healthy People 2000 is coordinated primarily by the Office of Disease Prevention and Health Promotion of the Department of Health and Human Services. It has released many publications, which are available to anyone who is interested.

Recognizing that it has become essential to take a stronger proactive stance in integrating preventive care into the community, Healthy People 2000 suggests that the most opportune arena for the promotion of wellness, and the reduction of risk, is within the ambulatory care environment.

Novell, a leader in network computing, provides us with a thought-provoking description of acceptable risk: "Last night you powered down a cholesterol-rich pasta with cream sauce. This morning you jaywalked across a busy four-lane street, and next weekend you're going to trust some 19-year-old who tells you there's no way the bungee cord can break."

Each of us has the authority, power, and control to diminish our own personal health risk. In addition, we are each in a position to influence the decrease of risk for our families and friends. We each are empowered to influence those risks affecting our food, water, and air quality. As our government becomes more responsible for payment of healthcare coverage, it seems obvious that elected officials should realize that they are, and have always been, in a position to decrease health risks by finally taking a stand against the tobacco industry and the manufacturers of child-oriented cereals and snacks. In addition (as is happening much too slowly), closer scrutiny of the labeling of food products, medicines, and topical applications is warranted.

According to the AHA's Annual Survey, 55.3 percent of healthcare organizations offered community health promotion programs in 1986, and that figure rose to 77.2 percent in the 1990s. This reaction to community demand reflects the population's search for healthier lifestyles. The AHA identified several developments that have resulted in an emphasis on prevention:

- Social recognition that absence of preventive care results in tragedies that need not have occurred
- Concern about ongoing increases in healthcare costs

- Increased knowledge of which interventions are effective
- Increased consumer interest and demand for information

These developments have helped refocus the emphasis for the U.S. healthcare system on addressing preventive care as the priority in any restructuring of healthcare delivery models.

Healthy People 2000 identified the following related priorities:

- *Health promotion:* physical activity/fitness; nutrition; tobacco; alcohol and other drugs; family planning; mental health; violent and abusive behavior; and education and community-based programs.
- *Preventive services:* maternal and child health; heart disease and stroke; cancer; other chronic and disabling conditions; HIV infection; sexually transmitted diseases; immunization and infectious diseases; and clinical preventive services (Figure 1–6).
- *Health protection:* unintentional injuries; occupational safety and health; environmental health; food and drug safety; and oral health.

Self-health as I mentioned a moment ago, is the concept that we each must enter into a participatory contract with healthcare providers, insurers, and regulators, to be proactive in our commitment to maintaining a healthy lifestyle. This agreement, passed on to our heirs through education and training, provides us the control today to ensure a better quality of life for our next generation.

The impact of such a participatory contract is as follows:

1. *Cholesterol.* What is it? It is a fatlike substance that is actually required by every cell in the body. It is derived from two sources: the liver and foods of other animal origin. It is a normal component of the blood but becomes of

◆ **FIGURE 1–6** Preventive care is the priority in any restructuring of our healthcare delivery models.

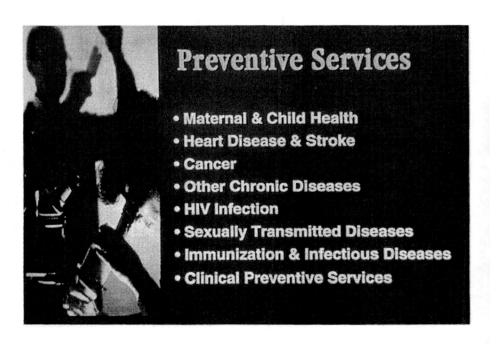

Preventive Services

- Maternal & Child Health
- Heart Disease & Stroke
- Cancer
- Other Chronic Diseases
- HIV Infection
- Sexually Transmitted Diseases
- Immunization & Infectious Diseases
- Clinical Preventive Services

concern when it is present in excessive amounts: greater than 200 mg/dl in adults and 140 mg/dl in preadolescents.

As stated by Abbott Laboratories, blood cholesterol is a direct cause of coronary heart disease, the number one killer in America. The National Institute of Health has proven that high cholesterol is a major cause of heart attacks. More than 1300 people die each day from coronary heart disease, which equals nearly one-half million people a year. This is more than the number of deaths occurring from all forms of cancer combined. This can be in our control, now!

2. *Smoking, alcohol, and drugs.* According to the Hospital Council of Southern California, cigarette smoking, air pollution, dietary excess and deficiency, alcohol and drug abuse, and hypertension are, together, the attributed causes of between 41 and 69 percent of all deaths in the United States. On the positive side, cigarette smoking has decreased to approximately one-fifth of the adult population, 21 percent; but with the increase of smoking by teenagers and younger children, thanks to the likes of Joe Camel and others, this rises to 27 percent of the population. It is of keen interest to me that no other industry can match the combined financial clout of tobacco and food companies. As of October 11th, just before the election, according to the *Los Angeles Times*, three tobacco companies were ranked within the top five political contributors, having given $1.6 and $.9 million to the Republican and Democratic Committees, respectively.

Alcohol consumption remains at approximately 57 percent, which is a decrease of five percent from 1986. Illegal drug use has risen in the past few years from 19 to 21 percent. Of interest, whites and those with higher educational levels are more likely to use illegal drugs. AIDS awareness has increased significantly. Almost one-quarter of all Californians report that they have been tested.

3. *Vitamins.* An article in the April 1992 issue of *Time* magazine focused on the power of vitamins in combating birth defects, cataracts, cancers, heart disease, and, yes, even aging. As the aging of our population usually associates with the chronic maladies of cancer and heart disease, greater attention is now paid to the benefits of these nutrients. Science has thus far identified 13 organic substances that are labeled vitamins. As *Time* reported, however, drug companies have as yet not committed great amounts of capital to studies of vitamin benefits, since the payoff is relatively small. Vitamin chemical formulas are in the public domain and therefore cannot be patented. This is a major dilemma for researchers, which must be recognized and given higher priority status. Again, we are faced with a focus on short-term economics, rather than a participatory approach to improving and maintaining health status.

According to the National Center for Health Statistics, the majority of Americans join President Bush in their dislike of most vegetables. This is most unfortunate, considering the established and potential benefits.

In his address at the AHA annual meeting, Dr. Koop suggested that public health need move from its after-the-fact teaching philosophy to one that focuses on changing behaviors. He also joined in the belief that each person needs to take charge of his or her own health, or to use our new phrase, to attend to "self-health."

When Emily Friedman received her AHA Honorary Life Membership

Award in July 1992, she focused her acceptance speech on healthcare reform. In making one of her points she stated that "going to church no more makes you a Christian than going to a garage makes you a car." I believe we can make a similar statement: that going to a hospital does not make you healthy. It may make you well, but it stops there. Our new healthcare system in the generation of 2022 will be different: placing much greater emphasis on education and prevention and on changing lifestyles. Keep well, not make well.

Services

I have spent time discussing the major impact of aging, genetics, and preventive healthcare or self-health on the new generation, so let us now attempt to foresee the types of services that will be most prevalent in our year 2022. From the information I have discussed and from the other programs presented at this Symposium, we can make several assumptions.

The first is in the area of genetic counseling and screening. One of the stated goals of the Human Genome Project with regard to research training is to attain an annual rate of 600 pre- and post-doctoral fellows by 1995. Genetic counselors are increasing their presence at many major medical centers. Their profession will become one of the highest in demand in the next generation of healthcare delivery. Unfortunately, this training is offered on a very limited basis at this time.

Concurrently, U.S. medical schools have continued their emphasis on primary care, although this appears to be changing. According to the May 1992 issue of *Hospitals* magazine, the number of primary care graduates did decrease by almost 20 percent. Internal medicine graduates also declined by 25 percent. The number of graduates in family practice decreased just slightly, and pediatrics actually appears to be increasing and has continued to do so over the past five years.

Another indicator of the shift in services is Hamilton/KSA's annual ranking of hospitals' total patient revenues. This survey ranks services by their success in generating a profit, or at least in breaking even. When we compare data from the past few years, we see that, as expected, outpatient surgery centers and outpatient diagnostic centers continue as the leaders. Also, as we have witnessed, women's services, along with psychiatric medicine and industrial medicine, both of which had continued to increase slightly, are now in a holding pattern due to an increase in competition and shifts in reimbursement. Of interest is the shift into the "winner's circle" of home health, pediatrics, wellness, and health promotion programs. The smaller and more rural the hospital, the greater the potential for reliance on ambulatory care revenues. This is different from hospitals with more than 400 beds and from teaching hospitals—which is to be expected considering their existing technological and inpatient facilities investments. This too will change by the year 2022.

Facilities

Now what does all this mean to the programmers, planners, designers, architects, manufacturers of equipment, finishes, and furnishings, and to the healthcare administrators and providers? What does all this mean with regard to the types of facilities and environments that will be required in 2022? As we have experienced in the past few years, continued emphasis will be placed on accessibility and on consumer convenience, as well as on consumer preference. The integration of design aesthetics and the philosophy of the healing environment will continue to be of importance. And of most significance will be functional efficiency—efficiency in planning and design of facilities to allow the caregivers to allocate their time to directing patient care, education, and counseling. Maximum facility adaptability for unforeseen uses and technology will continue to be a key to the survival of a facility and its ability to respond to change. The International Union of Architects' Eleventh International Public Health Seminar, in conjunction with the World Health Organization in Moscow, derived the following statement:

> Architecture for health must be more than economical, technical, sophisticated engineering of diagnostic and treatment performances of medicine. Architecture for health should mean being aware of the human and of the human environment. Humanizing the environment is not realized merely by designing a pleasant and colorful surrounding.

The American Institute of Architects (AIA) Committee on Architecture for Health identified the following characteristics of future healthcare facilities. These include:

- Clarity
- Shop-front healthcare
- Low technology
- Healthcare-driven fitness centers
- Creating urban spaces
- Data centers
- Integrated infracore
- "Character"-driven design
- Parking dock
- Adaptive re-use
- Vertically integrated campuses
- Tiering of campuses and systems
- Specialty-center proliferation

As we prepare to plan for the healthcare environments for the new generation of ambulatory care, we must first erase the presumption of today's healthcare delivery facility model as being a single place. We must dismiss the simplification of a strata of types of care based purely on level of acuity. This approach, which has served us well for the past three generations, will be modified for 2022. A new concept is emerging that far surpasses today's approach to patient-focused care. As Michael Brill states, we must rethink the healthcare physical environment not as a "place" but as a "tool." A new approach is required to address the myriad of interconnecting issues and considerations of the new generation. This concept is healthcare delivery through total integration into the personal conduct of life styles.

Decentralization of healthcare delivery sites is an essential strategic investment to bring services to the consumer and to the provider. The medical campus of 2022 will be an integrated community-focused healing environment, with increased attention being given to the wholeness of the individual as well as to the impact of body, mind, and spirit on health. The recent AHA "Management Advisory" discussed "Ethical Conduct for Health Care Institutions" and emphasized that they need to be concerned with the overall health status of their communities while continuing to provide direct patient services. Healthcare institutions will take even more of a leadership role. This role concentrates on enhancing public health and continuity of care within the community by communicating and working with other healthcare and social agencies to improve the availability and provision of health promotion, education, and patient care services.

With greater emphasis being placed on preventive care and health maintenance, there will be a much broader team approach between caregivers and educators, resulting in the utilization of preschool through high school for training and counseling. Greater attention to the value of preventive care by government regulators and insurers will result in more nutritious foods, properly labeled for the consumer's understanding and benefit. Greater attention will be placed on understanding the effects of the environment on health, resulting in better air and water quality control. Through continuing advances in technology, home health capabilities will soar, resulting in the increased utilization of the family as caregivers.

And people will not only live longer but will be healthier longer, with fewer years of illness and incapacitation. The retirement age will extend dramatically, providing an expanded work force of experienced, seasoned individuals. The emphasis within the ambulatory care environment, in addition to the expected increase in outpatient diagnosis and treatment procedures, will be on education and personal lifestyle training and self-health.

A healthier and more knowledgable new generation will exist in 2022. It is the responsibility of design professionals, as stakeholders, to enter into this participatory contract as educators and caregivers. We already have many of the answers and resources to address many of the issues. We now must work as a team with the providers, the owners, other planners and designers, the educators, and, most important, with the community as a whole. Not only have we the capacity to affect the physical environments of the next generation of ambulatory care, but we also have the power to actually change and decrease the need for many of the heathcare services that are required today.

In closing, I quote "There is no medicine like hope, no incentive so great, and no tonic so powerful, as the expectation of something tomorrow."

A planning and design consultant to the national and international healthcare community for over 25 years, George Pressler, AIA, is president of Planning Decisions Resources in Topanga, California. Since 1986, he has served on the faculty of the Department of Health Science at California State University, Northridge.

◆

◆

◆

◆

◆ Chapter

TWO

A   S E N S I T I V E   A P P R O A C H

◆ ◆ ◆

HISTORY OF HEALTHCARE ENVIRONMENTS

First Symposium on Healthcare Design, Carlsbad, CA, 1988

Neil Kellman, M. D., M. Arch.

I have been a healthcare facility consultant for about ten years. It has slowly become apparent to me that one of the reasons this industry is in such chaos is because we are in the throes of a new "religion" in our culture, or a religion substitute. I would like to introduce a whole new set of perspectives to think about. I believe there is a cultural madness, an obsession, with healthcare and wellness, disease and medicine, and machinery. It has become practically a national pastime. We have the appurtenances of a religion; we have temples and priests, and sometimes, unfortunately, we have sacrificial victims. There are certainly many rituals that we engage in. In studying the history of hospitals, I have noticed a rather odd correlation with religion.

Another interesting point is that modern architecture—the formal movement that started in the 1920s—was meant to symbolize and signify social progressiveness and equality. The movement that began in Germany between the Wars came to the United States and was embraced to a certain degree by hospital health systems. Many of the aesthetics born of the modern architecture movement can be seen in today's hospitals: the clean, sterile lines, lack of ornamentation, and so forth. Over a period of 50 or 60 years, many of these aesthetic standards have come to be accepted as the way hospitals ought to be.

So we have this curious correlation between modern architecture and modern medical technology. After about 50 years of that, starting about ten years ago, people began to tire of these kinds of medical environments. Something seemed to be missing, although people couldn't quite put their finger on it. It was almost as though there was a longing for some other kind of values in the healthcare setting—some kind of universal values that seemed to be totally lacking in the hospital setting. After all, we were dealing with issues that had to do with birthing, dying, or losing limbs or other body parts. This is the stuff that powerful myths in all cultures have been made of during the last 1000 years; myths often centered around the issue of health and disease. Thus we have a powerful symbolic content that no culture has been able to escape. On a certain level, our technology-laden culture has been striving to escape many inevitable things about human existence, and eventually the contradiction grew too strong. Unconsciously, people began to realize that the places they were going for their healthcare were not meeting a host of needs beyond the actual procedures rendered.

Three Issues Affecting Healthcare Environments

There are really three main ideas or issues I would like to discuss. The first is the connection between the past and the present. We heard from a futurist at this Symposium, but I think where we are today is in the future of yesterday. It's really a continuum, and my proposition is that basic human needs don't change—the details do, but the primary human needs don't. I think it's very healthful to look at the past and bring it up to the present.

The second point I would like to discuss is the difference between *caring* and *curing*. There's a one-letter difference in the two words, but a whole universe of expectations that are very different. We need to think about this when we are designing healthcare environments. What are our goals?

The third point I would like to discuss is what I call the concept of "health places." This brings to mind more than merely a room, a floor, a unit, a hospital, or a building. It has to do with the concept of "healing environments." There are a lot of concepts and words around, but I have chosen this concept to try to express the thought that, as designers, we have to create places that really are more; the sum total is more than any of the individual ingredients. We actually create a three-dimensional location in the universe in which health-related and healing-related activities occur. We do that as designers by manipulating certain tools such as light, color, materials, textures, patterns, sound, and so forth. We all know that if these tools are applied mechanically, one can come up with spaces (like those from government hospital guidelines); but there's really not a health "place" there.

Healthcare Facilities: Past and Present

In terms of the past and the present, these concepts began to form in my mind a few years ago when I was fortunate enough to receive a travel grant to Europe. I had researched a number of old hospitals and I thought that continuing this research would be a wonderful opportunity to go to Europe, which it was indeed. I really went expecting to see a lot of dry, dusty, boring buildings; but to my amazement every one of them, without exception, completely surprised me. Each building just whetted my appetite to go on and discover the next.

I found many concepts repeated over and over. For instance, there seems to be a trend in old healing or hospital environments that the initial purpose of the building is still retained in some way, either symbolically or in a real way. The original buildings by and large have not been abandoned and they have rarely been converted; they actually retain some kind of wonderful connection to their function of 400 or 1000 years ago. I found a level of caring and design in regard to detail that I had never before encountered in a healthcare environment. As noted in the recent book *Placeways,* by E.V. Walter, these buildings seemed to organize shapes, powers, feelings, and meanings into places such that one can merely walk in and be tremendously moved. People may not have been cured the way they are today, but surely they were cared for under incredibly adverse conditions.

One of the main thrusts for hospital development in Europe was the great plague that swept the continent for hundreds of years, followed by the pilgrimages and crusades that created a whole class of people in need. So these original institutions had a mission that was very profound, something that we might learn from looking at.

Another thing about the past is that, for the last 200 or 300 years the practice of medicine has been ruled in our culture by a concept called the "biomedical model." This is very different from Hippocrates and healers from Medieval times and from healers from other cultures. The biomedical model, developed in the book *The Turning Point,* by Fritz Capra, says that the human body is a machine and that we're going to get an NIH grant to study this machine—to learn about the molecules and the autoimmune system. Each time we learn something, we are going to apply a little cure to that piece of the machine and we are going to fix the machine. So we are in this pell-mell race for greater and greater cures, yet something seems to be going wrong. The biomedical model considers failure to fix the machine as a tremendous failure in medical treatment. A quote from *The Turning Point* amplifies this:

> Modern medicine sees death as a failure. The distinction between a good death and a poor death does not make sense. Death becomes simply the total standstill of the body machine. Healing will be excluded from medical science as long as researchers limit themselves to a framework that does not allow them to deal with the interplay of body, mind, and environment.

Caring and Curing

As far as *care* and *cure,* we couldn't have heard a more amazing personal example than what Sue Baier presented at this Symposium. Some of my experiences perhaps illustrate the same issues. For instance, my brother-in-law, who is in his early 30s, became suddenly ill last Christmas day. He ended up going to a very well-known, large California HMO chain, where he had emergency abdominal surgery. He recovered there after a somewhat stormy course. He remained in intensive care for nine weeks, during which he lost 50 pounds because of the combined effects of the surgery and the illness. He was finally sent home 50 pounds underweight (and he was not heavy to begin with) because he could not gain weight in the hospital. The reason he couldn't gain weight is because the hospital had closed its kitchen years ago and served only airplane-style meals. He could not eat this food; he had terrible trouble with his taste buds and digestion. The decision was made to send him home to eat.

So that was a situation in which a cure was readily available and was excellent in terms of mechanics and technology; but the basic nurturance and the basic care, which has of course been one of the mainstays of healing for years, was completely missing.

Another example is that after one of his bicycle accidents, my son emerged from a CAT scan and called out, "Dad, there's a rabbit in this big machine!" Since he jokes a lot, I asked him what he meant; so he suggested we take a look. Somebody had thoughtfully put stickers of rabbits inside the CAT scanner. This trite example of nurturing is so wonderful to me, because it tells us that our smallest efforts are appreciated. We should all be encouraged to persist in these little details and thoughts, particularly because there are so many pressures to turn them away.

Concept of Health Places

As to the last idea of healing places, I mention that designers have at their disposal a variety of tools with which to "weave" an environment. This can be illustrated by a quote from *Existence, Space, and Architecture,* by Christian Norgerg-Schultz. It states:

> Like the spider with its web, so every subject weaves relationships between itself and particular properties of objects. The many strands are then woven together and finally form the basis of the subject's very existence.

As designers, we create the environment for a sick person to enter. We create physiological and pyschological sets of relationships that have to do with all the senses, many of which are going to be discussed at this Symposium by other speakers. We assemble them and create a framework or web that supports the activity of healing and brings together a whole that is more than the sum of its parts.

The image of a Navajo sand painting in which there is a sick patient and a healer has always captured what I consider to be the essence of this idea of making a health place. In the painting, the curing person arranges, in a circumscribed area, an image of the patient, an image of the healer, and an image of all the powerful forces of nature. There is a balanced tension going on. Everything has a place within this framework of healing. I have always enjoyed that concept when thinking about creating spaces for people to get well in.

A number of years ago, I was consulting in a hospital that was a drab, dreary place. One day, I turned the corner and saw a striking luminosity in the corridor—I couldn't imagine what it was! I walked up to it and discovered a stunning piece of statuary. It was the only beautiful thing to look at in this entire miserable place. I was enthralled and asked about the history. Apparently 50 or 60 years before, a wealthy dowager patient had donated this Renaissance marble statue; and here it sat, sort of semidiscovered, for all these years, creating a wonderful glow at this intersection of corridors.

A hospital means different things to different people, because it has multiple origins. To some it means acute care or intensive care. Thinking of one of the healing-oriented environments of today, I can almost imagine a patient looking longingly and saying, "I wish I had been in that unit when I was sick." The intensive care unit I refer to has, among other esthetic touches, two-color carpeting on the floor, a multitiered lighting system so that the task levels can be adjusted, natural light from a skylight, and live plants.

During an interesting discussion at this Symposium with Ralph Nader about carpeting in healthcare facilities, I found that some are against it. But sometimes there are countervailing needs in the hospital environment, such as noise control. This is particularly true in intensive care, where there is a trade-off between noise control and potential bacterial contamination. As designers, we have to do the right investigating, take a stand, and then go to the regulatory agencies. They are beginning to listen to us.

Connotation of the Word "Hospital"

A hospital has different connotations for different people. To some, hospital means wellness, sports, and physical therapy. To others, it means laboratories, research, surgery, or chronic illness. So how can we design one setting for all these different expectations? One thing I want to share is that whatever the hospital is, physically and symbolically, it looms large in our landscape—both in the urban skyline and in the mental consciousness of our culture. It is still a very powerful, almost archetypal, element in our society.

The concept and word "hospital" has an interesting origin. It comes from the same word as "hospitality," "hotel," "hostel," and "hostelry." All these words have the same root, and the buildings are really the same type of building. Basically, hospitals started out as places of hospitality for pilgrims who were sick, tired, and poor. Hospitals also came from poor houses and churches. We can see in history that the line between hospitals and prisons became very thin and that the function of prisons was mixed within the whole framework of a hospital. More recently, we see that "hospitals" mean "laboratories and research" to some people and "spas" to others. So "hospital" has multiple origins and multiple meanings.

Design Elements that Promote Health

When we look to assemble some of our tools and elements as designers, how do we know what to use for criteria? There is aesthetics, which we all differ on (although there is some agreement). But we can also use science to learn about our physiology and biology and our reaction to light, water, sound, and color. We can really use science as a basis for part of what we do.

One of the hospital spaces I visited illustrates how natural light can be used as though it were a paint brush. This hospital had the most sophisticated natural lighting scheme I have seen in a modern facility. Natural light came in, bounced off the vinyl floor, hit a plaster wall, where it then rose upward and swept across a slightly textured plaster ceiling that diffracted and diffused the light. A hard-to-describe luminosity is created that really makes one feel special when one is in that space.

More specifically, the light that rebounds back up to the textured ceiling falls against the skylights and reduces the contrast between the skylight and the ceiling, thereby reducing the glare. That's a subtle side benefit that can also be experienced with textured walls—a design element that might be very hard to get past today's state code restrictions. As in the case of textured ceilings, textured walls help spread and diffract light into many small rays, as does plant material. Thus there is a whole symphony of thoughtfully designed elements working together to create a spectacular environment.

The basic healing elements we will see throughout architectural history are water, sky, earth, weather, direction, and so forth. All these elements recur, if not in our buildings, at least in our minds.

Historical Overview of Hospitals

Now I will present a kind of historical overview of healthcare facilities. In Europe, healthcare facilities emerged from buildings that often had a church on one side and a small hospital on the other. There were monasteries and churches that would have an outbuilding as an infirmary. Sometimes they would have two infirmaries: one for rich people and one for poor people. Gradually, the building that housed the hospital got bigger and bigger and finally overwhelmed the church. This change led to the development of hospitals being built primarily as hospitals, with a little chapel or church attached somewhere. In the last 30 or 40 years, the size of these chapels has shrunk and it is now very hard to find a hospital's chapel. But it's still there, reminding us of its origins.

The first place I visited on my European tour was in a tiny town in northern France. When I arrived, I took the only taxicab in town, a Citroen. The cabdriver picked me up, went home to pick up his son, who had cerebral palsy, and his wife, then drove off into the countryside. He dropped me off there and then took his son to a hospital somewhere else. Here I was at a deserted dirt road, not knowing what I would find.

Later I discovered this was a 15th-century monastery that I hadn't known was there. I walked through a series of gates, followed my nose, and came to a sort of Renaissance portal. I walked up to it and, to my amazement, there was a Gothic arch—one of a series. I walked through the arches and saw the small round window of a farther building. I was intrigued because these structures weren't what I had been looking for. I walked through the last Gothic arch and was suddenly at a basically Romanesque building (no pointy arches) that had been designed and built as a hospital—the earliest one I was able to visit. A beautiful piece of statuary marked the entrance. The statuary of the Romanesque period was very graceful and "embracing," like that in some of the earlier French cathedrals. Instead of the somewhat vindictive figures I was used to seeing, the statuary of this era was extremely embracing and caring.

I walked in, and as this was the first sunny day after a week of rain, the lighting was exquisite. I imagined being in that building as a patient. All the windows, about 84 of them, were situated above bed stations. When things got crowded, they put two people in a bed. This wasn't all bad because these buildings were very cold in the winter, and retaining body heat was always a problem.

The building and grounds showed a caring attention to detail as well as an incredible contrast of simplicity and complexity created with a limited palette of materials. An example is the typical thick window jamb, which is beveled, not just set straight into the wall. One of the results of the beveling is a gradation of lighting between the light source and the wall, an attempt to reduce contrast.

Another hospital I visited is in a town called Tonnerre and was built 80 years later than the monastary in response to a plague epidemic. In fact, the Queen of Burgundy personally subsidized this facility, which is typical of how earlier facilities were built. People became afraid of dying when the plague struck because they thought they were going to hell. If they had the means, they would erect a hospital or become a nurse as a way to salvation. This hospital was built for that reason. Its great roof is the biggest barrel vault in Europe. The interior has window sills that are eight feet from the ground. The queen used to come in through one of the windows and walk on a boardwalk that ran around the top of all the cubicles. We don't know whether she actually ministered to patients personally or merely gave orders to the sisters.

The chapel at the end of this facility was crafted with finer materials than the main hall, an example of how the builders got more mileage out of their materials: the lighting was different, the glass was different, and there was more glass. This particular hospital was 97 meters long, which is about the length of a professional football field.

The interesting thing is that behind this hospital is a district hospital from 1960, but they still use the old building in a symbolic way—for social and cultural events.

A drawing from around the year 1400 of a similar hospital in Belgium shows a rendition of what daily life was like. There is everything going on in this drawing—from birth to death: people flirting with the maids, surgeons holding up the result of their surgery, and so on. This is an example of hospital life as a whole, and we will see how that advanced over time.

An 1800s engraving from Massachusetts General Hospital can be compared with the hospital with the barrel vault ceiling. It shows the same idea of a hall with beds at the perimeter and curtains around cubicles constructed inside. The table in the center can be seen as a predecessor of the core-of-utilities function in today's modern nursing wings, with the corridor running around the central service core like a reversed doughnut. The only thing different here is the fireplace, the hearth. That's a function that we've lost in modern hospitals. It's been replaced by the television. (That's another interesting subject for designers to talk about—television and socialization.)

About 100 years later than the barrel-vault hospital, farther out in France, a hospice was built in the town of Beaunne. It is a wealthier town, as can be seen by polychrome roof tiles and the general high level of materials. When visiting there, I found myself in the midst of a tight crowd surging through a tiny constricted entry into the courtyard, not knowing quite what to expect. Suddenly I was thrown into a space where now the hospital hall is one part of a quadrangle. Around the other sides of the quadrangle are all the service areas, such as the kitchen, the pharmacy, and the fuel supply area. So the hospital begins to be organized in a more complex arrangement. Even so, exquisite care was taken with the detailing.

What is interesting about this town is its historical setting. The hospice was built around 1390, a time when civic governments instead of churches were beginning to take responsibility for hospitals and healthcare, because the problems were too big. With populations shifting, sanitary measures were required, so the problems became municipal. This hospice was funded by guilds and the city government instead of by the church. We begin to see that tendency more frequently.

Compared to the barrel vault we discussed, inside the hall of this hospice little Gothic points appear, so we can peg it as early Gothic. The chapel of the hospice has a little more money, materials, glass, and light lavished on it. The patients' spaces are cubicles, vestiges of which can be seen in the engraving of Massachusetts General (the patient curtains). Part of the function of cubicles was to keep people warm; there was no way to heat these buildings, so often a canvas fabric would be used across the top, providing insulation as well as privacy.

In the hospice, the ceiling timbers were exquisitely carved with demons, saints, and all kinds of vernacular characters. One can imagine lying on one's back looking at the ceiling and wondering if one is going to heaven or to hell. We've all seen little vignettes of the Middle Ages and later—there was a lot of humor in that period. I would imagine there was a lot of kibitzing that went on when people weren't mortally ill. Clear in my memory of this hospice is the layering of detail and elegance in the calmest, most subtle way, creating a sense of beauty and importance.

After the tour went home, I went through the last door. Through that door was another quadrangle. There I found two remarkable things. First, a garden had been planted the same colors as the roof tiles. It was a striking notion to me that one could express nature in the building as kind of a continuum. The second thing I found was that another building there was actually a current-day elderly care home. They had continued the same function in this place for 600 years.

The Foundling Hospital in Florence, Italy, supposedly inaugurated the Renaissance; the term Renaissance was coined after this building was created in 1420. On the building is a well-known logo, which unbeknownst to its inventor, has become a tremendous marketing tool over the last few hundred years for all kinds of children's and perinatal services. The logo was actually designed in an artistic competition funded by the city of Florence. The Renaissance uses Classical forms but expresses them in more delicate, refined ways and proportions.

To my amazement, the Foundling Hospital to this day is still an active child care center and public health station of the city. The building has a very plain and simple gallery, providing the feeling of a sheltering roof. There is simple lighting that obviously wasn't original. The single-loaded corridors are a luxury we can rarely afford in hospitals today, flooding the corridor with light. Part of the current child care area was once the location of patient wards and courtyards. There was also an area intended for unwed mothers to ambulate in. It is interesting that the same public health issue of foundlings and unwed mothers is a major health challenge still very much with us today.

The Cross-Shaped Plan

In a hospital built in England around 1500, we see the first major innovation in the hospital hall. Around that time, more and more people were coming to the cities, creating dense populations in which epidemics could, and did, readily occur. How were hospitals to care for the increased number of sick people? They could continually extend the vault, but it was already as long as a football field. Somebody said, "Why don't we make a cross in the plan, and that way we can take care of twice as many patients in the same amount of walking distance?" That was the original function of the cross-shaped plan. Of course, there was also a tremendous religious significance in the plan, and perhaps one got extra credit in heaven if one worked in one of these hospitals!

So cross-shaped plans have been a powerful originator of a lot of what we're still dealing with today. Whereas in a hospital in Milan in the 1450s, there is an altar at the crossing; in a hospital built in the 1950s, at the crossing is a nurse's station. Other than the function at the intersection of the cross, there isn't a tremendous difference between the plans.

Another hospital, built in Milan in 1450 as a result of a design competition, was the biggest hospital in Europe for hundreds of years. It was built as a result of plague epidemics and included an innovation to improve hygiene (at least the conception of it at the time), which was incredibly important. Every patient bed had access to a private latrine in the double exterior wall. A river was diverted through the basement of the hospital, irrigating the latrine system; and pipes to vent the latrines were part of the system.

Again, it's interesting that this structure was built in 1450, and yet a modern medical conference was being conducted there, which I attended. This is a place where one didn't have trouble finding the front door, because it is surrounded by statues of donors. Although it was very clear where one was supposed to enter, the problem was wayfinding, an issue still with us.

In that same hospital in Milan, when going into the main entry court, one may notice that the chapel from the original church is just barely visible. It's become vestigial—one has to get up on the second floor to see it. This hospital was based on two cross-shaped plans placed together in order to create delicacy of scale. Thus feelings of intimacy and location are created in a massive building.

Since the most recent courtyard of this building wasn't finished until about 1950, the hospital had a building program that lasted 350 years—a designer's dream, isn't it? One of my slides of that courtyard shows a gratuitous set of details that include old brick, newer brick, precast concrete lintel and jamb, the reflective glass with a window shade behind it, the reflections of the courtyard, and two cats sunning themselves. Upon seeing this slide, my landscape architect friend pointed out to me that the tree in the courtyard is a cypress tree, symbolic of health and life and associated with hospitals for thousands of years. He thought the specimen there was probably 200 years old.

I'll describe a couple of cross-shaped hospitals in the form that went to Spain for a few hundred years, but first a little digression. In a hospital that was built as a cloister in Venice there is a very irregular floor plan of the hospital, which is located on a canal. There is a drawing of a little boat on the bottom of the floor plan that says "Ambulance Entrance." The point of describing this is that even with this originally chaotic floor plan, 1960s planners created a fairly modern hospital out of seeming confusion and chaos. And, again, that's an issue we need to deal with as designers: how do we develop ways to organize space both vertically and horizontally so we can feel the overall plan in our mind's eye?

There is a cross-shaped hospital in Granada that one would never notice from the street. It's a former mental hospital two stories tall, with an entrance that is very clear. Even if one were crazy, one probably felt important going through those doors. In the patient space, the carved, wooden ceiling reflects the Moorish influence in Spain. Because the hospital is in a hot climate, the windows are small and high instead of big and low, as in France. In this hospital there is a stairwell filled with natural light. (I think stairwells are the lost opportunity of design. They're potentially wonderful, beautiful places. The staff of hospitals love to go up and down stairs, but hospital staircases are usually ugly and terrifying and can never be found). At the crossings in this hospital, there is always something special architecturally—for example, light that comes down through a big lantern, emphasizing a detail at the door of the administrator.

There is another very similar cross-shaped hospital built around the same time in the town of Toledo. At this hospital the entry is more highly elaborate in design and decoration. The style is called Plateresque, meaning "in the manner of the silversmith." The entrance appears to be formed of silver beaten with a hammer, then twisted and curved; but it's all done in stucco and stone. An amazing aside is that the ceiling of that hospital is based on the design of the ceiling of the Alhambra (which I visited on the same trip), which was done 150 years earlier. It was quite fascinating to see how the "real McCoy" was so far beyond the copies, when even the copies are wonderful.

Moving on now to hospitals that resemble prisons: In Paris in the 1600s Hospital Sal Petriere was built, named so because mineral salt peter was mined at this site for an arsenal. The hospital was built by King Louis, principally to confine vagrants and the intinerant and lumpen population that was invading Paris. Orphans, prostitutes, pickpockets, and the mentally insane were all thrown into the hospital, starting a trend that ended with the Bellevues of the modern era. Bellevue Hospital was where I happened to train, so I have a special place in my heart for Sal Petriere, the miserable-looking place. It's beautiful in a way, but it's very civic, monumental, and un-healing. It expresses the power of the state.

Another hospital by the same architect as Hospital Sal Petriere is the Hotel Des Invalides (where Napoleon's tomb is located). It is a military hospital and is also still in use today. As fate would have it, I walked up and all the vets, as if on cue, came rolling out in their wheelchairs and immediately started lighting Gauloises cigarettes, which is just what they'd do in VA hospitals in the United States. In fact, a television crew came up and started interviewing them about their old exploits and the First World War—very exciting.

From the plan of Florence Nightingale's hospital, it's clear that she took the hospital hall, strung eight or ten of them together, and connected them with long corridors. Her hospital was originally a military one, but it became a model for hospitals from the 1880s until 1950. Every city had a charity hospital, like San Francisco General, that was modeled on Florence Nightingale's hospital. They were great for expansion; if the hospital needed a new radiology department, it just "plunked on " another wing. They were also friendly buildings, the kind that people still, to this day, reminisce about and have personal feelings about the bricks and sticks. They were buildings in which one could feel comfortable with the scale and height. Trouble occurred when technology advanced, land prices got high, and land became congested; but for almost 100 years they worked.

The Hotel Dieu, the most infamous hospital in Europe, is in its fifth incarnation after several fires. It's now a very active, functioning city hospital. One walks through the gate and is greeted by a beautiful, planned vista. Instead of a chapel, at the axis of the plan is an intellectual meeting place—the auditorium. So we find that here, logic and science have taken over from religion in the hospital setting.

The last hospital I visited was the most fun. It's the same kind of hospital as Hotel Dieu but elaborated in the most zany way because it came from Barcelona. We all know about Gaudi, the architect, but Pablo Casals, Savadore Dali, Joan Miro, and a host of incredibly creative people were active in Barcelona at the same time this hospital was being built. It's a fantasy of architectural forms, having a little bit of everything. It may be the first post-modern hospital. There are Gothic arches and Celtic crosses and half-carved-out domes with the other halves missing, and spires, and Moorish influence.

The lobby is an indoor/outdoor space. The best part about this space is not the architecture but the little ladies hired by the hospital to greet patients when they come in. They know many people by name and they'll ask "How are your kidneys this week?" and "Can I help you to the clinic?"

Upon walking into the hospital, one is basically in a city within a city, and each space has been elaborated in a unique style for a particular medical subspecialty. There's a streetscape inside the grounds, which are about 25 acres.

In one building, there's a very interesting experiment in trying to put new technology into an old building—a modern obstetrical service inside one of the original pavilions. So the closing image from my journey is a combination of the old and the new. As designers, we can draw some lessons and integrate into the present some of the things we've seen in the past.

Humanizing the Healthcare Environment

In conclusion, I'd like to personally encourage designers to push forward in trying to humanize the environment and deal with the challenges that come from state codes and from traditions that are no longer valid. Some of the specific issues we need to look at are the avoidance of fatigue from monotony (or from its reverse, sensory overload), the control of lighting and the ability to modify it for whatever the task is at the spot, the articulation of entries and circulation points so that we know where we are in these scary buildings, and the really persistent effort that's required to hang on to nature. I think we're finding that as our external environment becomes more and more eroded we desperately need pieces of nature in our healing environments—in our homes, hospitals, and workplaces. Another issue we need to look at is the control of patterns such that the placement of them becomes as important as the pattern itself. We also must give clients a choice, taking care not to overwhelm them with our ideas of what fashion or design might be. Lastly, we must tame the television and seek another substitute for the hearth as a symbolic design element.

If we look to human values, we'll find good design that acknowledges the worth of the individual. If we look to science, we can find not only technical excellence in machinery, but also a biological basis for caring design. And if we look to the past, we can find confidence that beauty still has a place in our field.

I would like to close with a short quote from Albert Einstein:

> The most beautiful experience we can have is the mysterious. It is the fundamental emotion which stands at the cradle of true art and true science.

Footnote

Much of my European itinerary was developed from the book *The Hospital, A Social and Architectural History,* by J.D. Thompson and G. Goldin (Yale University Press, 1975).

Neil Kellman, M.D., M. Arch., is principal of Neil Kellman & Associates, a firm based in Berkeley, California, that offers environmental consulting and health facility planning and design. Trained in architecture and medicine, Dr. Kellman is a distinguished author, speaker, and lecturer who has done extensive research and documentation on the origin and history of the hospital in society.

FUTURE TRENDS IN HEALING

Second Symposium on Healthcare Design, Orlando, FL, 1989

Richard Gerber, M.D.

I would like to talk to you about an entirely new approach to healing: vibrational medicine. But before we begin, let's examine the traditional approach to healing.

We use models and metaphors to explain how everything in our world operates. We try to visualize an image or choose a reference point that explains how our world functions. Our ability to conceptualize the human body functions is based on technological models of how the world functions. Since the inception of modern healthcare in the 16th century, human beings have been treated as mechanistic systems, clockwork organisms that function with gears and levers, pumps, pulleys, and pistons. It was thought that the heart functioned like a pump, the kidney functioned like a filtration system, and the locomotion muscles functioned like pulleys and levers.

Newtonian Physics

During the early days of science and medicine, pioneer Isaac Newton discovered not only gravity, but some basic laws about how the universe works: laws of acceleration and mass action. These Newtonian laws offered a different view of how the world operated.

Newtonian physics allowed us to predict how mechanistic systems operated according to certain laws of physics. Until Newtonian physics provided us with a predictable, orderly way of understanding the world, we were at the mercy of mystics, who felt that divine supernatural forces, over which we had little control, operated the universe. Newtonian physics provided us with a comfortable sense of control over our world.

Unfortunately, modern medicine remains rooted in the Newtonian model. This model, known as billiard-ball mechanics in college physics courses, advocates that if one knows the mass of two balls on a billiard table and the angle between them, one can predict how they will bounce off of each other and which billiard pocket they will go into.

Today's medicine remains rooted in this simplistic, 200-year-old concept of Newtonian physics. We still think of ourselves as machines operated by cogs, pistons, and gears. The recent emergence of sophisticated examination tools has allowed us to peer deeper and deeper into the human body and discover smaller parts of the machinery. Today, instead of explaining the body's functioning as the gross interaction of cogs and pistons and gears, we now explain its operation as the interaction of molecules or hormones.

When medicine was rooted in the mechanistic model of human physiology, healing approaches were fairly simple. A "bad part" could be either removed surgically or treated with herbal or gross chemical substances. As medicine has become more sophisticated, however, it has developed a molecular biology model of human physiology. We are focusing on smaller and smaller parts of the body. First, we realized that the body consisted of smaller subunits called "organs," each having its own function. With the discovery of the microscope, we found that organs themselves consisted of tiny chemical factories called "cells." Focusing further, we discovered that these tiny chemical factories housed their own miniature organs called "organelles." Now, we know that individual peptides, proteins, and molecules are the chemical messengers that run the entire show.

But are peptides, proteins, and molecules really running the entire show? This is the question we ask today. Molecular biology has resulted in marvelous medical advances. It has enabled us to develop cancer chemotherapy drugs that improve the survival rate—up to a 90 percent cure rate—for patients with formerly fatal illnesses like Hodgkin's disease. It has enabled us to produce antibiotics and heart medicines that achieve specific reactions in the body. Conversely, molecular biology has enabled us to produce drugs that bind in a body site and block a disease from spreading. Although in theory these drugs were designed to be site specific, they do affect other parts of the body. So today's medicine produces modern cures and modern side effects as well.

Today's surgical approach to curing disease also has become more sophisticated. Not only can we remove a diseased part, we can replace it with a new mechanical part. In a sense, today's surgeons have become bioplumbers; they cut into the body and reroute plumbing. If an organ system like the intestine gets blocked, surgeons remove the blockage and reconnect the pieces.

Although modern medicine remains rooted in the mechanistic medical model that considers the body a grand machine, we have become more sophisticated. Science and medicine are making marvelous advances with drug–receptor interactions and computer-designed drugs. However, we are finding that the mechanistic approach does not tell us how to heal humanity's industrial-caused diseases. We are finding that even the molecular biology model is not a comprehensive explanation for the way living systems function.

Energy Flow

Because the mechanistic medical model provides an incomplete picture of how the human body works, we are researching the missing pieces of the physiological puzzle. One of the missing pieces is energy flow.

The type of energy we are most familiar with is electricity. We have known about the principles of lightning from time immemorial. Batteries were one of the first manufactured devices that allowed us to harness and channel electrical current.

Within the human body are also electrical regulatory systems that operate with the cellular biological mechanisms I have discussed. The heart, for example, is a tirelessly beating organ with its own natural pacemaker that electrically stimulates the organ to expand and contract. The same type of electrical pacemaker exists in other organs of the body as well. The intestines have a natural pacemaker that electrically stimulates food to move peristaltically through the entire organ. Even the brain may have pacemakers that monitor electrical activity to increase or decrease physiological function.

The pacemaker is one type of physiological electrical control, but the brain itself originates electrical impulses that communicate with the rest of the body via the nervous system. The brain sends tiny electrical signals to our arms and legs to instruct them what to do. (We hope the signals work well enough to get us where we want to go!) Our electrical nerve connections are more extensive than we dreamed. Not only do our nerves connect with the major organs of our body, such as the heart, lungs, and intestines, but they actually extend to the lymph nodes and lymphatic organs.

Immune System

For many years, researchers felt that the immune system was an autonomous system. One famous experiment seemed to confirm this erroneous notion. In the experiment, researchers injected a small animal's arm with an allergy-producing chemical. They took another animal and cut off it's head, injecting the same allergin into this animal's arm before it died. Both the living and the dead animal developed an allergic reaction to the allergin. This caused researchers to believe that the immune system functioned independently of the brain.

When this theory was later found to be incorrect, as many of our initial assumptions tend to be, we discovered that the immune system is an integral component of what is known as the body/mind connection. Modern medicine now feels that the mind regulates the functions of the body, many of which were thought to be autonomic or beyond conscious control. With the advent of biofeedback technology, which allows monitoring of the electrical action of the muscle and cell, we can now consciously regulate activities once thought to be regulated only by the subconscious mind.

Current of Injury

There is one human energy regulation system I find fascinating—the current of injury that occurs whenever the body receives trauma. When a human cell is injured, the body creates an electrical voltage at the injury site to stimulate cellular mechanisms to repair damage. When a person cuts his or her finger, for instance, an electrical signal at the injury site stimulates the body's self-healing mechanism to activate immediately blood platelets and clotting factors. Initially, researchers thought the exposure of tissue chemicals stimulated repair, but apparently this current of injury is more critical to healing than we thought.

Dr. Robert Becker, like many orthopedic surgeons, could be considered one of today's biomechanics or biocarpenters; he cuts into the body with sophisticated mechanical tools like sterile drills, saws, hammers, and screws. Becker, however, is considered somewhat of a radical in conventional orthopedic medical circles. He began researching the body's electrical regulatory systems, particularly the current of injury as applied to regeneration—the ability of the body to regrow parts.

Becker performed his regeneration research on salamanders, very unique organisms. He learned that if the arm of a salamander is amputated, it will grow an entirely new arm complete with nerve, muscle, and bone. Yet if the arm of a frog—which is a more evolved amphibian—is amputated, it will not grow a new arm but instead exhibits a nicely healed stump.

Becker further studied regeneration in relation to the current of injury theory. He measured the electrical potential across the surgical amputation site in frogs and found that it began at a positive voltage potential similar to the plus pole in a battery. As the wound healed over a 20-day period, the positive electrical current at the amputation site gradually drifted back to zero. The electrical stimulus at the injury site seemed to be strongest at the time of injury before the body began to repair itself. This current gradually diminished as repair neared completion.

When Becker performed the same experiment on a salamander, he found a positive voltage potential at the injury site during the first several days. After this period, however, he found a negative voltage potential. The voltage measure had reversed polarity and begun showing a negatively charged electrical current at the amputation site.

Because Becker thought the negative electrical current might be a clue to the salamander's ability to regenerate, he used a battery to artificially create a negative current at the frog's amputation site. The artificial stimulation resulted in the frog growing an entirely new arm—fingers, nerves, muscles, and bone! This phenomenal discovery prodded Becker to study whether artificial electrical stimulation could cause regeneration in the salamander's cells and organs. If the experiment proved fruitful, Becker hoped to research whether the human heart, for instance, could be electrically stimulated to regrow heart muscle cells after a heart attack. Unfortunately, his work is still experimental and it has not progressed as far with mammals as it has with amphibians.

The electrical stimulus phenomenon does exist to some extent in human beings, however. One British study found that if the finger of a child under the age of five is amputated and the wound simply cleaned and dressed with suturing, an entirely new fingertip—nail bed, bone, muscle, and nerve—will regrow. Therefore, humans do have the ability to stimulate regeneration electrically up to a certain point.

But we have not really examined the possibilities of the body's electrical regulatory system because we have been so focused on molecular biology. Becker carried his work to its conclusion when he found that when electrodes were implanted on adjacent sides of a slow-healing broken bone and an electrical current applied across the site, the bone would heal. This experiment was first performed successfully on valuable racehorses with broken legs. Usually, a horse with a broken leg is destroyed. But Becker's study revealed that when battery-powered electrical stimulation was applied to the bone fracture of a horse, complete healing occurred and the racehorse could actually return to racing.

Gradually, Becker teamed up with Dr. Andrew Bassett to develop a noninvasive electrical system that used pulsed electromagnetic fields instead of electrical currents around the cast supporting a broken bone. When a person's leg bone, which supports the body's entire weight, breaks and is not healing properly, the situation is called nonunion of fracture. Until ten years ago, a bone with nonunion of fracture that didn't heal within a year was possible cause for amputating the body part. To prevent this situation, Becker and Bassett found that they could place a coil around the cast protecting the bone and while the person slept, plug the coil into an electrical outlet to stimulate bone fracture healing. The electrical frequency of the stimulus was important because the wrong frequency could cause the bone fracture to get worse. So, they found the exact frequency of pulsed electromagnetic field that would stimulate the bone cells to create more calcium and to knit.

This is just one example of how we are using energy rather than drugs or surgery for healing the body. We're beginning to examine human physiology from an energetic perspective rather than a mechanistic one. Another application of energetic medicine has been discovered in Sweden. Bjorn Nordenstrom, a radiologist at the Karolinska Institute, won a Nobel Prize for pioneering work in developing the technique of needle biopsy. He was the first physician to suggest using a needle to enter a lung cavity exhibiting a suspicious mass and draw out enough cells to place under a microscope and determine whether the mass was malignant or benign. As Nordenstrom studied the chest X-rays of patients with a variety of malignant lung tumors, he found that a circular shadow, or electrical field, often surrounded the tumors as if the tumors were electrically charged to attract disease-fighting cells.

Nordenstrom's research ultimately led him to believe that within the body, there is an entire electrical circulatory system based on the flow of ions and currents generated by both normal metabolism and diseases and infections. This hypothesis is somewhat different from the current-of-injury theory. According to Nordenstrom, the tumor-fighting cells—the white blood cells—are positively charged. Knowing that positive poles are attracted to negative poles, Nordenstrom inserted a thin platinum needle electrode into the chest tumors of terminal cancer patients and another electrode in the patients' abdomens to create positive and negative electrical poles. When he attached the needles to an electrical circuit and turned on a low-voltage current of five to ten volts, he found that the electrical charge around the tumor attracted tumor-fighting cells to the diseased site.

Nordenstrom eventually cured 40 or 50 patients with irreversible lung cancer using his model of electrotherapy. Unfortunately, this technique can be used only on patients whose cancerous site can be penetrated by a needle and the biopsy guided by X-ray.

To further explore the electrical model of medicine, we've discovered that the cell has some peculiar electrical characteristics. In an idealized cell, the genes, the chromosomes, and the DNA reside in the control center, or nucleus. In fact, each body cell is like a small being; it has its own brain, central control system, and a series of tiny organs called "organelles." For many years, scientists have attempted to discover the function of these different organelles. Many seem to be involved in protein synthesis. Some organelles are similar to microcrystalline bodies. Some, such as the cell membrane, perform like electrical capacitors to retain an electrical charge. Other organelles, called "mitochondria," operate like tiny electrical batteries, suing oxygen to generate energy.

Albert Szent-Gyorgi, the discoverer of vitamin C, found in his early research that many of the behavioral and electrical characteristics of the cell are similar to a tiny, integrated electrical circuit. He discovered that the cell has semiconductor properties such that the human body may be one giant integrated circuit in which each cell has the ability to manipulate electron flow. Szent-Gyorgi suggested that the body has electronic switching mechanisms that activate or deactivate the growth process in cells.

Szent-Gyorgi believed that cancer was the result of cells becoming stuck in an "on" mode rather than the result of cells reproducing too many times, which is a normal cellular function. Instead of using today's molecular approach to heal cancer by interfering with the DNA of rapidly dividing cells and killing them, we might consider Szent-Gyorgi's approach and reset the electronic switch that controls cell division. This approach may be similar to today's electrotherapy methods for healing cancer.

Besides researching how electrical currents and electronic switching in the body can cure disease, we also should be researching how other forms of energy—such as light, a type of electromagnetic radiation—might affect healing. Light affects us daily. Light cycles regulate our waking and sleeping cycles. Light directly penetrates the body through the skull, the eyes and the nerve pathways leading to the brain affect the pineal gland, which regulates the onset of puberty and sexual maturation. Some theorists suggest that with the advent of electrical lighting in the early 1900s and longer exposure to daylight because of daylight savings time, we are experiencing longer light cycles—thus gradually lowering the age puberty begins.

Medical science now uses light in healing. Children born with jaundice are placed under blue light to rid the system of bilirubin. Patients with seasonal-affective disorder (SAD), or "the winter blues," are healed with doses of natural or full-spectrum light. This cure was found when researchers noted that some people become inexplicably depressed during the winter months, yet when they travel to tropical, summer climes, their depression lifts until they return home. The key cure factor appeared to be light and the light cycle, so doctors now recommend that SAD patients sit in front of a lightbox emitting full-spectrum light during various times of the day.

Cellular Energy Communication

We know that people are affected by light hormonally, behaviorally, and psychologically; but it also is possible that we may be affected by light cellularly. Our bodies may actually generate and emit light. In the 1940s, Russian researcher Alexander Gurvitch studied cellular communication via an unusual experiment. He placed two identical cell cultures in two quartz dishes side by side. Even though the containers were sealed to avoid a physical connection between the cultures, he found that if he put a drop of poison in one cell culture, the other cell culture died a mirror-image death. When he conducted the same experiment in glass culture tubes, however, the second culture was unaffected. From this information, he theorized that some kind of communication must exist between the cells in quartz dishes, an energy transmission that occurs without physical, chemical, or hormonal communication. This interculture communication or energy transmission was absent between the cells in the glass tubes. He called this cellular communication mitogenetic radiation.

In the 1980s, Gurvitch's work was updated by a German researcher, Fritz Popp. Working with photomultiplier tubes so sensitive they could measure one photon, one quanta of light, he found that cells emit photons of ultraviolet light that allow them to communicate with each other. Gurvitch was able to show communication between cultures in quartz, because quartz transmits UV light. Conversely, Gurvitch was unable to obtain the same results in glass dishes because glass blocks ultraviolet light transmission. Therefore, glass does not allow cellular communication.

Studies like these indicate that humans have very sophisticated energy regulatory systems that transmit bioinformation via very weak electrical currents inside and between cells, between organ systems, and even through the emission of photons—weak light impulses that stimulate intercellular communication. This means that the human body is a lot more complex than we thought.

Besides the existence of electromagnetic communication within the body, there is now extremely good evidence that other energy systems, life energy systems, exist in the body. Although less easily quantifiable than electromagnetic systems, life energy systems can be measured. The life energy system model began with the Vitalists, who believed the human body was animated by a spirit that endows the body with the characteristic of light. They believed that all living energy inhabits the body until departing at the point of death.

Ancient Chinese philosophers and physicians also believed that people were both matter and spirit, a microcosm within a macrocosm called the universe. They believed that occurrences in the universe were mirrored by the principles governing the body—that if one studied the macrocosm, one could understand the microcosm. Because they observed a natural energy exchange between the sun, water, and wind in the environment, they believed people also had a natural energy exchange within the body. This energy flow, called "chi," was absorbed into the body through certain pores in the skin. From these pores, which became known as acupuncture points, life energy flowed to different organ systems of the body. When this energy flowed evenly and in a balanced manner throughout the body, it was considered healthy. Thereby, the Chinese developed acupuncture, a form of medical treatment by which these energy pores could be activated by extremely thin needles and cause the life energy to flow evenly throughout the body. For those who haven't experienced acupuncture, be assured that, as frightening as it may sound, it is a fairly painless procedure when practiced by a good acupuncturist.

Acupuncture has additional medical applications other than maintaining health. It also can be used as an anesthetic. In Michigan during the 1950s, surgeons performed a radical neck dissection on a woman without using traditional anesthesia. Instead, surgeons placed acupuncture needles in the patient's forehead and connected the needles to an electrical wire. Although the woman was awake through a surgical procedure that would have left most of us screaming, she felt no pain!

For many years, acupuncture has been used for surgical anesthesia by the Chinese. The West only learned about this technique after Richard Nixon's trip to China. Among Nixon's press entourage was the *New York Times* reporter Richard Reston who had the fortune, or misfortune, to contract acute appendicitis in Beijing. After being rushed to the hospital to have his appendix removed, Reston was given acupuncture anesthesia to numb the surgical pain. To his horror, he was awake during the entire surgery. But he was so amazed by the lack of pain, he summarized his experience in a newspaper article that hit the front page of the *New York Times*. Suddenly, acupuncture became a subject of great curiosity in Western circles.

Even with experiences like Reston's, the Western medical community did not accept the validity of acupuncture until the discovery of the endorphin system—a series of morphinelike chemicals secreted by the brain. The first ground-breaking studies in animals—and ultimately in humans—proved that when people were given acupuncture treatment for pain relief, measurable quantities of endorphins could be extracted from their spinal fluid. When these same people were given an endorphin-blocking agent, acupuncture anesthesia did not work. The initial simplistic result of the study was that acupuncture released endorphins.

Suddenly, Western medicine was comfortable with the fact that acupuncture was based on scientific data it could accept. But this data was interpreted to mean that when acupuncture needles were inserted into the body at certain points, they stimulated the nerves to stop pain—even though nerves

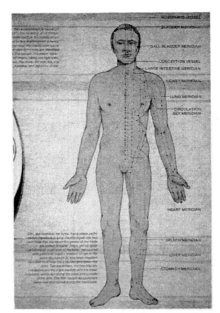

◆ **FIGURE 2–1** In this diagram of the acupuncture meridian system, body meridians can be seen as energy circuits leading to different organ systems.

were not always found near acupuncture points! But in the West, we move slowly to embrace new ideas.

Western medicine also could not accept the Chinese idea that throughout the body were meridian channels and energy pathways that were affected by stimulation of acupuncture points. This seemed a bit exotic because no Western pathologist had ever seen a meridian under the microscope. But let's take a look at the Chinese model of meridians. The body meridians can be seen as energy circuits leading to different organ systems (Figure 2–1). A majority of the meridians are bilaterally symmetric; there is a right lung meridian and a left lung meridian, a right gallbladder meridian and a left gallbladder meridian. This symmetry is in accordance with the Chinese theory of Yin/Yang, which holds that life is a series of polarities that balance one another—light and dark, left and right. The polar energies between the two sides of the body must be balanced for a person to be healthy, according to Chinese theory; an abnormally deficient or excessive flow of chi energy to any organ system results in illness. So the Chinese tried to correct any imbalance by inserting very fine acupuncture needles into the body at points that would serve as relay stations, diverting energy away from an area of energy excess or sending energy to an area lacking a sufficient amount.

Although the endorphin theory explained pain relief, enough to be acceptable to the West, it did not explain how acupuncture also was able to cure malaria, reverse blindness, or cause accelerated healing from a stroke. In addition, the West felt that the release of endorphins in pain anesthesia experiments might be the result of the placebo effect. They felt that because the Chinese believed so strongly in the positive results of acupuncture, their bodies were positively affected.

This theory, however, denies that any good can arise from the placebo affect, which is really an innate capacity for self-healing. For today's drugs to be effective, they have to perform better than a placebo because placebos are effective 50 to 60 percent of the time. But acupuncture has been found to cure disabilities that placebos don't, such as blindness and hearing loss. And there is now documented evidence that nerve regeneration can take place after acupuncture treatment.

Body Meridians: Energy Pathways

The real question for modern medicine, however, is what is behind the Chinese acupuncture theory of meridians and energy channels? In the early 1960s, Korean researcher Kim Bong Han experimented with acupuncture on animals in an attempt to visualize their meridians. Acupuncture had been successfully used in veterinary medicine for hundreds of years without doubting its validity or invoking the placebo effect. After all, how can a horse believe in the healing properties of an acupuncture needle enough to actually heal itself? I would like to see someone stick a needle in a horse and get it to believe it's going to get better. That person is more likely to get kicked!

In his experiment with acupuncture and animals, Bong Han injected a radioactive tracer into an acupuncture point of a rabbit. He found that the tracer diffused into surrounding tissues very weakly, but concentrated along pathways that are the same as those in the classical acupuncture meridian system. In fact, Bong Han claimed he could actually see these pathways under a microscope even though they were only a half a micron in diameter. This study is considered highly controversial because it was carried out in the 1960s, researchers had difficulty locating Bong Han, and no one else replicated the experiment until decades later.

It was Dr. Claude Derras, a French physician working in the nuclear medicine department at Necker Hospital in Paris and president of the French Acupuncture Society, who replicated Bong Han's experiment with human beings in the mid-1980s. Working with Dr. De Vernejoul, Dr. Derras injected a radioactive tracer into a human acupuncture point to observe its path via imaging with a typical gamma camera. A patient lay on a table with the scanner above him, and the two researchers injected dye into the acupuncture point—the same safe radioactive technetium used in today's bone and thyroid scans. They found that the tracer followed the classical acupuncture meridian exactly as it had in the animal experiments Bong Han conducted 20 years earlier. This experiment has been replicated a number of times by Dr. Derras, who found that the tracers even followed zigzag pathways when classic acupuncture meridians zigzagged. In other experiments by the two men, acupuncture needles were inserted at a point distant from the injection site and manipulated; this increased the flow rate of the technetium along the meridian, substantiating the Chinese belief that acupuncture does change energy flow through the meridians with needle stimulation.

In other experiments, the two doctors injected the same tracer into an area one-half inch away from the acupuncture point, so it entered surrounding tissue close to the point. Or they injected the tracer into a blood vessel, an artery, a vein, or a lymphatic vessel. When injected into normal tissue, the tracer would remain localized. When injected into an artery, vein, or lymphatic vessel, the tracer quickly diffused out of the area.

These experiments confirm that there is an entirely new anatomical system that may open up new avenues for medical research, diagnosis, and treatment. We can now locate acupuncture points electrically. There is a zero to 20-volt drop in electrical resistance on the skin over an acupuncture point. When energy travels along paths of least resistance, acupuncture points become energy pores that are synchronized with our electromagnetic environment. A variety of devices called "pointfinders" allow us to locate electronically acupuncture points on the body via electrical skin resistance.

Devices other than pointfinders also can measure electrical energy on the body. A map shows electrical conductivity on the skin over acupuncture points. The small zone in the middle is the area of highest conductivity. From this zone outward are zones of gradually increasing skin resistance. So, the skin has a very special electrical integrity.

An early model of an AMI device was built by Dr. Motoyama of Japan. Motoyama wanted to confirm technologically the Chinese belief that body meridians are connected to the organs. His experiment concluded that all of the major body meridians end at the fingers and toes. A photo shows a gentleman sitting passively while Motoyama inserted acupuncture needles in the man's fingers and toes, then attached a microclip to each needle, which in turn was connected to a computer. The computer compared the electrical activity of the meridians on one side of the body to the other. For instance, the computer measured and compared the electrical balance of the right lung meridian to the left lung meridian and provided a comparative printout.

Motoyama conducted his study on patients with known illnesses so that he could compare the computer's diagnosis to the traditional medical diagnosis.

But he performed the experiment without knowing what specific illness each patient had. When computer profiles were completed, they were highly accurate predictors of which organ system was unbalanced or diseased. If a person had heart disease, the printout showed the heart meridian to be unbalanced 90 percent of the time. If a person had a disease of the digestive tract, the printout indicated that the small or large intestine meridian was unbalanced.

Motoyama's meridian diagnosis system has since become more sophisticated, and needles no longer are used. Today, adhesive circular metal pads are placed over the acupuncture points, and a technician touches a metallic probe lightly to each point. The probe, which is connected to a computer, plots a graph for each point, providing an instant, nine-page readout. In addition, the computer prints out the orientation of the spine to determine whether scoliosis or abnormal spinal curvature exists. At one conference I attended where this was demonstrated, a staff member sitting in the audience was hooked up to the machine. The printout indicated she had a certain degree of scoliosis. A doubting neurosurgeon in the audience then offered to examine the accuracy of the printout. To his amazement, he discovered the staff member had the exact degree of spinal scoliosis indicated by the computer printout. There definitely seems to be a correlation between the meridian system and the organs of the body.

Europe is way ahead of us in using sophisticated machinery to make meridian diagnoses. One European machine, the electroacupuncture diagnostic device, has been perfected in Germany and is now being incorporated into the German medical education system. The advancement of the European medical system over ours is not unusual. Even the drugs used and approved in the United States by the Food and Drug Administration have been in use for seven to ten years in Europe.

The AMI device, long used in Europe, is now being used to study Parkinson's disease in the Bob Hope Parkinson's Research Institute in Miami, Florida. Here they have noted that people with neurological disease often have imbalanced intestinal meridians. Poor digestive tract barriers and permeable digestive linings might allow certain neurotoxins that cause the disease to be selectively absorbed and rerouted to the brain, where it affects the body.

Another type of energetic diagnostic device—the Voll Machine—was created by Dr. Rheinhold Voll, a German physician who studied the use of acupuncture in medicine. The machine provides a readout of stress points along acupuncture meridians that correspond to the organs where disease is. Although patients underwent typical X-ray examinations and standard blood tests before being tested by the machine, there was a very high correlation between the Voll Machine meridian diagnosis and the conventional medical diagnosis. This would not be surprising to the Chinese, who believed that when an acupuncture point is touched, the point is linked via a meridian circuit to a body organ. If the organ is diseased, the abnormal flow of chi energy in the corresponding meridian would appear as an indicator drop over the acupuncture point correlating to the area of disease.

The Voll Machine method of meridian diagnosis can be used for more than finding areas of disease in the body. It also can be used for testing various types of food sensitivities, food allergies, and other natural allergies and deficiencies. When a medicine vial is placed on the meridian circuitry, an energetic aspect of the medication seems to be transmitted to the patient.

The Voll Machine measures this transmission, and the printout provides a lie-detector response from the patient's meridian system or autonomic nervous system. This diagnostic method has proven as accurate as conventional blood testing in pinpointing allergies or in discovering when elements in the environment are affecting the general population.

This device is called the Interro, a computerized version of the Voll Machine. Instead of testing the reaction of acupuncture points to different medications, environmental toxins, or various natural elements like ragweed, researchers test the body's reaction to many allergic sensitivities at once using a magnetic hard disc with an energetic coding of many different allergins.

The human body is a biomechanism, this is true. But through the body flow energy currents that can be used for disease diagnosis and detection. Although a classical acupuncture needling is highly useful in pain relief, electrical stimulation of the acupuncture points provides even better pain relief. This electrical stimulation is now being provided with ultrasound and magnetic fields. In the Soviet Union, the United States, and Europe, solid-state neon lasers, rather than surgical burning lasers, are being directed into the body's acupuncture points to cure a variety of illnesses.

Energy Plus Matter Equals the Whole

At the turn of the century, with the equation $E = MC^2$ Albert Einstein proved that matter and energy are interconvertible, one and the same. What does this mean? It means that when the energy in a teaspoon of uranium is released, for instance, a tremendous nuclear explosion occurs—enough to level a city. This discovery has influenced our thinking about matter and energy since we entered the atomic age in the 1940s. It proved that matter is really a form of energy. The converse also is true; we have observed that energy becomes matter, although we still can't make it happen.

In one matter/energy experiment in a cloud chamber in which ionization trails from charged particles appeared as small, spiral trails traveling in opposite directions, the unplanned result was that a cosmic ray in the vicinity of heavy lead foil suddenly became a particle/antiparticle pair. In laymen's terms, a high-energy photon, a quanta of light, became two solid particles.

Does this experiment indicate that it is possible for something to change from one state to another? Perhaps. Water, for instance, exists in a number of different states. Water can be liquid. Water can be solid in the form of ice. Water can be gaseous vapor, after liquid is heated. So perhaps this experiment simply proves that matter is actually frozen energy that can be transformed from a gaseous state and frozen and compressed to form a solid particle of energy field.

Recently, physicists have demonstrated that the constituents of matter—electrons, neutrons, and protons—have a double personality called a "wave/particle duality." Theoretically, electrons might act like particles on Mondays, Wednesdays, and Fridays; and like waves on Tuesdays, Thursdays, and Saturdays; and like either on Sundays. In some physics experiments, beams of electrons aimed at each other will bounce off each other like billiard balls. In electron microscope experiments, electrons focused on an object as light will illuminate the object. Physicists know that the particles of matter are actually miniature, frozen energy fields—literally frozen light. Since all the molecules that make up the body are made of these same particles, we are made of miniature, frozen energy fields. We are literally made of frozen light.

The Hologram

Although today's physicists believe we are living energy systems, today's physicians do not. But there are some interesting aspects to the idea of matter as simply frozen energy fields. If the body is simply a frozen energy field, then the characteristics of energy fields should apply to us. One of those characteristics is the hologram, which is comprised of energy interference patterns. Most of us are familiar with holograms. They are stamped on our Visa Cards and MasterCards; they are everywhere in our man-made environment.

A hologram is comprised of energy interference patterns created when a single laser beam—mathematically pure light whose waves march in step like little soldiers in a parade—is split into two beams with the aid of a beam splitter. One beam, the reference beam, is shone onto a photographic plate. The other beam, the working beam, is shone onto the object being photographed.

A hologram is created when light bouncing off the object being photographed hits the photographic plate at the same time as the light from the working beam, producing a mixing of beams that causes an energy interference pattern. (The interference pattern is much like one created when a pebble is dropped into the water in a kitchen sink and an expanding circle of waves occurs. However, when two pebbles are dropped into the water at the same time, two series of waves occur. The cross-hatched pattern caused by the meeting wave fronts is an energy interference pattern.) These energy interference patterns then are recorded on film to make the original hologram. If one holds the hologram in front of regular light, it looks like a smokey haze. But if one holds that same hologram in front of laser light, it will recreate the entire image in perfect three-dimensional characteristics. If one were creating a hologram of an apple, for instance, and there was a worm on the underside of the apple that couldn't be seen from one angle, the viewing angle can be changed so that one could actually see the worm. I've seen a hologram of a microscope that had a tiny integrated circuit with a light shining on it inside. If I looked at the hologram from one angle, I could see only the microscope. Then I could change angles and actually look through the eyepiece of the microscope and see the integrated circuit magnified.

Another interesting aspect of holograms is that the original photograph can be cut into 50 different pieces and each of those pieces would contain the complete, original three-dimensional image (Figure 2–2). Or, a circular hole could be cut in the middle of a hologram and by holding the circular piece up to laser light, one could still see a complete, albeit smaller, version of the original image.

The holographic principle, wherein every piece of the hologram contains the information of the whole, may apply to other life principles. Remember that our ability to explain physiology depends on what we know to be true about the world. Now that we've discovered the holographic phenomenon, is there some way it functions in nature? If we observe human beings, we need go no further. We are made up of literally billions of cells. Yet each of these cells contains the master DNA template for creating an entirely new

THE HOLOGRAPHIC PRINCIPLE:
EACH PIECE CONTAINS THE WHOLE

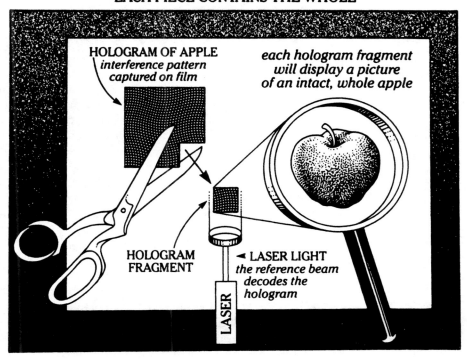

"As Above, So Below":
The Holographic Principle in Nature

"us" from scratch. Every cell in our body holds the body's complete master library. Therefore, we are literally a representation of the holographic principle, wherein each piece contains the information of the whole.

The holographic principle can also apply to energy. In the 1940s, Dr. Harold Saxton Burr at Yale University mapped the shape of electrical fields that surround living beings. In doing so, he found that salamanders not only had an electrical field that was identical to their physical shape, but they had a positive and a negative pole—an electrical axis. To find out at what stage the salamander developed this electrical axis, Burr tested earlier and earlier stages of the salamander's embryology. He discovered that even the unfertilized salamander egg had an electrical axis. Confused, Burr then injected black India ink into both sides of the electrical axis of a salamander egg, allowed the egg to be fertilized, and traced the results as the egg developed. As he expected, all the ink remained in the areas of the brain and spinal cord, along the electrical axis.

Burr's discovery that an electrical field not only existed but oriented the behavior of fetal cells as to where they would organize was remarkable. When he experimented on plants, however, he found an even more remarkable discovery: The shape of the electrical field around a seedling was the shape of the adult plant, the shape the seedling was destined to become. This convinced him that living matter contained some sort of organizing energy template, which he called the L-field or Life-field, predetermining where cells migrated in the developing fetus or seedling.

Kirlian Photography

Russian Semyon Kirlian, founder of an unusual form of electrical photography that now bears his name, also discovered that living matter emitted energy fields. Kirlian photography consists of photographing an image on top of an insulator, or dielectric, under which is placed a metal plate or electrode. As the photograph is taken, a high-frequency, high-voltage current is shot into the insulated plate, setting up an electrical field that bathes the film and creates sparks around the object being photographed. The sparks create a corona discharge, an aura, around the photographed object.

A famous Kirlian-type photograph taken by Thelma Moss of UCLA illustrates the corona discharge of a leaf. Before this picture was taken, the upper third of the leaf was amputated and destroyed. Yet the corona discharge is in the shape of the complete, intact, three-dimensional leaf. This phantom leaf effect, as the phenomena is now called, shows that even when the physical tip of the leaf no longer exists, its electrical field does.

When Kirlian photography was first introduced, the results were questioned. Skeptics felt that the phantom leaf effect was caused by moisture seeping from the spot where the leaf was amputated. To prove that the coronas were not caused by moisture, Kirlian photography researcher Robert Wagner first photographed a leaf via the Kirlian process and got an image of the entire leaf. Then he took the same leaf to a separate table and amputated the upper third of the leaf. He place an acrylic block on top of the amputated area to prevent existing moisture from bouncing off the acrylic; then he took a photograph. He found that the amputated portion of the leaf materialized in the photograph even through the acrylic block. He then photographed the same leaf five minutes later, and the amputated portion no longer existed. This tells us that the phantom leaf effect seems to be a fleeting phenomenon difficult to capture. But it has been captured enough times to make us question whether a similar organizing energy template exists in the human body as well.

The most convincing evidence I have seen for the holographic characteristic was provided by Romanian Dr. Dumitrescu using an electronographic process similar to Kirlian photography. After photographing a whole leaf, he cut a hole in the middle of the leaf and rephotographed it. This produced a picture of a leaf with a hole in the center, but there also was a picture of a smaller leaf with a hole in the center—inside the hole. This is exactly the result one would expect when looking at a hologram: If a hole is cut in the middle of a leaf hologram and held up to laser light, one would see a tiny, intact leaf in the film piece cut from the hole. This is fairly strong evidence for the holographic nature of the energy body.

In esoteric U.S. and European literature, the energy body—often referred to as the etheric body—is considered a template that guides embryological development and repairs damaged or diseased organisms. If this energy template is indeed a road map for cellular change in the physical form, then it is possible that disease may first appear in the energy template. If so, we might be able to develop an etheric body scanner than can detect disease in the etheric body before physical symptoms appear. If we could detect cancer at the one-cell stage, for instance, we could change our current lifestyle and nutritional habits before the illness manifests as a serious physical disease. I think the creation of an etheric body scanner is a distinct possibility in the next 10 to 15 years.

Therapeutic Touch

Let's talk about another type of life energy therapy called "therapeutic touch," a term coined by nurse-researcher Dr. Dolores Krieger, who followed in the footsteps of Montreal gerontologist Dr. Bernard Grad. Grad was interested in the phenomenon of psychic healing or laying-on-of-hands healing. (Many may know this type of healing as one where charismatic public healers in huge public auditoriums ask the sick to come up on stage. The healers say "Heal!" and the sick swoon and fall over backward and are carried away by the healers' assistants.) Being a hard-minded physiologist, Grad wondered if psychic healing was the result of the placebo effect or if it was a way to document the healing process. To discover an answer, he began experimenting on sick plants. First he soaked barley seeds in growth-retarding saltwater to create a sick "plant patient." Then he employed the services of local psychic healer Oscar Estebany, who had been successful in healing. He asked Estebany to perform a laying-on-of-hands healing on a large flask of saltwater. This water was then transferred to another flask and labeled Brand X, while an identical flask was filled with non–healer-treated saltwater and labeled Brand Y. Lab technicians, who were unaware which flask was which, watered the barley seeds. When the seeds sprouted, the technicians tabulated the percentage rate of germination. Then they placed both sets of sprouts in identical environments.

In comparing the two sets after 14 days, technicians found that the healer-treated plants were approximately 30 to 40 percent larger than the non–healer-treated plants, contained more chlorophyll, had larger leaves, and were much heavier. This experiment was replicated in different laboratories with different healers, and the results were always the same.

Grad later performed variations of his experiment. In one, he replaced barley seed with animals—an experiment that ironically won him an award from the CIBA Foundation, a foundation associated with a drug company! The experiment showed that healers could accelerate wound healing. In another, psychotically and neurotically depressed patients held the flask of saltwater. Grad found that although normal and neurotically depressed people did not affect the saltwater, the psychotically depressed patients imbued the water with something that retarded growth—just as some people have "green thumbs" and others "brown thumbs."

Grad's experiment leads us to believe that energy was exchanged in the laying-on-of-hands healing of the saltwater and that the water acted as a repository for that energy, having both a positive and negative influence on living systems. Other researchers repeating Grad's experiment found that laying-on-of-hands healers contained more chlorophyll. Since chlorophyll is structurally similar to hemoglobin, Dr. Krieger measured amounts of hemoglobin in patients after healing. She found that healers using therapeutic touch therapy on patients caused a statistically significant increase in patients' hemoglobin levels, even if they were on bone-marrow-suppressive drugs that induced anemia.

Dr. Krieger eventually teamed up with Dora Kunz, who believed that everyone has the gift of healing. Together they created a graduate-level course in therapeutic touch called "Frontiers of Nursing: Therapeutic Human Field Interactions" at the New York University College of Nursing. Sixty nurses who graduated from the course were asked to participate in an in-hospital study replicating experiments with healers. The study indicated that nurse-healers could actually increase hemoglobin levels in patients regardless of the patients' medical condition. This provides strong evidence that we all have the ability to be natural healers of others, in addition to having the ability to heal ourselves.

Since Dr. Krieger's study, thousands of U.S. and European healthcare practitioners—doctors, nurses, and allied healthcare workers—have been trained in therapeutic touch. The National Institute of Health has actually funded studies in therapeutic touch that proved this form of therapy helps decrease patient anxiety in coronary care units and other systems. In the future, I feel this course will be incorporated into healthcare practice to augment the effect of conventional medical and surgical therapy.

Electricity: A Cancer Cure?

Another energetic therapy to consider is the use of electricity for healing cancer. We use electrical currents in such devices as transcutaneous nerve stimulators (TNSs) for healing various types of pain from a variety of disorders. We use electroshock therapy for depression. Europeans use brain tuners to rebalance brain chemistry in patients with addiction disorders. (It is interesting that even though this therapy has cured addictive patients within days far better than do traditional medical cures, it is fairly inexpensive. So traditional medical practitioners prefer not to introduce the therapy to the United States because of their own profit motives.) We use sound in physical therapy. We use ultrasound to cure back pain. We use shockwave lithotripsy to shatter kidney stones. Polish physicians use pulsed magnetic fields to assist in rheumatoid arthritic and osteoarthritic remission.

We use subtler life-energy therapies, such as acupuncture, to redirect the flow of life energy in the body. We use therapeutic touch, including traditional massage, for a variety of illnesses. We use homeopathy, an unusual treatment method that uses extremely minute doses of herbal and other substances absorbed into water to extract certain healing frequencies of energy from plants. We use body/mind therapies like biofeedback and visualization to reroute and regulate natural electrical mechanisms controlled by the brain.

The Healthcare Environment

How does energetic medicine relate to the healthcare environment? We know now that human beings are more than just mechanistic systems of nerves, muscles, and bones; we are extremely complex biomolecular mechanisms in tune and controlled by higher energy regulatory systems. Some of these systems are electrical in nature. Some of these systems may be similar to a holographic energy template that appears to guide growth and development.

We are exquisitely sensitive to the energy fields in our environment—color, light, sound; electrical currents and magnetic and electromagnetic fields. All of these energies can be used for healing. However, they also can cause illness. Unfortunately, we have introduced so many frequencies of electromagnetic fields into our environment—from high-tension power lines and microwave ovens to video display terminals—that energy is often looked upon as illness-producing. In fact, preliminary data now suggests that high-voltage tension wires and power transformers may actually contribute to childhood leukemia. Other data shows that those working as electricians or around radar installations have a higher incidence of various types of cancer. Women with long-term exposure to video display terminals or electric blankets have shown a higher rate of miscarriage.

In a recent series of *New Yorker* articles, titled the "Annals of Radiation," author Paul Brodeur details how researchers have tried to validate that U.S. power lobbies suppressed information on the cancer-causing properties of our energy production systems. This issue is highly controversial, however, because of its economic consequences. If high-tension wires and transformers cause cancer, then it will cost power companies enormous expense to reroute and change the system—because it means changing the entire world.

The other area I want to discuss is our personal environment. What we place in our environment—whether it be a hair dryer, video display terminal, or microwave oven—affects our health. But the location of our environment also affects our health. In a drawing of a small town in France, gray areas and dotted lines indicate the location of underground streams. Black stars indicate areas in which people have contracted cancer over the last 10 to 15 years. About 90 percent of these areas are over underground streams. These areas are known as zones of geopathic stress.

The Chinese, who are masters in working with energy, avoid geopathic stress by using Feng Shui, a science that determines whether man-made environments are in balance and harmony with the natural environment. Major industries and businesses in Japan and China consult with Feng Shui experts before designing and building their hotels, offices, and homes to guarantee favorable results.

The converse of Feng Shui is geopathic stress, or building in areas where natural energies work against people. In one recent study, researchers found that people with a high incidence of cancer were sleeping in beds directly over crossing underground streams with a major flow rate. These same locations also may cause other illnesses, such as arthritis, major types of rheumatic disease, spinal disorders, deformities, and miscarriages.

Further results of geopathic stress can be found in the French town I mentioned that has an underground stream. A hedge shows abnormal growth where the underground stream crosses it 60 feet below the soil. A road is the site of recurring accidents where the underground stream crosses it. A tree with a cancerous nodule is directly over the stream.

The strangest evidence of geopathic stress yet is that lightning does strike twice, particularly a tree directly over a geopathic stress zone—a fact that has literally been confirmed over a thousand times by European researchers. And fruit trees over a geopathic stress zone will produce abnormal fruit and grow away from the stress zone, almost as if they sense negative energy (Figure 2–3). According to farmers, pigs living in a geopathic stress zone will eat their young, have many miscarriages, and behave abnormally; yet when moved to another site, the pigs will revert to normal behavior.

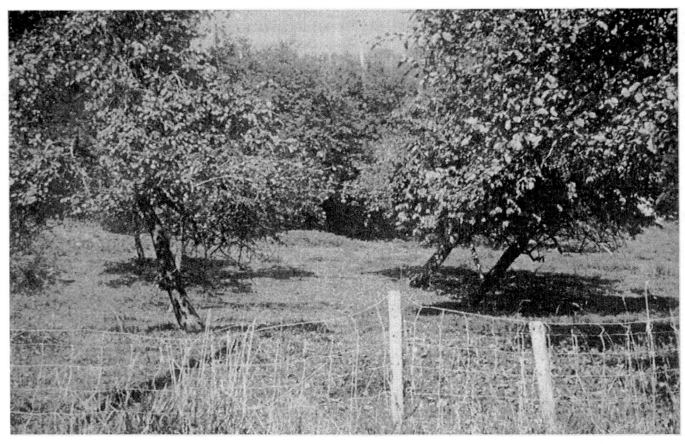

◆ **FIGURE 2–3** Fruit trees over a geopathic stress zone will produce abnormal fruit and grow away from the stress zone.

French researcher Pierre Cody studied the cause of geopathic stress zones, which was found to be ionizing radiation. When electroscopes that measure ionization in the air were placed directly over a geopathic stress zone, they indicated high ionization associated with some type of radiation. When electroscopes were placed three feet away from the stress zone, it showed a drop in radiation. Whatever this noxious radiation was, it formed a vertical column from the source. This radiation can be eliminated by placing lead sheets on the floor over the area of geopathic stress. When lead sheets were placed in the basements of homes in which patients suffered from illnesses that did not respond to conventional medical therapy, patients would have an initial week of exacerbating symptoms and thereafter their symptoms would disappear. But the lead sheets would age and discolor and have to be replaced within two or three months.

Ionizing Radiation

Today's ionization research has become more sophisticated. Scientists have found an increase in both ionized radiation and gamma rays—a by-product of natural radioactivity—directly over areas of geopathic stress. A special scintillation detector on wheels was used in Germany and Switzerland to detect ionizing radiation. Researchers, noting that high-accident areas on the German autobahn also were geopathic stress zones, installed special interrupter-type field devices to change the energetic environment, and the areas no longer cause problems. The ion ring radiation detected by the machine also was found to be greater in areas showing high cancer death rates. Interestingly enough, people living in geopathic stress zones tend to resist acupuncture therapy, homeopathy, and even conventional medical therapies. So there seems to be some correlation between physiological disturbances, physical trauma, and negative stress from the earth.

The question is, what causes geopathic stress? The causes may be abnormal gradients and densities of magnetic fields, the same culprits found in electromagnetic radiation.

Dr. Ludger Mersmann, who has done research with a special magnetometer, has registered large peaks in magnetic activity directly over the beds of patients suffering from diseases related to geopathic stress. One patient had severe recurrent arthritis of the hip, and the biggest fluctuation in the magnetic field was found directly over the hip zone (Figure 2–4).

◆ **FIGURE 2–4** Dr. Mersmann's work with one patient showed that the biggest fluctuation in the magnetic field was found directly over the hip zone.

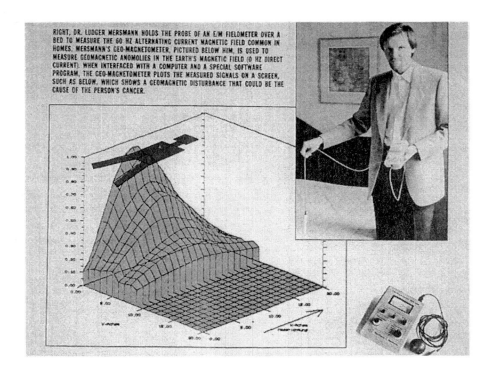

Research also has discovered the existence of a discharging field—a downward change in the magnetic current—over crossing underground streams. Another type of geopathic stress is found along geological fault lines that abut each other where crystalline deposits create a charging field.

Healthcare Design

The bottom line is that as we design future healthcare facilities in which people will be spending more time, we need to be aware of the potential hazards caused by negative electromagnetic fields, geopathic stress, and lighting. The Habechtswald Clinic in Castle Willems, West Germany, was specifically designed to eliminate geopathic stress. The rooms are crafted with natural woods; no metal can be found. Floors are covered with natural-fiber carpeting. Mattresses are filled with natural materials. Each room contains live plants. Heat is generated by natural, underground thermal pools. Results were favorable when each room was checked for signs of geopathic stress. Again, Europeans are far ahead of us in dealing with geopathic stress. I suspect as this information filters into America in the next 10 years, we will begin incorporating it into our healthcare interior design.

What I have presented may sound unreal to many design professionals and even more unreal to the majority of orthodox medical practitioners in this country. But it may not be. To be on the cutting edge of healthcare design, we need to use this information to perform solid research on the subject of energetic medicine. We need a multidisciplinary healing research center of the caliber of a Mayo Clinic.

I am now working with the World Research Foundation, an organization based in Sherman Oaks, California, which has started a fund to create just such a healing research center. The center will not only fund research, but also create an interactive healing research database that will allow those needing information to access healing data via their computers. In addition, the healing research center will promote and sponsor educational symposia on energetic healing.

Richard Gerber, M.D., is a physician, author, and teacher. He is board certified in Internal Medicine and is currently in private practice in Warren, Michigan. Author of the book Vibrational Medicine: New Choices for Healing Ourselves *(Bear & Co., Santa Fe, NM), Dr. Gerber has studied and researched alternative/complementary medical approaches for the past 17 years. His personal vision is the creation of an international, multidisciplinary healing research center that would help to validate ancient healing approaches and assist in integrating complementary and modern medical therapies.*

◆

◆

◆

◆

◆ Chapter

THREE

P A T I E N T - F O C U S E D   C A R E

PATIENT PERSPECTIVE

*First Symposium on
Healthcare Design,
Carlsbad, CA, 1988*

Sue Baier

I t is not only a privilege, but a challenge to speak to you about the design of healthcare environments. As you know, I have spent many months getting to know healthcare facilities as a patient. During this time, I have grown familiar with, almost expert at, the operation of healthcare environments. Yet, when I was asked to speak about healthcare design, I wasn't sure I could contribute any expertise. Then I realized that I had experienced every single facet of the healthcare environment.

We are here because environment is so important to our well-being. It even plays a role in helping patients maintain the will to live. Because a great deal of knowledge is represented by the design and healthcare experts present today, my thoughts may not sound original. But perhaps I can shed new light on some thought that may have been recognized, but not yet realized.

Until December 1980, I was a very active wife, mother, and community volunteer, who when I had time enjoyed a good game of tennis. Suddenly, an abrupt change in my being rendered me paralyzed with the exception of my eyelids; I was diagnosed as having an extreme case of Guillain-Barre Syndrome. Within 48 hours of the diagnosis I was placed on a respirator. I remained on the respirator in an intensive care unit for four-and-a-half months. I spent seven more months in the hospital before returning to my home and family.

When I finally returned home, I was barely able to stand alone. The attending orthopedic physician was amazed that I was walking even with the aid of leg braces and crutches because I had not yet redeveloped the muscles necessary for walking.

Today, seven years later, I am still recuperating from that devastating illness. It is still necessary for me to wear leg braces away from home because of foot drop and a certain lack of balance. And the dexterity in my hands is not as fine as I would like. But I have made great improvement.

When you are as ill as I was, comfort and security are paramount. You become almost childlike in your need for them. Although my body was paralyzed at the onset of my illness, my mind was not. I was still able to feel, hear, and see. Because I could do nothing but think, my mind was exceptionally alert. I remember everything! I felt a strong need to continue my role as wife and mother by keeping up with the activities of my family. A friend who is a professional counselor expressed surprise that I hadn't become disoriented in the intensive care unit and that I didn't require counseling after my recovery. This was due in large part to my interest and involvement in the activities of those around me. It was also due to the help of my husband, Bill. He researched Guillain-Barre Syndrome in a local medical school library after we discovered that few people in the hospital were familiar with the malady. More importantly, he constantly assured me I could get well.

Many people have told me they just cannot bring themselves to visit anyone in intensive care. I can well understand why. It's difficult enough for patients to be attached to millions of monitors without also knowing that their loved ones had to get themselves "psyched up" to visit the hospital. ICU is frightening. There I was on the respirator, unable to speak or move. Yet the hospital staff reminded me that because I was stable, they would probably

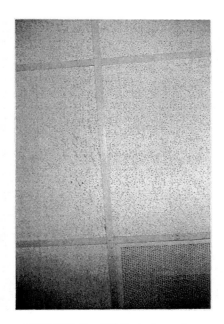

◆ **FIGURE 3–1** While in intensive care for four-and-a-half months, Baier stared at nothing but a white acoustical ceiling. (*Photo:* William E. Baier, Jr.)

spend most of their time taking care of other patients who really needed them.

Several years ago, a good friend of mine—an intelligent man who had become a corporate vice president—had a serious operation. After spending a few days in ICU after surgery, he could stand his surroundings no longer. He pulled off all his monitors and walked out into a hallway where he was later found collapsed on a pile of laundry, unconscious. His unique complaint worked: They moved him to a private room the next day!

As I continue to hear such stories, I realize that dramatic changes need to be made in our healthcare environment to help the healing process or ease the dying process, or even influence those who work in the environment. When I share this thought with people in the medical profession, I receive a most favorable response.

People generally think intensive care patients are in a state of unconsciousness. This just isn't true. Often patients are simply resting or have closed their eyes because there is nothing to see or do. Patients may not even remember the time they spent in ICU, but that doesn't mean the environment had no effect on their recovery. One woman who had spent many months in an intensive care unit was never spoken to by the staff. One day, a very caring nurse patted her and said, "I'll see you later." The little woman added, "Alligator." I wonder how she must have felt about having gone without communication for so long.

I think I know how she felt. For four-and-a-half months I stared at nothing but a white acoustical ceiling. The holes in the ceiling were not patterned so that they could be counted. Occasionally, I felt something like a particle of dust falling in my eyes. Otherwise, the boredom was pervasive.

My eyes often wandered from the ceiling to a large clock situated on the side of the nurses' station, which was literally at the foot of my bed. That clock was very important to me. Although a watched clock can be like a watched pot, it made me aware of the time of day and enabled me to count the minutes before an important visit or a test or procedure.

The clock made me think I was doing something for myself. Most impor-

◆ **FIGURE 3–2** The clock on the wall stimulated Baier to think—about the time of day and what her family and friends might be doing. (*Photo:* William E. Baier, Jr.)

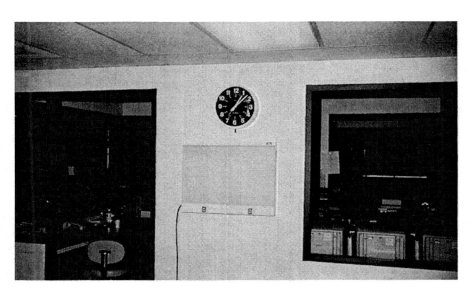

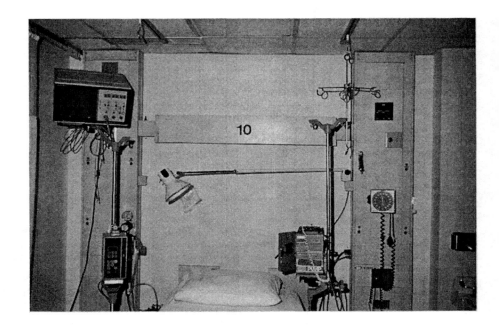

◆ **FIGURE 3–3** Baier wrote a book about her experiences as a patient, appropriately titled, *Bed Number 10,* where she spent four-and-a-half months in intensive care. (*Photo:* William E. Baier, Jr.)

tant, it made me think—period. Depending on the day of the week, I imagined what my daughters might be doing, thought about a meeting taking place, or visualized church activities. When I was later moved to another room on the same floor, the first thing I requested was a clock. Many former patients who have read my book, *Bed Number Ten,* have also commented on the importance of a clock.

A window is as important to a patient as a clock. In my intensive care unit, the only window visible from my bed was across the room. Yet it was so small I couldn't even enjoy the scenery beyond it. One day a radio announcer talked about possible snow flurries—an unusual occurrence in Houston, Texas. I was excited about it, but I wasn't alone in my enthusiasm. One of the nurses couldn't wait to go home and share the snow with her toddler. How I, too, would have loved to share the snow with my family, not to mention see the flurries from my window. It would have made my day eventful and genuinely improved my outlook.

Nature is an important factor in helping heal a patient. I love plants, flowers, and the outdoors. During the first week of my illness, my husband brought me a beautiful holiday arrangement of poinsettias from a friend. A nurse abruptly took it way explaining that plants were not allowed in intensive care. I understood, but I would have given anything to have kept it to replace the sad little plastic tree that was in the room. I didn't realize what the sight of a tree—any tree—meant to me until I saw one for the first time in months. Plants may not be allowed in intensive care units or even in some patient rooms for understandable reasons, but couldn't they be provided under skylights or in atriums? The landscaping for a medical building is always very important. That's why plants are placed in waiting rooms and lobbies. But that same link to nature provides a special relaxing effect, even a kind of healing power, for patients who must spend lots of time in a hospital room.

Think about how to bring the outdoors in. I spent three to four hours a day in physical therapy during the last few months of my hospital stay. It was almost always painful, very difficult, and tiring. Being able to see the out-of-doors during the process was very helpful. A well person likes to run, bike, and swim outdoors, so being able to see nature while working out can have beneficial effects.

Fresh air can also be important to a patient. I know, because one day a thoughtful physical therapist opened the window behind my bed for a few minutes to allow me to feel the fresh air. It was so therapeutic! Since I was on a respirator, I could not breathe in the fresh air, but I could feel it, and it was wonderful. A respiratory therapist in Galveston, Texas, called to tell me that when he rolled a patient of his—respirator and all—outdoors the man reacted favorably. I understand there is a facility in California that allows intensive care patients access to an outdoor rooftop terrace. More of this type of amenity would be beneficial.

A radio can also be beneficial to patient recovery. My husband brought me a small portable radio on the first full day of my hospitalization. I selected an easy-listening FM music station that provided highlights of the news and weather. Although it was difficult to find people who were willing to turn the radio on for me every day, I now realize what an important role that little radio played in the early days of my recovery. It not only helped me pass the time, but it gave me very normal things to think about. From my own experience, I feel we may too often deprive patients of any association with the outside world in our well-meaning desire to protect them or keep their environment quiet. I know only too well what too much quiet can do.

From the beginning of my hospitalization, I could communicate with my husband via a system in which I blinked my eyes to denote letters of the alphabet. Bill explained this to the hospital staff. Some of them would use the system to talk with me, but others would complete an entire eight-hour shift without ever speaking to me, touching me, or looking me in the eye. Therefore, even though I could communicate, I often felt ignored and very much alone. Yet, recent research published in a neurological journal shows that comatose and anesthesia patients do react to noise in their environments and that positive sounds produce positive results.

Having a feeling of control over your environment is important to recovery, yet I had little over even the light in my room. There was a lamp at the edge of my cubicle that could be dimmed or brightened depending on the needs of those tending me. A respiratory therapist discovered that this light could never be completely turned off, causing days and nights to appear the same—not at all a healthy situation. In other hospital units, this same lamp was installed directly over the bed. These large lamps may be needed when a patient is being cared for, but that need is not constant.

The noise level in an intensive care unit is another factor patients should have some control over. A hospital has constant emergencies that require hospital staff to rush around with all kinds of noisy lifesaving equipment. There should be some kind of material or barrier to absorb this noise.

Color can play a psychologically healing role for a patient. In children's healthcare facilities you often find colorful rooms decorated with balloons and other serendipitous patterns. This type of color application would be appropriate for and very much appreciated by everyone.

Temperature control is of particular importance for the very ill. Many hospital staff members assume that the average patient is cold and needs lots of heat and blankets for warmth. But being too warm is as unhealthy as being too cold. I was consistently warm during my hospital stay. Only later did I learn this was not only a symptom of my illness, but a symptom of being on a respirator as well. Yet few, if any, of the nursing staff were aware of this. Often I mentioned being too warm. I was told, however, that there were many elderly people with poor circulation in the unit and I would just have to accept the situation. Access to an individual temperature control mechanism would have made me more comfortable.

I would also like to touch upon the importance of properly located electrical outlets. An electrical air mattress was used on my bed to prevent bedsores. The mattress plugged into an outlet that was continually hit by a floor mop, disconnecting the mattress. Because I couldn't speak it was often hours before I could get someone to reconnect the mattress plug. How would an unconscious or comatose patient deal with a similar problem?

Hospital mattresses and bed frames in general should be longer. I am six feet tall, as are a good number of other people. Yet the beds in most ICUs are no longer than I am. What does a hospital do with people over six feet tall?

Personal amenities also are important in a healthcare environment. A bulletin board or shelf provides a place to hang favorite greeting cards or original artwork from a child or grandchild. This display area needs to be fully visible to the patient from his own eye level instead of being placed behind the bed where it is usually located.

Another important factor to consider when designing a healthcare facility is access to a restroom, particularly in a semiprivate room. Because restrooms are usually near available pipe systems, they are not always conveniently located for the patient. Because many patients must use their arms for leverage in a hospital restroom, commodes should be a reasonable height and a safety bar should be available. Railings should be placed on both sides of a patient restroom. Two years after my release from the hospital, I broke my left arm and again required hospitalization. The railing in the orthopedic floor restroom was located only on the left side of the commode. This made it necessary for me to drag a chair into the narrow restroom, even though I could barely walk, and use it as a substitute railing. Few of the nurses or aides understood the problem, but it was a monumental one for me to overcome.

Although many patients require a bedside commode, there is seldom a good place to put one. The bed table, chairs, and other furnishings usually need to be moved to accommodate a portable commode and placement of the equipment is often awkward. When using a restroom, we all take privacy for granted. But how would one feel about having to perform this function in the middle of a room with all sorts of strangers milling about?

Appropriate bath fixtures are also important in a healthcare facility restroom. My hands are now bent in an abnormal fashion, but they are strong; they can be likened to those of someone with arthritis. Yet, it is difficult for me to manipulate nonleverage-type faucet handles. The leverage-type handles are so much easier to manipulate than knobs.

While discussing grasp, I would like to mention the importance of handrails. Many handrails are attractive, but they obviously aren't meant for use by healthcare patients or anyone else! Can you imagine anyone trying to grasp a square rail whose four sides are five or six inches wide? Handrails are often too large or too small to grasp, causing a sense of insecurity. The finish of a handrail is as important to safety as the size when a patient's hands perspire. And the height of handrails should take into consideration patients of all heights.

Ambulation

Pretty, shiny floors may look attractive, but they can appear slippery to someone who is weak or lacks balance. This creates fear, which may in itself cause a fall. Rough-surface flooring, on the other hand, might cause the same person to stub a toe or fall.

Fear of falling can also be caused by stairways and steps. I cannot use steps without a railing to provide balance. Yet, there are many areas of a hospital that have one-, two-, or three-step areas without railings nearby. I can't tell you how many fingerprints I've left on stairway walls to prevent myself from slipping. Falls can be caused by visual problems as well as lack of balance. A person who has had cataract surgery, for instance, cannot see a step up or down unless it is distinctly marked with a contrasting color.

The type of steps designed for a healthcare facility are also terribly important. It's actually exciting to see a stairwell with wide, flat steps! They can almost be maneuvered without a railing, and they are so much easier to handle for someone who uses a cane or crutches. Stairways should not be too steep to maneuver because even when elevators are available, patients are often encouraged to use stairways to increase their circulation.

I also must say a few words about elevators. The newer ones are wonderful; they often "talk" to you while they carry you from floor to floor. But their doors often close so quickly it is frightening. If the elevator cage does not stop evenly with the floor, there should be a color differentiation to provide guidance. Elevator buttons need large print so everyone, including the elderly, can read them. The "open door" button and "lock" button should also be easier to find, and handrails should be a must.

As for entering and exiting a medical building, a patient who is alone often has a problem. An acquaintance of mine with MS was being trained to be independent before returning home from the hospital. From a wheelchair she could transfer to her car, store the chair, and drive away. Yet, she couldn't reenter the hospital and return to her room alone. She teased the staff about this until the hospital finally installed a sliding magnetic door at the entrance.

Ramps are replacing stairs to facilitate wheelchair use, but people confined to wheelchairs do not feel secure on ramps that have no railings. Too often, as is true of stairs, these ramps are narrow, steep, and appear slippery.

Healthcare Furnishings

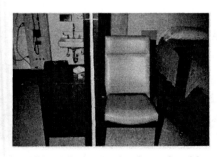

◆ **FIGURE 3–4** Lack of comfortable visitor's chairs was the biggest complaint of Baier's husband during her stay. (*Photo:* William E. Baier, Jr.)

Hospital furniture should be selected with patients in mind. Seating areas, lobbies, and waiting rooms generally provide low, comfortable seating that is inviting to sit in but difficult to get out of. As is true for a commode, many weak and elderly people appreciate higher seating surfaces with arms for leverage. People laughingly say that the furniture in patient rooms is meant to be uncomfortable to keep well-meaning visitors from overstaying their welcome. But what about the comfort of family members, friends, and hospital staff who must spend hours at a patient's bedside? A patient may even use these chairs for any given number of reasons, and a very firm seating surface is uncomfortable for someone who is quite thin. I weighed only 85 pounds in the hospital and when I sat in a chair, I became bruised where my skin rubbed against my pelvic bones. That same chair never put my husband in a comfortable position to hold my hand, something that gave me a great deal of security when he was able to do so. With all of the things my husband had to manage during my hospitalization, including three hospital visits a day, the lack of comfortable hospital seating was his biggest complaint.

Furniture arrangement is as important as the furnishings themselves. In physical therapy, for instance, there was a definite lack of privacy. A therapist usually works with several patients at a time and needs to keep an eye on all of them. A patient trying to motivate a broken limb is often placed on a work table in a large room to make the therapist's job easier and to provide the incentive of competition for patients. But stroke patients or those with catheters or nasal gastric tubes attached don't need to feel more obvious than they already are, which can detract from the effectiveness of therapy. Therapy tables might be placed in corners and turned in opposite directions to create a feeling of privacy.

In Houston, a new rehabilitation facility in a residence building for senior citizens provides several "practice rooms," where patients can live before returning home. These rooms help patients relearn everyday activities before the moving-home adjustment. I would love to see more of these practice rooms in regular hospitals where orthopedic rehabilitation takes place. They would help the patient more easily adjust to daily living with the guidance of a supportive therapist.

The arts can help contribute to the healing environment. Patients using back halls of a hospital on their way to required testing, X-ray, etc. find themselves in areas as drab as intensive care units. A patient may be fasting or apprehensive about a forthcoming test or pushed into a test area and left, alone, until time to be tested. Waiting time could be made so much easier with the aid of piped-in stereo music and interesting artwork.

Bed Number Ten

The only way I could have written *Bed Number Ten* or do what I'm doing today is with the support of my family, friends, and staff of the hospital I was in. The staff even organized my first autograph party after the book was published.

Let me describe to you how "bed number ten" and the environment in which I spent much time with that hospital staff has changed. When I returned to the hospital since, many things had been altered. Some for the better, some not. The small window that was behind my bed has been eliminated. (I immediately thought of the nurse who had told me that if there were ever a fire, the window would be used as an exit for me!) The window on the opposite side of my room had been enlarged to give patients more than just a glimpse of the outdoors. Clocks had been placed in every intensive care unit, but the chairs in the semiprivate rooms had not been changed; they were the same uncomfortable ones as before.

A few weeks ago, I saw an article in the Sunday paper headlined in solid caps: WELLNESS APPROACH BENEFICIAL. The article said that with increased awareness people can help prevent their own illness and that the number of people requiring medical attention seems to be dropping. The head of physical therapy in the facility where I was treated said that I nearly drove the staff crazy by staying two steps ahead of them but that I probably got myself out of the hospital sooner.

I have had, and still do have, lots of love and support from many sources. For those who do not, a healthcare environment can make a difference in their healing rate. As I mentioned earlier, this presentation has been a challenge. I hope some of that challenge can now become yours. Creating this Symposium is an exciting advancement for healthcare because the possibilities for change in the field are numerous. Your response [a standing ovation] is the kind of love and support I continue to have. It gives me the encouragement to go on.

Sue Baier graduated from Southern Methodist University in 1958 with degrees in business and home economics. She and her husband, Bill, reside in Houston, Texas, where they have spent most of their married lives raising their two daughters. In late 1980, Baier was stricken with Guillian-Barre Syndrome, which resulted in temporary total paralysis, requiring four-and-a-half months in intensive care and seven additional months of hospitalization. She recounted her experience in the book, Bed Number Ten *(CRC Press), which has been well received by healthcare designers and practitioners. Baier serves on the Board of Directors of the Guillian-Barre Syndrome Foundation International and was honored as its 1993 "Citizen of the Year."*

◆ ◆ ◆

THE PLANETREE PHILOSOPHY

Fourth Symposium on Healthcare Design, Boston, MA, 1991

Robin Orr, M.P.H.

The Planetree Organization is a nonprofit, consumer healthcare organization based in San Francisco, Calif. The organization is dedicated to working with progressive organizations and institutions to create models that offer a more patient/consumer-oriented approach to the delivery of healthcare. Our mission, simply put, is to redirect and restructure the healthcare system from the patient's perspective by focusing on humanizing, personalizing, and demystifying the healthcare experience. Our efforts are not directed at attempting to fix the hospital or to enhance or improve the quality of outdated, ineffective systems. Rather, our goal is to change profoundly the very nature of the healthcare system.

Perhaps some background information on myself and Planetree will give some perspective on our motivation. I was a hospital administrator for seven long years, which were basically wrought with frustration and a strong sense of helplessness. After years of sitting in boardrooms, I left the field of hospital administration, tired and cynical, believing that hospitals were dinosaurs and impossible to change. At that point, I decided to return to school and pursue a Master's Degree, hoping that a break from hospital administration would give me an opportunity to renew the strength, attitudes, and idealism I had when I first went into the field. My goal was someday to reenter the healthcare arena.

I began my studies at the University of Hawaii and later transferred to the University of California at Berkeley. David Starkweather, a professor of hospital administration at the University of California—a man considered to be the "guru" of hospital administration—was my mentor. One day, he called me into his office and said, "Robin, I've been approached by a nonprofit organization in San Francisco called Planetree. I'm not quite sure what they're up to—something about consumers and healthcare and trying to change the hospital. Sounds like they're doing some interesting things, but they need some help. They need somebody who has experience as a hospital administrator and who can help them translate some of the philosophy and ideals that they have. I tell you what, I'll give you credit for a class if you go and help them out."

I told him I'd be happy to and decided that it didn't really matter what Planetree was doing; if I didn't have to sit in another classroom, I would be more than delighted to go and talk to these folks in San Francisco.

He gave me an address for the Planetree Health Resource Center on Webster Street. When I walked through the front door, I was on the ground floor of a large, beautiful, historical building, which also houses the Health Sciences Library of California Pacific Medical Center—the second largest biomedical library in northern California, which, by the way, is restricted to the lay public. Upon entering the Planetree Resource Center in this building, I immediately recognized that something different was going on. The center was a very small room with a lot of books and shelves. It looked much like the libraries I had been spending a lot of time in recently at the university. All sorts of people—young and old, males and females—were engaged in research, looking up information on diagnosis, different diseases, and health topics.

I noticed, however, that the people sitting in this room were just ordinary people—they weren't health professionals. And not only did the Resource Center have all the usual medical and health books, but it also had many books written by the lay public on health (such as how to treat somebody in the home and what to do with a loved one dying of a terminal illness). The classification scheme organized books in a way different from any that I'd ever seen in a regular library. In addition, the center had a clipping file of the current research and information from the world literature. It had an information and reference system of physicians that included physicians' questionnaires, covering not just information from physicians about what they charge for their services but also information on the philosophy of care of each particular physician. There were thousands of listings of support groups, agencies, and clinics all over the world that made up a consumer network of people who have health problems and who are interested in talking to other people with similar problems. It also had a health information service that accessed a world data base from the National Library of Medicine and Physician's Desk Query of the National Cancer Institute.

Needless to say, I was immediately intrigued by an organization that had created this very special Resource Center. I was then introduced to Planetree's founder, Angie Thieriot, who told me the story of why she had begun this organization. To this day, her story stays with me as one of the prime motivations to continue Planetree's work.

Angie was a young woman who had been sick with an undiagnosed virus. She had been admitted to a hospital in San Francisco, and anyone who has ever been admitted to a hospital for any reason knows it can be very frightening. Angie remembers that during her stay, she was sent down to the radiology department and left out in the hallway for 45 minutes, no one asked her if she were okay, offered her a blanket, or explained that someone would be with her in a moment. She remembers lying in bed, totally disoriented and having a very high temperature, with nothing pretty to look at. Finally, she spoke up and got somebody to pay attention to her. But it made her think about what the same experience would be like for an elderly person or for somebody who is too frightened or intimidated to speak up.

Around that same period of time, Angie's son was also hospitalized in San Francisco; so she became the mother of a patient in a hospital. Her son was scared and she didn't want to leave him alone. She was granted permission to spend the night in the hospital in a chair in a corner of the room. During the night, she walked to the nurses' station and tried to get someone's attention. Because the nurses' station was both a physical and symbolical barrier that served to separate sick people and others from the people who work there, she had difficulty.

Finally, after getting the attention of a nurse who was seated behind a glass barrier, she was told, "I'm sorry, I cannot answer that question because I'm a float nurse from Orthopedics." Angie had wanted to see her son's medical record because she wanted to know what was happening with the various tests and procedures that he was having. She was told she could not see that medical record.

Also around that same period of time, Angie's father-in-law, a powerful, influential man in San Francisco who was used to making major decisions every day of his life, was admitted to one of the finest medical institutions in the world. The experience she and her family recount of that institution is also less than dignified.

As Angie was telling me this story, I, as a good hospital administrator, immediately became defensive. I started to think, "Well, of course hospitals are like that, and of course people are busy. Hospitals have to protect confidentiality. Hospitals are not restaurants, so why should patients expect good food? Things can't be pretty in a hospital because people will steal and wreck them."

But as I began to listen to and understand the very naive, honest experience that this woman had, I said, "You're right!"

"Robin, why does it have to be that way?" Angie asked. "Why is it that we have created a healthcare system that has some of the finest technology— we can save people's lives; we can substitute artificial organs for diseased ones; we can do all these wonderful things in the name of scientific medicine. But somewhere along the line, what we know about human beings, about health and healing (words you don't even hear in hospitals), the importance of families, diet, and nutrition, and the impact of the environment on our well-being have been lost?"

At that point, the Planetree Organization captured my intellectual curiosity, as well as my feelings and dedication. I decided that I wanted to work with this wonderful organization in San Francisco.

Health Resource Center

The Health Resource Center in San Francisco was the first project Planetree did. It was very clear to Angie that of all the things she spoke about, the main reason that patients are disempowered by the healthcare system is because they do not have access to information in order to make informed healthcare decisions. The Health Resource Center offers patients access to information they need when they are in the hospital, and people in the community information on how to stay well and not end up in the hospital.

After we got the Planetree Health Resource Center off the ground, we focused on our original intention, which was the hospital. That is what Angie really cared about. She wanted to approach hospitals and say, "Listen, let's really be creative here. Let's dream, let's look about, let's listen to the things patients say about their experiences." Our intentions were and continue to be to infuse a more humanistic, holistic healing philosophy into the heart of the healthcare system, which is the hospital. We want to change the very image and nature of hospitals from the patients' perspective and focus on the experience of healthcare.

Our first project in 1985 was a 13-bed medical/surgical unit at a 310-bed tertiary hospital in San Francisco that has now merged with Children's Hospital. The Henry J. Kaiser Family Foundation gave us money to implement the Planetree philosophy as a model within the acute care environment as a three-year demonstration project. Obviously, it still exists today and now includes patients with a variety of diagnoses—everything from asthma to AIDS. These days, we have more AIDS patients than chronic obstructive pulmonary disease.

The second project, at San Jose Medical Center in San Jose, California, was completed in 1989.

We are currently working on the Mid-Columbia Medical Center, which is outside Portland in a small town called The Dalles. We're redoing the entire hospital, which is very exciting. It's going to have a 30-foot waterfall cascading off one side of the new atrium, which patients can experience from the activities room on each floor.

We are also working on a 50-bed pavilion at Delano Regional Medical Center in the central valley of California, which has many migrant workers and is a culturally rich community. The unit will include a subacute care unit and a skilled nursing unit.

Our most ambitious project to date is the one we're doing at Beth Israel Medical Center in New York City—1,050 beds, of which we have 34. We were told that these "weird, flaky" ideas will work in California, but not in New York—we shall see.

The Planetree Blueprint

Continuity, accountability, and education make up the cornerstone of the Planetree model philosophy. These are the areas we looked at as we began to explore creating a new blueprint for healthcare:

1. *Nurse Training.* As an administrator, I had very little appreciation for the nursing staff and the incredible work they do every day. When I began working with Planetree, I took the time to listen to and understand the nurses. What I heard was shocking. Most told me that if they had a choice of going into the nursing profession or choosing another profession at this point in their lives, they would choose another profession.

Now, one of the most admirable, wonderful professions I can think of is nursing. So what were the nurses saying? They were saying exactly what Angie was saying: "I want to participate in what happens in the hospital."

We learned very soon that if we were going to empower patients—if we

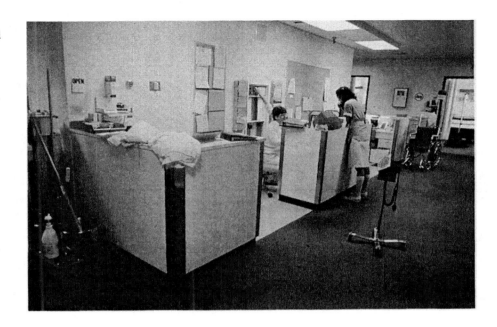

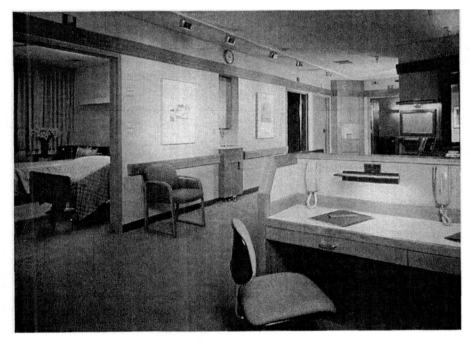

were going to create a new blueprint for the delivery of healthcare that paid
attention to the human side of the equation, we were going to have to empower everyone who works in the institution. If we were going to empower
patients, we had to empower nurses. Who did we hire and how did we train
them? Our nurses called it "untraining." What happens to these wonderful
individuals (who go into the nursing profession for all the right reasons, to
become healers) is that they walk through the front doors of these institu-

tions and are forced to become clerical workers. As such, they are truly not empowered to be part of the decision-making process.

We looked at primary nursing as a delivery system in terms of nursing care. The only thing that made any sense was for patients to have a nurse co-ordinate who is responsible for their care from admission to discharge.

2. *Access to Information.* One of the nicest things we can do for our patients, in creating the institutions that serve people who are sick, is to provide them with information. We have to say to patients and others who come to our institutions, "We trust you, we have no secrets here, we want to demystify this experience for you; we want you to be part of the process of making decisions about your care, your health. We want you to read your medical record. In fact, not only do we want you to read your medical record, we want you to write your own progress notes, your own observations about what's happening."

We have found that diagnostic fact sheets are useful in answering questions. What does it mean to have asthma? What about the tests and the procedures? Does the medication taste like a milkshake?

We also know that as many as 40 percent of the patients who are readmitted to hospitals are there because of medication mismanagement and noncompliance. Noncompliance, in most cases, comes from a lack of information and understanding. What do you do if you miss a dosage of that medication? What are the side effects of that medication? What about taking this medication with that medication, or with this food? In most hospitals, discharge planning and teaching occur just as patients are ready to walk out the door, when all they are worried about is how to find the parking lot. How are we preparing patients to go home in a way that they know how to take care of themselves—to change a surgical dressing or flush a Hickman catheter?

Most procedures that patients are doing in their homes are very compli-

◆ **FIGURE 3–7** A resource library and open chart areas allow patients and families access to information.

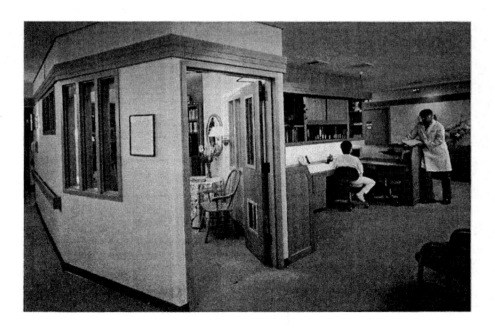

cated. The hospital provides that "teachable" moment when staff has the responsibility to make sure patients are prepared to go home. But, giving our patients a free membership to the Planetree Health Resource Center says, "Maybe right now you're so confused and sick that this is not the right time for you to understand. If your family members don't understand what's going on either, when you leave the hospital you can come back to this Resource Center that's right across the street from the hospital." People can get information, books, fact sheets, or research literature on topics of interest, or find out what they need to know so that they can take care of themselves. It is the link back to the community that makes the hospital the health resource for the community.

Now, we know that not only do these things make sense, but we also know that so much of the lack of information and lack of trust in the healthcare system today ends up in litigation because of that lack of trust. Also, if we're ever going to get people to be good consumers of healthcare, they have to have access to information in whatever way that makes sense.

3. *Nutrition.* Angie recounted stories about nutrition; one of the major complaints is usually about how bad the food is in hospitals. Most hospital food is so bad that if it were served to me in a second-class restaurant, I would send it back. This is one of the obvious examples of how many healthcare institutions have lost track of what their responsibility is all about. We know that many of the diseases we are faced with today are lifestyle-related. On the human side, having a kitchen on a unit in a hospital is one of the most nurturing, friendly things that can be done. When people have parties in their houses, guests usually end up in the kitchen. At Planetree, we have cooking demonstrations in the kitchen. We do counseling on diet and nutrition, focusing on the importance of diet not just for patients who are at risk or suffer from malnourishment, but for all patients.

4. *Families.* Research shows that people who have support systems, whether a family or a network of friends, don't get sick as frequently and they get well faster. Most hospitals or places that are supposed to be about healing only allow family and friends to be there for a certain period of time. Hospital administrators tell me they have relaxed these rules. But we're not talking about giving permission for a husband, wife, or little child to be in the hospital visiting a mother, father, or aunt. We're talking about encouraging them to be part of what happens there and providing an environment supportive of families and friends.

There should be unlimited, unrestricted visiting hours. I don't care what time of day it is, if a husband or a wife wants to be with a patient, we will make arrangements for it to happen. If we didn't have the environment in which that can happen, it wouldn't work.

That is why the work design professionals do is so very important. We believe that the physical environment does enhance the well-being of patients, family, and staff. The focus is not just to make the hospital a nicer place, or less institutional. It is an acknowledgement that the physical environment must change in order to enable the Planetree philosophy to work.

5. *Physicians.* Just as I, as a hospital administrator, had opinions about nurses, I also had opinions about physicians. I was told by others that physicians will never buy this concept. I could hear their complaints: "Patients having access to the world literature, including information on complementary therapies? Patients reading their medical records, writing their own progress notes? Nutrition and education happening right in the hospital? Families running amok? People in kitchens cooking things, smelling up the place, wrecking the place?"

We did not get every physician to buy into the Planetree philosophy, but we got 15 to start. Fifteen role models, physicians who recognized the value of having patients involved in their own care. One of the first physicians whom Angie talked to was Dr. John Gamble, the chairman of the Department of Medicine at California Pacific Medical Center. He'd been practicing medicine for a long time. When she approached him about Planetree, he said, "Angie you're right. Not only are *you* angry and frustrated, but so am I. I used to know my patients. I used to be able to trust that when my patients left the hospital they knew what they were doing. They were prepared to go home. This whole system is out of whack. We have to focus on making sure that the quality of care is the best and that we really look at this from the patient's perspective to make sure that patients are part of the process and know what's going on."

Physicians have to have special admitting privileges to get patients into a Planetree Unit. In San Jose, we ask them to sign an acknowledgment form that says they understand what the expectations and differences are. We started with 15, and now have more than 300 physicians vying to admit patients to 13 beds at California Pacific Medical Center in San Francisco.

The reason why we have so many physicians now is because they love it and their patients love it. A study done by the University of Washington showed that physicians rated the California Pacific Medical Center Planetree unit experience significantly higher than other units in the facility. They were more satisfied with the environment, unit nurses, and patient care. The study also showed clearly that physicians were noticeably more pleased with the quality of care resulting from collaboration. And believe me, when I first mentioned the word "collaboration" to physicians, they were ready to throw me out of the room. They are willing to collaborate with other MDs, but I was talking about collaborating with a nutritionist, a nurse, a patient. The other thing that is absolutely wonderful, but not surprising, was that the physical environment truly enhanced the physician's perception of the quality of care that was delivered.

Other Planetree Values

The keynote speaker at the Fourth Symposium, Ben Franklin-impersonator William Meikle, emphasized that we shouldn't forget the good things that are part of our history as we are moving forward and doing new, exciting things. When we did our original research into exemplary models, such as the New York University Cooperative Care Program (which has been successful since the mid-1970s in educating patients and getting families more involved), we went a little bit farther back in time and studied the first hospital—the Epidaurus in ancient Greece.

In 5 B.C., there wasn't much to offer people in terms of modern medicine. When people got sick, they went to an Epidaurus, which was a beautiful healing environment. There were waterfalls, music, and amphitheaters with plays. When people came to an Epidaurus, they were given a potion (proba-

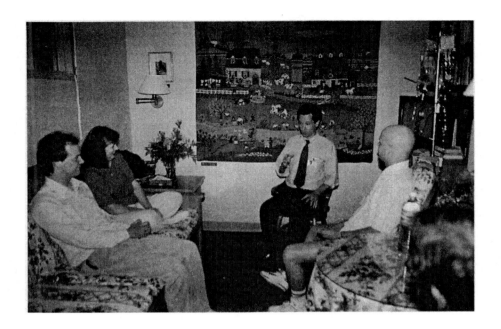

bly an herbal tea of some sort) and were told that Æsclepius, the god of healing, was going to enter their bodies and help heal them. A true healing environment. Think about the research now being done in the area of psychoneuroimmunology and the shift that's happening in our society in which people are finally getting in touch with the connection between mind and body. That is what was happening at the Epidaurus and that is why we must begin to think of music, massage, movies, relaxation, beautiful artwork, and humor not as amenities in hospitals, but as necessities. As a patient lying in a bed knowing that she had nothing pretty to look at, Angie intuitively knew this. She knew that if she did have something pretty to look at, it was not only going to make her time more pleasant, but it was going to help her get well sooner.

To incorporate some of these values in a Planetree unit, we have a storyteller. Imagine a sick patient, lying in bed worrying about the next test or procedure, trying to overhear conversations because maybe they might be talking about the patient, and it's something he or she might want to hear. Instead, somebody comes into the patient's room and tells him or her a wonderful story about climbing a mountain. Or somebody comes into the room with a Sony Walkman and encourages the patient to listen to beautiful music. Planetree has a library of music for all tastes.

We also have a massage therapist, who touches people. The only time patients ever get touched in a hospital is when somebody is going to hurt them or do something invasive. The massage therapist is there to give massages to patients, family members, or staff. It took us two years to get a massage therapy program started at California Pacific Presbyterian Medical Center. We were told that physical therapists or nurses do that. We now have an all-volunteer massage therapy program comprised of certified massage therapists who go through training at our hospital to learn how to provide massages for people who are acutely ill and lying in bed with restrictions on movement.

This was not easy to do. A perfect example of how difficult it is to change

◆ **FIGURE 3–9** The view from the patient's bed can be a positive or negative influence on the healing process. (Schematic drawing is by Marc Schweitzer Architect.)

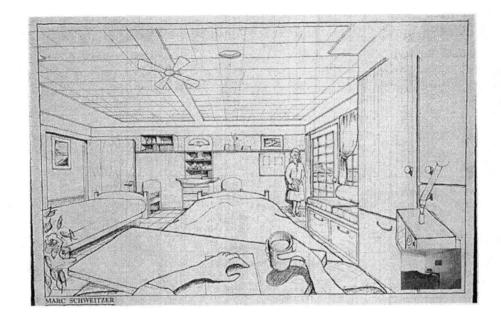

hospitals and deal with hospital protocols, is to introduce something as simple as a massage therapy program. We didn't stop when hospital administrators said, "You can't do that because these therapists are not recognized by the Inner Disciplinary Practice Committee of the hospital." We did not stop because we had the Planetree model and were committed to its values. We were creating a healing environment. And one of the most wonderful things we can do for people who are sick, or well, is to touch them.

This therapy program is one of the best things that we have done. It's so obvious. I think about what we had to go through to make it happen. That's why it's so important to have models, to be able to prove that these ideals can be implemented in hospitals and will make them better places for everyone.

Robin Orr is president of The Robin Orr Group in Los Angeles, California, an international consulting firm providing planning and implementation strategies for "patient-centered" operational restructuring, product development, and environmental design. Prior to creating her own consulting firm, Orr was National Director of Hospital Projects for the internationally acclaimed Planetree Organization and an administrator at the Children's Asthma Research Institute and Hospital.

Chapter

FOUR

D E S I G N   I M P A C T

EFFECTS OF HEALTHCARE INTERIOR DESIGN ON WELLNESS: THEORY AND RECENT SCIENTIFIC RESEARCH

Third Symposium on Healthcare Design, San Francisco, CA, 1990

Roger S. Ulrich, Ph.D.

The design of healthcare facilities traditionally has emphasized the functional delivery of healthcare, as expressed in such concerns as providing efficient spaces for laboratories or doors wide enough to accommodate beds. This emphasis has often produced facilities that are functionally effective but psychologically "hard." There is a growing recognition that hard designs are unsatisfactory from the standpoint of marketing facilities to patients. More fundamentally, hard facilities usually fail because they are stressful or otherwise unsuited to the psychological needs of patients, visitors, and staff. There is increasing scientific evidence that poor design works against the well-being of patients and in certain instances can have negative effects on physiological indicators of wellness. Research has linked poor design to such negative consequences for patients as, for instance, anxiety, delirium, elevated blood pressure, and increased intake of pain drugs (Wilson, 1972; Ulrich, 1984).

In this context, design should do more than produce health facilities that are satisfactory in terms of functional efficiency, marketing, cost, and codes. Another critically important goal of designers should be to promote wellness by creating physical surroundings that are "psychologically supportive" (Ruga, 1989). Supportive surroundings facilitate patients' coping with the major stress accompanying illness. The effects of supportive design are complementary to the healing effects of drugs and other medical technology, and foster the process of recovery. By comparison, hard settings raise obstacles to coping with stress, contain features that are in themselves stressors, and accordingly add to the total burden of illness. Unsupportive design has effects that work against the process of healing.

Against the background of these comments, a major objective of this presentation is to discuss, from my perspective as an environmental psychologist, ways in which health facility design can be psychologically supportive and accordingly promote wellness. Another major purpose is to describe examples of scientific research that show how certain design choices or strategies can foster or hinder wellness. Such scientific research on health interiors can be useful in informing the design process, and can help designers achieve solutions that are successful in meeting the needs of patients. Much of the research surveyed will focus on the effects of interior visual attributes of health facilities on physiological indicators of well-being and on health-related indicators.

Scientific research findings can also help designers in other ways. For example, compared to insights derived from intuition, they have more credibility in the medical profession and carry greater weight with healthcare decision makers. This is especially the case for research that evaluates the effects of design in terms of *physiological* well-being and health. Further, there are instances when research findings concerning health-related effects of good design can be linked to dollar savings in healthcare costs. Therefore, research that yields credible evidence of the role of design in fostering or hindering wellness can create a greater awareness among healthcare decision makers of the need to give high priority to psychologically supportive design in constructing or renovating new facilities.

The amount of scientific research to date on psychologically supportive health design is limited, however; and studies still need to be done on many important issues. For many design questions, there is no sound research yet available to inform the designer's personal intuition, sensitivity, and experience. But in recent decades a large body of "indirectly" relevant research and theory has appeared in fields such as health psychology, behavioral medicine, and clinical psychology that suggests well-founded general directions for successful health design.

Another major objective of this presentation is to relate this work directly to issues in health facilities design and to integrate it with new findings and theory from health design research. This makes it possible to outline the basic elements of a research-based theory of health facility design for promoting wellness. The theory proposed here is intended to help increase understanding of the needs of patients, visitors, and staff in relation to physical environments. The theory also suggests flexible strategies for achieving supportive design. For design questions where specific research findings are lacking, the theory should help designers steer their creativity and intuition in the general direction of solutions that promote wellness.

The next section discusses a key concept in the theory, stress. Subsequent sections describe the theory of supportive design and give examples of design strategies suggested by the theory that should prove successful in promoting wellness. The theory also serves as an organizing framework for discussing findings obtained from scientific research.

Stress: A Major Obstacle to Healing

A starting point for a theory of psychologically supportive design is the well-documented fact that most patients experience considerable stress. In very general terms, there are two major sources of stress for patients: illnesses that involve, for instance, reduced physical capabilities, uncertainty, and painful medical procedures; and physical-social environments that, for instance, can be noisy, invade privacy, or provide little social support. Patient stress has a variety of negative psychological, physiological, and behavioral manifestations that work against wellness.

- Psychologically, stress can be manifested, for instance, in a sense of helplessness and feelings of anxiety and depression.
- Physiologically, stress involves changes in bodily systems, such as increased blood pressure, higher muscle tension, and high levels of circulating stress hormones (Frankenhaeuser, 1980). A considerable body of research has shown that stress responses can have suppressive effects on immune system functioning (Kennedy et al., 1990). Reduced immune functioning can increase susceptibility to disease and work against recovery.
- Behaviorally, stress is associated with a wide variety of reactions that adversely affect wellness, including verbal outbursts, social withdrawal, passivity, sleeplessness, alcohol or drug abuse, and noncompliance with medication regimes. To the extent that prolonged stress sometimes may be linked with lower compliance with medication regimes, this can be a significant problem working against wellness, especially for patients with chronic disease.

In addition to patients, stress is a problem for families of patients, visitors in health facilities, and for healthcare staff. As an example of the deleterious effects of stress on families of patients, recent research suggests that the severe stress experienced by caregivers of Alzheimer's patients has suppressive effects on their immune system functioning (Kiecolt-Glaser and Glaser, 1990). When health facility staff experience considerable stress, this can in several ways reduce the quality of healthcare and adversely affect patient wellness. Job-related stress is a widespread problem among health facility personnel (Pardes, 1982). It is associated with low levels of job satisfaction, high rates of burnout (Shumaker and Pequegnat, 1989), absenteeism, notoriously high turnover rates, and possibly has been a factor—along with such economic issues as salaries—in strikes at health facilities. In recent years, I have toured hospitals that reflect laudable attempts to design attractive, supportive settings for patients, and in some cases, visitors, but reflect little concern for the design of staff areas. If health facilities are to be successful in delivering high-quality care, it is vitally important to attract and retain high-quality healthcare personnel. It is probably the case that supportive design in staff areas can be a positive factor in marketing a facility to prospective employees, increasing productivity or efficiency (Sundstrom, 1986), enhancing job satisfaction, and perhaps reducing turnover.

To promote wellness, it is fundamentally important that healthcare facilities be designed to foster coping with stress. At the very least, facilities should *not* raise obstacles to coping with stress or contain features that are in themselves stressors, and thereby add to the total burden of illness. Further, healthcare environments should be designed to facilitate access or exposure to physical features and social situations that scientific studies suggest can have a therapeutic, stress-reducing influence. Target groups should include patients, visitors, and healthcare staff.

A Theory of Supportive Design

In outlining a theory of supportive design centered on the concept of stress, there is no suggestion here that the theory is comprehensive or that it includes in some complete way all factors that might influence wellness. For instance, it is conceivable that a patient's psychological well-being might also be positively influenced if he/she thinks, say, that the hospital room furniture is high in quality or attractive; and this in turn somewhat enhances the individual's self-esteem or self-image. However, the reality is that there is a lack of sound research on this and many other possible mechanisms through which design might promote wellness. A related point is that many studies on health design have obtained data from verbally expressed patient reactions that have at best tenuous, weak links with wellness—such as data on expressed satisfactions, preferences, and attitudes. If a researcher administered a questionnaire to patients and learned, for example, that they preferred or were satisfied with, say, a certain bedside table or chair, this finding would not justify the conclusion that the furniture reduced anxiety, lowered blood pressure, or in some other way had an effect that was linked directly to wellness. By comparison, stress is a well-established concept in health-related fields, and a very large amount of scientific research has shown that stress is linked with psychological, physiological, and behavioral dimensions of wellness. By focusing on the concept of stress, a theory of supportive design can be developed that conceptualizes design impacts on humans in ways that are related directly to scientifically credible indicators or interpretations of wellness.

If healthcare facilities should be designed to foster coping with stress, what theory or principles can be suggested that are most likely to prove to be sound, general guideposts for designers? Research and theory in the behavioral sciences and health-related fields suggest that healthcare environments will likely support dealing with stress and thereby promote wellness if they are designed to foster:

- A sense of control with respect to physical/social surroundings
- Access to social support
- Access to positive distractions in physical surroundings

What criteria were used to select these three components of supportive design? First, in the case of each component there is evidence from different scientific studies that it can influence wellness down to the level of physiological effects and health-related indicators. Further, these components, especially control and social support, have been found to affect stress and wellness across a wide range of groups of people and situations. Also, these concepts are sufficiently broad or overarching to subsume many other important issues and patient needs. For instance, control subsumes the issue of privacy, which can be interpreted as the need to control or regulate access to the self (Altman, 1976).

One: Sense of Control

This well-established concept is familiar to many designers. A great deal of research has shown that, for diverse groups and situations (e.g., hospital patients and employees in workplaces), sense of control is an important factor influencing stress levels and wellness (Steptoe and Appels, 1989). Scientific evidence indicates that humans have a strong need for control and the related need of self-efficacy with respect to environments and situations. Many studies have found that lack of control is associated with such negative consequences as depression, passivity, elevated blood pressure, and reduced immune system functioning. Situations or conditions that are uncontrollable usually are aversive and stressful. As an everyday facility example, music that can be heard coming through the wall of a neighbor's apartment is likely to be perceived as stressful noise; however, the same music that one has chosen to play in one's own apartment, at much higher decibel levels, is perceived as positive. As this example suggests, a consistent finding in stress research has been that if an individual has a sense of control with respect to a potential stressor, the negative effects of the stressor are markedly reduced or even eliminated (Evans and Cohen, 1987).

In healthcare contexts, lack of control is a pervasive problem that increases stress and adversely affects wellness. As noted earlier, patients are exposed to two general sources of stressors: illnesses and physical/social environments. Illness confronts patients with a number of problems that are quite stressful, in part because they are either uncontrollable or reduce a sense of control. Examples are chronic pain, reduced physical capabilities, and restrictive diets that dictate what is eaten. At the same time, patients' sense of control can be markedly reduced by health facilities that are, for instance, often noisy or confusing from the standpoint of wayfinding (Carpman et al., 1986) or that invade privacy or prevent personal control over lighting and temperature (Winkel and Holahan, 1985). In addition to patients, nurses and other healthcare staff experience stress and often burnout because their work is characterized by low control and high responsibility (Shumaker and Pequegnat, 1989). This problem can be aggravated by poorly designed work environments that, for instance, lack adequate lounge or break areas. This shortcoming reduces the sense of control among staff by making it difficult to escape briefly from work demands.

A few examples of design approaches that should increase control and thereby reduce stress include providing: (1) access to visual privacy for gown-clad patients in an imaging area; controllable television in patient rooms and visitor areas; gardens or grounds that are accessible to patients; (2) a setting in a nursing home that allows residents to pursue personal interests and hobbies (Lawton, 1979); (3) control of room temperature by hemodialysis patients who typically feel cold; (4) break or "escape" areas for staff; (5) and staff work areas designed and located so as to be accessible to patients yet not produce noise that invades patient rooms.

Although links among control, stress, and wellness have been established in many scientific studies, only a small amount of design research has directly tested the extent to which specific design strategies in healthcare facilities actually increase sense of control and accordingly reduce stress. With respect to the example design strategies listed above, theory suggests that such approaches should prove successful; yet research is needed to determine whether these and other strategies actually are effective in promoting wellness. One research project that is currently in progress at Texas A&M University should shed light on the effectiveness of certain interior design approaches in increasing control, reducing stress, and promoting wellness. A major objective of this study, which is funded by the National Institutes of Health, is to investigate how interior design characteristics of kidney dialysis clinics influence patient stress and compliance indicators, and affect staff satisfaction and turnover. (The multidisciplinary team of researchers, led by Dr. Sherry Bame, includes two architects, an interior designer, an environmental psychologist, a health planner, a nephrologist, and an expert on employee job satisfaction and turnover.)

Patients with chronic kidney disease typically experience pronounced loss of control and endure substantial stress for years. Among the many factors that reduce sense of control are restrictive diets, fatigue, pain, and complex medication regimes. Patients typically require frequent and lengthy visits to the dialysis facility, usually needing two to four treatments per week with each treatment lasting three to five hours. In rural areas, much of a patient's time is scheduled around the lengthy dialysis sessions and long distance commutes to and from the clinic. Inside the clinic, control is further undermined by, among other factors: noise; crowding; arrangements that prevent self-regulation of privacy or social interaction (Olsen, 1973); blocked access to window views; uncontrollable television; and the inability of patients to control air temperature (most patients are cold during a dialysis session because their blood is circulated externally through an artificial kidney).

The initial phase of the study, which was directed by Dr. Bame, examined design characteristics for a sample of 16 urban and rural clinics. These findings indicated that the interior environments of several clinics approached theoretical perfection from the standpoint, unfortunately, of *denying* control to patients. The current phase of the Texas A&M project is investigating whether such features as controllable television and privacy partitions are in fact associated with greater sense of control and reduced stress. Importantly, this research is also determining whether stress levels are in turn related to scientifically credible indicators of dialysis patient compliance and wellness, such as blood urea nitrogen levels.

Two: Social Support

Patients derive important benefits from frequent or prolonged contact with family and friends who are helpful, caring, or otherwise supportive. Many studies in the fields of behavioral medicine and clinical psychology have found across a wide variety of health and nonhealth situations (e.g., work situations) that individuals with high social support, compared to those with low support, experience less stress and have higher levels of wellness (Cohen and Syme, 1985; Sarason and Sarason, 1985). For instance, employees in demanding positions who have supportive family or friends evidence less stress than people with similar jobs but low social support. Studies have found links between low social support and both higher rates of illness and less favorable recovery indicators following serious illness (Berkman and Syme, 1979). As an example, myocardial infarction patients with high social support have more favorable long-term survival rates. The fact that social support has been found rather consistently to be an important factor in stress and wellness suggests that it should be included in a contemporary theory of stress-reducing design.

Unfortunately, only a few studies have directly examined how health facility design can facilitate or hinder access to social support. Nearly all research has focused on psychiatric units and nursing homes. These studies have typically investigated how furniture arrangements and floor/room layouts affect levels of social interaction among patients (Sommer and Ross, 1958; Holahan, 1972). For example, studies of day rooms or lounges have found that social interaction is reduced considerably when chairs are arranged side-by-side, especially along the walls of the room. Also, heavy, unmovable furniture usually inhibits social interaction. These studies indicate that the interior designer can considerably increase social interaction among patients by specifying comfortable, movable furniture that can be arranged in small, flexible groupings.

Despite these and other useful findings, there is a lack of research that has examined whether design that increases levels of social interaction actually reduces patient stress or in other ways promotes wellness. Although a few studies have linked increased social interaction with such positive indicators of patient well-being as alertness (Knight et al., 1978), there is a conspicuous need for sound, controlled studies that examine whether increased social interaction over prolonged periods is also manifested, for instance, in positive changes in physiological indicators of well-being and in health-related behaviors. Remarkably, there is even a lack of scientific research concerning the extent to which patients' social interaction with visitors in hospitals actually promotes wellness. In this regard, it seems conceivable that in some situations visitors may increase rather than reduce patient stress.

Despite the gaps in research on health facilities, the findings on health benefits of social support for other types of contexts are so convincing that it seems justified to assume that design strategies that facilitate access to social support will probably tend to lower stress and promote wellness. A few examples of design strategies that should foster social support include: convenient overnight accommodations for families of patients who live considerable distances from health facilities; comfortable visitor waiting areas with movable seating that allow family or friends of seriously ill patients to support one another; outdoor gardens or sitting areas that foster patient/visitor social interaction (Calkins, 1988); and, in nursing homes, designing one wing so that companion animals can be accommodated (in this regard, research suggests that pets facilitate social interaction among pet owners). Finally, as a caution to designers, it should be emphasized that designs should be avoided that strongly promote social interaction to the point of denying access to privacy. An interior arrangement that enforces social contacts but denies privacy will be stressful and work against wellness. The earlier section on control implies that providing patients with some degree of control over their contacts both with other patients and perhaps with visitors will help ensure that social contacts will be positive and stress reducing rather than stressful.

Three: Positive Distractions in Physical Environments

Research in environmental psychology suggests that human well-being is usually fostered when physical surroundings provide a moderate degree of positive stimulation—that is, levels of stimulation that are neither too high nor too low (Wohlwill, 1968; Berlyne, 1971). If stimulation levels are high due to sounds, intense lighting, bright colors, and other environmental elements, the cumulative impact on patients will most likely be stressful. At the other extreme, prolonged exposure to low levels of environmental stimulation produces boredom and often such negative feelings as depression. Also, when there is a lack of external positive stimulation or distractions, patients may focus to a greater degree on their own worries or stressful thoughts, which can further increase stress. In the case of certain groups, such as many elderly in nursing homes and long-term hospital patients, chronic understimulation can be a significant threat to wellness.

Some of the most striking scientific evidence regarding negative human consequences of poor design has emerged from studies of patients exposed to low stimulation or sensory deprivation in health facilities. For instance, research on intensive care units has shown that sensory deprivation stemming, for instance, from lack of windows is associated with high levels of anxiety and depression and with high rates of delirium and even psychosis (Wilson, 1972; Parker and Hodge, 1967; Keep et al., 1980). In intensive care units, windowlessness appears to aggravate the deleterious effects of low levels of environmental stimulation associated with such conditions as unvarying lighting and the repetitive sounds of respirators and other equipment. In addition to research on patients, several studies of employees in different types of workplaces in the United States and Europe have found that windowless rooms are consistently disliked and can be stressful (Heerwagen and Orians, 1986; Collins, 1975).

The concept of a positive distraction implies that, apart from stimulation levels per se, certain types of environmental elements are especially important in reducing patient stress and promoting wellness. A "positive distraction" is an environmental feature or element that elicits positive feelings, holds attention and interest without taxing or stressing the individual, and therefore may block or reduce worrisome thoughts (Ulrich, 1981). Findings from a growing number of studies indicate that responses to positive distractions also involve positive changes across different physiological systems, such as reduced blood pressure. The most effective positive distractions are mainly elements that have been important to humans throughout millions of years of evolution: (1) happy, laughing, or caring faces; (2) pets or unthreatening animals; and (3) nature elements such as trees, plants, and water. In recent years, theory advanced by authors in different fields has tended to converge in contending that a combination of evolutionary/biological influences, as well as learned effects such as cultural conditioning, account for positive human responses to such elements as trees, water, animals, and happy faces (Ulrich and Parsons, 1992; Ulrich, 1983; Kaplan and Kaplan, 1989; Orians, 1986; Katcher and Beck, 1989; Öhman, 1986). A premise shared by most authors is that the long evolutionary development of humans in natural and social environments has left its mark on our species in the form of unlearned predispositions to pay attention, and respond positively, to these specific types of content and elements.

Nature as Positive Distraction: Stress-Reducing Effects

The intuition-based belief that visual exposure to trees, water, and other nature tends to produce restoration or recovery from stress dates as far back as the earliest large cities, such as ancient Rome (Ulrich and Parsons, 1992). In the United States in the 19th century, intuition-based arguments about stress reducing, healthful effects of viewing nature were influential in establishing urban pastoral parks, such as New York's Central Park, and later in preserving wilderness for public use (Olmsted, 1865, 1976). Historically, a theme running through these beliefs is the notion that if individuals are stressed, views of most natural settings will have stress-reducing influences; whereas views of urban or built settings will tend to impede recuperation, especially if they lack nature content such as vegetation and water. More recently, my associates and I have theroized that acquiring a capacity for restorative or stress-reducing responses to certain natural content and configurations (e.g., water, savannahlike settings) had important survival advantages for humans during evolution (Ulrich et al., 1991).

A small but rapidly expanding body of research on *nonpatient* groups has tested the old belief that visual contacts with nature have restorative or stress-reducing influences (for survey of research see Ulrich and Parsons, 1992). Findings from a sequence of studies on groups such as university students suggest that views of everyday, unspectacular nature, compared to urban scenes lacking nature, are significantly more effective in promoting recovery in the psychological component of stress (Ulrich, 1979; Ulrich and Simons, 1986; Honeyman, 1987). This research suggests that many nature scenes or elements foster stress recovery because they elicit positive feelings, reduce negatively toned emotions such as fear, anger, and sadness; effectively hold attention/interest; and accordingly might block or reduce stressful thoughts. New research also indicates that views dominated by nature content, in contrast to built or urban scenes lacking nature, foster more rapid and complete

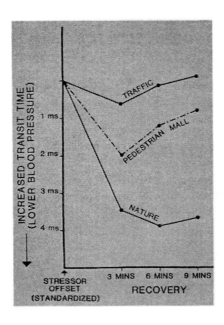

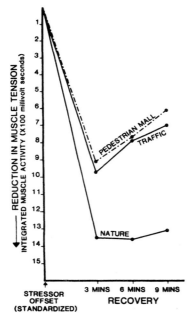

◆ **FIGURES 4–1 and 4–2** Visual exposure to everyday nature has produced significant recovery from stress within only five minutes or less, as indicated by positive changes in physiological measures, such as blood pressure and muscle tension.

restoration in terms of another critical component of stress, the physiological. In laboratory research, visual exposure to everyday nature has produced significant recovery from stress within only five minutes or less, as indicated by positive changes in physiological measures such as blood pressure and muscle tension (Ulrich and Simons, 1986; Ulrich et al., 1991). (See Figures 4–1 and 4–2.)

Also, a study of unstressed individuals found that slides of nature sustained attention much more effectively through a lengthy viewing session, and produced more positive feeling states, than did built scenes (Ulrich, 1981). In the same study, recordings of brain electrical activity in the alpha frequency range suggested that individuals were more wakefully relaxed during the nature exposures (Ulrich, 1981). In sum, these and other studies indicate that for stressed individuals, restorative influences of viewing nature involve, among other responses, a broad shift in feelings toward a more positive-toned feeling state, positive changes in activity levels in different physiological systems, and moderately high levels of sustained attention.

Effects of Nature in Healthcare Environments

The research surveyed above suggests that short-term visual contacts with nature can be effective in promoting recovery from stress. This has also been found in a few studies in which patients in healthcare settings were exposed for comparatively short periods, such as ten minutes, to views of nature. For instance, in research by Heerwagen and Orians on patient anxiety in a dental clinic (Heerwagen, 1990), questionnaire data suggested that patients felt less stressed on days when a large mural depicting a natural scene was hung on a wall of the waiting room, in contrast to days when the wall was blank. Likewise, heart rate measurements also indicated that individuals were less stressed or tense when the nature mural was visible. In a study of patients who were about to undergo dental surgery, Katcher and his associates (Katcher et al., 1984) found that contemplation of a different configuration of nature content—an aquarium with fish—significantly reduced anxiety and discomfort, and increased scores for patient compliance during surgery. Coss (1990) studied the effects of displaying different types of ceiling-mounted pictures to acutely stressed patients who were on gurneys in a presurgical holding room. His findings indicated that patients exposed to "serene" pictures (primarily displaying water or other nature) had lower systolic blood pressure levels 10–15 points lower than patients exposed to either aesthetically pleasing "arousing" pictures (e.g., a sailboarder leaning into the wind) or to a control condition of no picture. Despite the fact that the arousing pictures were rated as aesthetically pleasing, Coss concluded that such pictures were inappropriate for highly stressed patients.

While short-term exposures to nature can foster impressive stress recovery, it seems possible that wellness benefits tend to be greatest in certain situations involving long-duration exposures to nature, especially when individuals who experience considerable stress are required to spend long periods in a confined setting (Ulrich, 1979, 1984; Clearwater and Coss, 1990). Apart from many healthcare situations, such long-term contexts also include prisons and certain high-stress work environments (Ulrich and Parsons, 1992; Clearwater and Coss, 1990). In these types of settings, prolonged visual contact with nature may have persistent positive effects on psychological, physio-

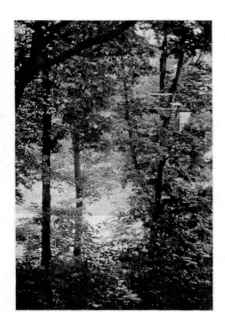

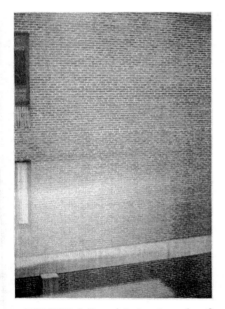

◆ **FIGURES 4–3 and 4–4** A study of hospital patients recovering from gall bladder surgery found that individuals had more favorable postoperative courses if windows in their rooms overlooked a small stand of trees rather than a brick building wall.

logical, and possibly behavioral components of stress. Over time, these effects may be manifested in higher levels of wellness or health.

In this regard, findings from a few studies of hospitals and prisons suggest that prolonged exposure to window views of nature can have important health-related benefits. A study of hospital patients recovering from gallbladder surgery found that individuals had more favorable postoperative courses if windows in their rooms overlooked a small stand of trees rather than a brick building wall (Ulrich, 1984). Patients with the natural window view had shorter postoperative hospital stays, had far fewer negative evaluative comments in nurses' notes (e.g., "patient is upset," "needs much encouragement"), and tended to have lower scores for minor postsurgical complications such as persistent headache or nausea. Further, the wall-view patients needed more doses of strong narcotic pain drugs, whereas the nature view patients more frequently received weak analgesics such as acetaminophen (Figures 4–3 and 4–4).

Likewise, a questionnaire study of patients who were severely disabled by accidents or illness (and presumably stressed) found that a highly preferred category of hospital window views included scenes of natural content such as trees (Verderber, 1986). These results are echoed in findings from studies on prisons suggesting that prison cell window views of nature, compared to such views as walls and buildings, are associated with higher levels of prisoner wellness, as indicated by lower frequencies of stress symptoms, such as headaches and digestive illness, and fewer sick calls (Moore, 1982; West, 1986).

In an extension of this direction of research, Outi Lundén and I recently completed a two-year study at Uppsala University Hospital in Sweden that investigated whether exposure to visual stimulation in intensive care units, including views of nature, promotes wellness with respect to the postoperative courses of open heart surgery patients (Ulrich and Lundén, 1990). One hundred and sixty-six patients who had undergone open heart surgery involving a heart pump were randomly assigned to a visual stimulation condition consisting of a nature picture (dominated either by water or trees), an abstract picture dominated by either curvilinear or rectilinear forms, or a control condition consisting either of a white panel or no picture. Previous research suggests that surgery involving a heart pump produces mild temporary brain injury and cognitive impairment in 50 to 60 percent of patients. To evaluate effects on the patients of the different visual conditions, a wide variety of questionnaire, physiological, and behavioral data were collected before surgery and at different times following surgery.

Findings from this heart patient study suggested that the individuals exposed to the nature with water picture experienced less postoperative anxiety than the control groups and the groups exposed to the other types of pictures. Designers should note that the rectilinear abstract pictures were associated with higher anxiety than were the control or no picture conditions. Also, four days after surgery, patients who had been exposed to any type of picture (either nature or abstract) were able to complete a visual/perceptual functioning test faster than individuals in the control groups. This finding is important because it suggests that by providing exposure to visual stimulation, it may be possible to facilitate recovery from mild reversible brain injury, especially with respect to visual/perceptual, but not necessarily verbal, functioning. Future articles stemming from this project will report findings based on physiological and behavioral indicators of wellness, such as drug intake.

Economic Implications

Some of this research that has linked nature to health-related effects raises the possibility that supportive design can be credibly related to dollar savings in healthcare costs. For instance, the study of gallbladder surgery patients (Ulrich, 1984) found that individuals with attractive window views required fewer moderate and strong analgesic injections, but received more tablets of weak pain drugs. In hospital charge schedules, injections of strong analgesics usually are more expensive than oral doses of acetaminophen. Because patients with the window views of nature needed far fewer of the costly doses, this suggests a dollar savings benefit for the positive distraction of the view. Likewise, it seems conceivable that large dollar savings might eventually be linked to such possible benefits of good design as somewhat shorter stays in intensive care units for certain categories of patients.

Negative Distractions

In contrast to positive distractions, negative distractions are environmental elements that assert their presence, are difficult to ignore, and are stressful. In general, elements are more likely to be negative distractions if they are imposed on patients without possibility of personal choice or control. Also, designed features are more likely to be negative and stressful if the patient is stressed and needs calming distraction, but the designed distraction (e.g, wall art mounted directly in a patient's line of vision) is stimulating, arousing, and characterized by uncertainty.

Research Example: Uncontrollable Television in a Waiting Room

In 1986, psychologist Robert Simons and I conducted a study of a blood bank that yielded some insights concerning the effects on stress of one of the most common and important distractions that is placed intentionally in healthcare facilities—television. Donor stress is an important problem for blood banks because most people consider giving blood to be painful and unpleasant. Apparently, many health facility administrators and designers assume on the basis of intuition or common sense that a television playing continuously in a waiting room, whether in a blood donor clinic or a hospital, is a positive distraction that benefits stressed patients or visitors. The well-intentioned policy of the blood bank we studied was to have daytime television playing continuously in the waiting area where donors typically spent 10 to 15 minutes before the phlebotomy phase. The waiting room contained appealing, comfortable seating, many well-maintained plants, and a wall that was covered by a mural of an attractive forest setting. We expected that the nature decor in the waiting area would tend to reduce stress among donors. Permission was obtained to turn the television off on randomly selected days and to have it on continuously during other days. New data obtained for the waiting room phase for 440 donors indicated that for days when the television was on, donor stress was actually higher than for days when the television was off. Greater stress associated with daytime television was indicated by *higher* heart rate and systolic blood pressure. In view of the pervasive use of television as a distraction in healthcare facilities, much more research is needed that examines under what conditions television can be either a positive, stress-reducing distraction or a negative, stressful feature. As a tentative guideline for designers, it seems advisable to consider providing television in spaces for stressed individuals only if the television is controllable or easily avoidable.

Research Example: Abstract Art as Negative Distraction in a Psychiatric Ward

A widespread assumption is that virtually all paintings and other visual art are positive distractions for patients. This notion is formally expressed, for instance, in the policies adopted by different European countries of devoting 1 to 2 percent of the budgets for health facility construction to interior art. Given the fact that the style and content of paintings and other art varies enormously and that the content of many paintings is strongly emotional, it seems important to investigate scientifically whether some types of art tend to have especially positive influences on patients and if certain categories of content might even have stressful effects (Ulrich, 1986).

I explored these issues in a small-scale, preliminary study of the effects of wall art in a psychiatric ward at a Swedish hospital (Ulrich, 1986). Nearly all the patients could engage in meaningful conversation. The ward was extensively decorated with paintings and prints reflecting a wide variety of styles and subject matter. Unstructured interviews suggested that patients had positive attitudes to paintings dominated by nature content (e.g., rural landscape, vase of flowers). By contrast, abstract paintings and prints, where the content was ambiguous or completely unclear, elicited many negative comments, and some patients reported that this type of wall art disturbed them.

More convincing evidence emerged from an analysis of paintings and prints in the ward that during the previous 15 years had elicited overt negative responses or actions from patients. These actions included: physical attacks (e.g., tearing the picture from the wall and smashing the frame) and unsolicited strong complaints to the staff (e.g., "the painting disturbs me terribly—take it away"). The physical attacks were dramatic actions given that these patient were considered to be unaggressive and not at all prone to violence (the ward was not locked).

Seven paintings and prints were identified as having been the targets of physical attacks; five had been attacked more than once and therefore had been removed. None of the total of seven paintings showed a natural landscape or was dominated by nature content such as flowers. In the case of the attacked art, there was a consistent pattern of abstract content. These paintings and prints lacked clarity of content and portrayed disordered, comparatively chaotic arrays of contrasting colors and abstract elements. To many mental patients, the world may seem chaotic, uncertain, or frightening, and they may have great difficulty perceiving order and security in their surroundings and lives. Perhaps for some patients, an abstract painting of unintelligible disorder displayed prominently in their room might threaten whatever fragile security and sense of order they retain (Ulrich, 1986).

Accordingly, the art could be profoundly disturbing and might elicit an extreme response such as a physical attack.

Although this study was preliminary, and the findings should be interpreted with caution, the results nonetheless raise the possibility that some types of wall art may sometimes have distinctly unhealthful effects. Along with the research of Coss and Clearwater (Coss, 1990; Clearwater and Coss, 1990) and the study of heart surgery patients in Sweden (Ulrich and Lundén, 1990), this psychiatric ward study implies the need for research to establish scientific guidelines to help interior designers select art that is reliably stress reducing and psychologically supportive for different patient groups. It appears that art and posters can indeed have important effects on patients: appropriate visual distractions can have positive influences, but inappropriate art can be stressful.

As tentative guidelines, the safest course for the present may be to choose representational pictures showing serene, spatially open nature settings containing water or parklike areas and to avoid chaotic abstract art, surreal art, works containing incongruous elements, and scenes containing little depth or openness (Ulrich, 1986; Ulrich and Lundén, 1990; Coss, 1990; Clearwater and Coss, 1990). Further, it seems prudent to avoid pictures depicting close-ups of animals that are staring directly at the observer (Coss and Towers, 1990). It also seems likely that many "cheerful," arousing pictures that may be aesthetically pleasing to designers and healthcare staff can be stressful to anxious patients for whom calming stimulation is more psychologically supportive. Some interior designers may be disappointed by these tentative guidelines, since the recommended style and types of content might be considered pedestrian, unimaginative, or even low brow. However, these studies imply that when designers or hospital art committees select art styles or content for patient areas that would pass critical muster in, say, a New York gallery, such art in many cases will increase stress and work against wellness.

Summary and Discussion

To summarize briefly, general key points in this presentation include the following:

- To promote wellness, healthcare facilities should be designed to support patients in coping with stress.
- As general compass points for designers, scientific research suggests that healthcare environments will support coping with stress and promote wellness if they are designed to foster: (1) a sense of control; (2) access to social support; and (3) access to positive distractions, and lack of exposure to negative distractions.
- A growing amount of scientific evidence suggests that nature elements or views can be effective as stress-reducing, positive distractions that promote wellness in healthcare environments.

In considering the needs of different types of users of healthcare facilities—patients, visitors, staff—it should be kept in mind that these groups sometimes have conflicting needs or orientations with respect to control, social support, and positive distractions. It is important for designers to recognize such differing orientations as potential sources of conflict and stress in health facilities (Schumaker and Pequegnat, 1989). For instance, a receptionist in a waiting area may understandably wish to control the programs on a television that he/she is continuously exposed to; however, patients in the waiting area may experience some stress if they cannot select the programs or elect to turn off the television.

In the case of art, some staff may prefer bright, arousing pictures for corridors and patient rooms where they spend much of their time; however, for many patients, such art may increase rather than reduce stress. A difficult but important challenge for designers is to be sensitive to such group differences in orientations and to try to assess the gains or losses for one group vis-à-vis the other in attempting to achieve the goal of psychologically supportive design.

Designers should also consider programs or strategies that combine or mesh different stress-reducing components. For example, it seems possible that a program enabling patients to select at least some of their wall art or pictures would foster both control and access to positive distraction. As another example, the theory outlined in this presentation suggests that an "artist-in-residence" program—wherein an artist with a caring, supportive disposition would work with patients—might foster social support in addition to control and access to positive distraction.

Running through this presentation is the conviction that scientific research can be useful in informing the intuition, sensitivity, and creativity of designers and can thereby help to create psychologically supportive healthcare environments. Scientific research and design are complementary activities from the standpoint of the common goal of creating healthcare facilities that promote wellness. While the amount of scientific research on supportive design is limited, studies to date indicate that good design can have important beneficial influences on patients; whereas poor design can aggravate stress and add considerably to the burden of illness. One need is for more research that goes beyond collecting information obtained from questionnaires and interviews to include information on physiological, behavioral, and health-related effects of design. Apart from deepening our understanding of the characteristics of design that foster well-being, findings from such research will have more credibility in the medical community and carry greater weight with healthcare decision makers. Further, this presentation pointed to instances when scientific findings concerning health-related effects of good design can be linked to dollar savings in healthcare costs. Future research that contributes tangible, credible evidence of the role of design in facilitating or hindering wellness will most likely be effective in creating greater awareness among both health care decision makers and the public of the need to give high priority to psychologically supportive design.

Acknowledgments

Portions of the research reported here were supported by National Science Foundation grant SE-8317803. Other portions were funded by Cooperative Agreements 28–C7–424 and 28–C7–420 with the USDA Forest Service, Rocky Mountain Forest & Ranger Experiment Station, Fort Collins, CO.

References

Altman, I. 1976. *The Environment and Social Behavior*. Monterey, CA: Brooks/Cole.

Berlyne, D.E. 1971. *Aesthetics and Psychobiology*. New York: Appleton-Century-Crofts.

Berkman, L.F. and Syme, S.L. 1979. Social Networks, Host Resistance, and Mortality: A Nine-Year Follow-Up Study of Alameda County Residents. *American Journal of Epidemiology* 109: 186–204.

Calkins, M.P. 1988. *Design for Dementia: Planning Environments for the Elderly and Confused*. Owings Mills, MD: National Health Publishing.

Carpman, J.R., Grant, M.A., and Simmons, D.A. 1986. *Design That Cares: Planning Health Facilities for Patients and Visitors*. Chicago: American Hospital Association.

Clearwater, Y.A., and Coss, R.G. 1990. Functional Aesthetics to Enhance Well-Being in Isolated and Confined Settings. In A. Harrison, Y.A. Clearwater, and C. McKay (eds.), *The Human Experience in Antarctica: Applications to Life in Space*. New York: Springer-Verlag.

Cohen, S., and Syme, S.L. (eds.). 1985. *Social Support and Health*. New York: Academic Press.

Collins, B.L. 1975. *Windows and People: A Literature Survey*. NBS Building Science Series 70. Washington, D.C.: National Bureau of Standards.

Coss, R.G. 1990. Picture Perception and Patient Stress: A Study of Anxiety Reduction and Postoperative Stability. Unpublished paper, Department of Psychology, University of California at Davis, Davis, CA.

Coss, R.G., and Towers, S.R. 1990. "Provocative Aspects of Pictures of Animals in Confined Settings. *Anthrozoös* 3: 162–70.

Evans, G.W., and Cohen, S. 1987. Environmental Stress. In D. Stokols and I. Altman (eds.), *Handbook of Environmental Psychology* (2 vols.). New York: John Wiley.

Frankenhaeuser, M. 1980. Psychoneuroendocrine Approaches to the Study of Stressful Person–Environment Transactions. In H. Selye (ed.), *Selye's Guide to Stress Research, Vol. 1*. New York: Van Nostrand Reinhold.

Heerwagen, J.H. 1990. "Psychological Aspect of Windows and Window Design." In R.I. Selby, K.H. Anthony, J. Choi, and B. Orland (eds.), *Proceedings of the 21st Annual Conference of the Environmental Design Research Association*. Oklahoma City: EDRA, pp. 269–80.

Heerwagen, J.H., and Orians, G. 1986. Adaptations to Windowlessness: A Study of the Use of Visual Decor in Windowed and Windowless Offices. *Environment and Behavior* 18: 623–39.

Holahan, C.J. 1972. Seating Patterns and Patient Behavior in an Experimental Dayroom. *Journal of Abnormal Psychology* 80: 115–24.

Honeyman, M. 1987. Vegetation and Stress: A Comparison Study of Varying Amounts of Vegetation in Countryside and Urban Scenes. Unpublished Master's Thesis, Department of Landscape Architecture, Kansas State University, Manhattan, KS.

Kaplan, R., and Kaplan, S. 1989. *The Experience of Nature*. New York: Cambridge University Press.

Katcher, A., Segal, H., and Beck, A. 1984. Comparison of Contemplation and Hypnosis for the Reduction of Anxiety and Discomfort During Dental Surgery. *American Journal of Clinical Hypnosis* 27: 14–21.

Katcher, A., and Beck, A. 1989. Human-Animal Communication. In E. Barnow (ed.), *International Encyclopedia of Communications*. London: Oxford University Press.

Keep, P.J., James, J., and Inman, M. 1980. Windows in the Intensive Therapy Unit. *Anesthesia* 35: 257–62.

Kennedy, S., Glaser, R., and Kiecolt-Glaser, J. 1990. Psychoneuroimmunology. In J.T. Cacioppo and L.G. Tassinary (eds.), *Principles of Psychophysiology: Physical, Social, and Inferential Elements*. New York: Cambridge University Press.

Kiecolt-Glaser, J., and Glaser, R. 1990. *Chronic Stress and Immunity in Older Adults.* Paper presented at the International Congress of Behavioral Medicine, Uppsala, Sweden, June 1990.

Knight, R.C., Zimring, C.M., Weitzer, W.H., and Wheeler, H.C. 1978. Effects of the Living Environment on the Mentally Retarded. In A. Friedman, C. Zimring, and E. Zube (eds.), *Environmental Design Evaluation*. New York: Plenum.

Lawton, M.P. 1979. Therapeutic Environments for the Aged. In D. Canter. and S. Canter (eds.), *Designing for Therapeutic Environments: A Review of Research*. Chichester, England: Wiley.

Moore, E.O. 1982. A Prison Environment's Effect on Health Care Service Demands. *Journal of Environmental Systems* 11: 17–34.

Öhman, A. 1986. Face the Beast and Fear the Face: Animal and Social Fears as Prototypes for Evolutionary Analyses of Emotion. *Psychophysiology* 23: 123–45.

Olmsted, F.L. 1865, 1976. *The Value and Care of Parks.* Report to the Congress of the State of California. [Reprinted in Nash, R. (ed.) (1976), *The American Environment*. Reading, MA: Addison-Wesley, pp. 18–24.]

Olsen, R. 1973. Design for Dialysis: A New Blueprint for Treating Emotions as Well as Disease. *Modern Hospital* 121 (3).

Orians, G.H., 1986. An Ecological and Evolutionary Approach to Landscape Aesthetics. In E.C. Penning-Rowsell and D. Lowenthal (eds.), *Meanings and Values in the Landscape*. London: Allen and Unwin.

Pardes, K.R. 1982. Occupational Stress Among Student Nurses: A National Experiment. *Journal of Applied Psychology* 67: 784–96.

Parker, D.L. and Hodge, J.R. 1967. Delirium in a Coronary Unit. *JAMA* 201: 132–33.

Ruga, W. 1989. Designing for the Six Senses. *Journal of Health Care Interior Design* 1: 29–34.

Sarason, I.G., and Sarason, B.R. (eds.) 1985. *Social Support: Theory, Research, and Applications*. The Hague: Nijhoff.

Shumaker, S.A., and Pequegnat, W. 1989. Hospital Design, Health Providers, and the Delivery of Effective Health Care. In E.H. Zube and G.T. Moore (eds.), *Advances in Environment, Behavior, and Design, Vol. 2*. New York: Plenum.

Sommer, R., and Ross, H. 1958. Social Interaction on a Geriatrics Ward. *International Journal of Social Psychiatry* 4: 128–33.

Steptoe, A., and Appels, A. (eds.) 1989. *Stress, Personal Control, and Health*. Chichester, UK: John Wiley.

Sundstrom, E. 1986. *Work Places: The Psychology of the Physical Environment in Offices and Factories*. New York: Cambridge University Press.

Ulrich, R.S. 1979. Visual Landscapes and Psychological Well-Being. *Landscape Research* 4: 17–23.

————. 1981. Natural Versus Urban Scenes: Some Psychophysiological Effects. *Environment and Behavior* 13: 523–56.

————. 1983. Aesthetic and Affective Response to Natural Environment. In I. Altman and J.F. Wohlwill (eds.), *Human Behavior and Environment, Vol. 6: Behavior and the Natural Environment*. New York: Plenum, pp. 85–125.

————. 1984. View Through a Window May Influence Recovery from Surgery. *Science* 224: 420–21.

————. 1986. Effects of Hospital Environments on Patient Well-Being. Department of Psychiatry and Behavioral Medicine, *Research Report Series* 9 (55). University of Trondheim, Norway.

Ulrich, R.S., and Lundén, O. 1990. *Effects of Nature and Abstract Pictures on Patients Recovering from Open Heart Surgery*. Paper presented at the International Congress of Behavioral Medicine, Uppsala, Sweden, June 1990.

Ulrich, R.S., and Parsons, R. 1992. Influences of Passive Experiences with Plants on Individual Well-Being and Health. In D. Relf (ed.), *The Role of Horticulture in Human Well-Being and Social Development*. Portland, OR: Timber Press.

Ulrich, R.S., and Simons, R.F. 1986. Recovery from Stress During Exposure to Everyday Outdoor Environments. In J. Wineman, R. Barnes, and C. Zimring (eds.), *Proceedings of the Seventeenth Annual Conference of the Environmental Design Research Association*. Washington, D.C.: EDRA.

Ulrich, R.S., Simons, R.F., Losito, B., Fiorito, E., Miles, M.A., and Zelson, M. 1991. Stress Recovery During Exposure to Natural and Urban Environments. *Journal of Environmental Psychology* 11: 201–30.

Verderber, S. 1986. Dimensions of Person-Window Transactions in the Hospital Environment. *Environment and Behavior* 18: 450–66.

West, M.J. 1985. Landscape Views and Stress Response in the Prison Environment. Unpublished M.L.A. thesis, Department of Landscape Architecture, University of Washington, Seattle.

Wilson, L.M. 1972. Intensive Care Delirium: The Effect of Outside Deprivation in a Windowless Unit. *Archives of Internal Medicine* 130: 225–26.

Winkel, G.H., and Holahan, C.J. 1986. The Environmental Psychology of the Hospital: Is the Cure Worse than the Illness? *Prevention in Human Services* 4: 11–33.

Wohlwill, J.F. 1968. The Physical Environment: A Problem for a Psychology of Stimulation. *Journal of Social Issues* 22: 29–38.

Roger S. Ulrich is a professor and associate dean for research in the College of Architecture at Texas A&M University. He has several years' experience conducting scientific research on the influences of healthcare facilities and other designed surroundings on human well-being and health. Ulrich's research was the first to document the health-related benefits for hospital patients of viewing nature. His work has been widely published and is cited often by designers and scientists.

◆ ◆ ◆

DESIGN FOR THERAPEUTIC OUTCOMES

Fourth Symposium on Healthcare Design, Boston, MA, 1991

Margaret A. Williams, Ph.D., R.N., FAAN

Good design in healthcare facilities is, like much of life, a trade-off. There are simply too many users with too many divergent needs to arrive at solutions optimal for patients, nurses, physicians, families, housekeeping, dietary, diagnostic services, etc. The rallying point, however, is that good design should serve to support activities essential to achieving desired patient outcomes without imposing stresses on the patient beyond those that already exist because of illness and its treatment. Good design also serves a symbolic function in conveying to patients and families that the people in the institution care about their comfort and welfare. In fact, it is possible for design that is poor in terms of supporting therapeutic processes to play a positive symbolic role. There are many healthcare institutions in which the design and furnishings convey an initial positive symbolism to users of that institution, but the actual processes of care are not enhanced or may be impeded by that same design.

Obviously, then, aesthetics are important. Current literature, however, indicates that there has been no neglect of symbolism and aesthetics—there is a good deal of "show and tell" but considerably less of how design can support care that leads to therapeutic outcomes.

Design that can support therapeutic processes also may be undone by inflexible organization policies and procedures, poorly trained staff, or a rancorous social environment. It is a tribute to the resilience of human beings that recovery still occurs in the presence of some of these features.

Before we go further, it is best to make the differentiation between therapeutic environments and therapeutic outcomes. A *therapeutic environment* has been variously defined as "a location in which therapy occurs," to "a major therapeutic agent" (Canter and Canter, 1979). A middle-ground meaning of the term "therapeutic environment" is that both the physical design of the setting and the social environment are oriented toward enhancing therapeutic goals and activities. Somewhat akin to this concept is that of the prosthetic environment, in which prostheses are provided to compensate for deficits in physical and social skills. A therapeutic environment, however, moves people beyond a compensatory environment.

Therapeutic outcome, in contrast, indicates an intermediate or end result of treatment and care. If the desirable outcome results, it may be because of characteristics of the setting, the patient, medical or surgical procedures used, or the quality of direct care given. Therapeutic environments, however, logically should be associated with therapeutic outcomes. Two historical examples in which the emphasis has been on therapeutic environment as the major agent follow.

Historical Example #1

The first example is the grand experiment to construct asylums for the mentally ill beginning in the Jacksonian period (roughly 1829–1837). During that period, a belief arose that mental illness was caused by a breakdown in social institutions in the community; therefore, for cure, the patient was taken out of that community and placed into an environment that was opposite in its characteristics. The institutions for such treatment thus came to be located in pastoral settings; schedules were regular and regulated; and physical labor in the garden, kitchen, and farm was valued. Visits from family and friends were discouraged. The buildings themselves were constructed in a manner to facilitate this regularity of living. One of the earliest and most famous of this type of asylum was the Pennsylvania Hospital for the Insane, of which Thomas Kirkbride was the superintendent. The emphasis on the institution and its total environment as the vehicle of treatment was exemplified in the title of his book, *On the Construction, Organization, and General Arrangements of Hospitals for the Insane, with Some Remarks on Insanity and Its Treatment* (1880).

The asylum was a grand experiment and early results reported were positive; but an economic recession and an influx of poor, usually immigrant, persons gradually began to make the asylums less attractive as objects of community support. They became custodial in nature. Superintendents began to base their claims for retaining the institutions on their ability to provide clean and hygienic conditions, not their treatment effectiveness (Rothman, 1971).

Historical Example #2

The second example is that of Florence Nightingale, the founder of modern nursing, who was an outspoken advocate for the use of the environment for therapeutic purposes. Her book, *Notes on Nursing* published in 1859, describes the importance to the health of patients of adequate ventilation, warmth, noise control, light, cleanliness, and variety in a sick room—as well as a social environment free of "chattering hopes and advice" and characterized by orderliness and good management.

A set of two papers, "Notes on Hospitals" (1859), is introduced by the statement, "It may seem a strange principle to enunciate as the very first requirement in a hospital that it should do the sick no harm," referring to the fact that, at the time, mortality rates for the same disease were higher for patients in hospitals than for patients cared for at home. In Nightingale's view, this was due to the dangers arising from details of hospital buildings and fittings, through defective ventilation, drainage, sanitary arrangements, kitchens, and ward furniture (Rogers, 1972).

Notes on Hospitals and other writings had enormous influences on hospital architecture throughout the world. In their work on the architectural and social history of the hospital (1975), Thompson and Goldin state that Nightingale was the single greatest influence upon that architecture for more than 100 years. The advent of antibiotics and construction material that enabled the erection of high-rise hospitals inaugurated the demise of the open, airy, cross-ventilated wards and the pavilion hospitals that she advocated (Figure 4–5). This type of building and ward configuration arose largely because Nightingale was a staunch miasmatist. Miasmatists believed that disease arose from the miasma, or exhalations, surrounding ill persons. That belief logically led to emphasis on hygiene, cleanliness, maintenance of certain distances between beds, and above all, generous exchanges of air.

As hospitals became less hazardous to health, and housekeeping and maintenance tasks were delegated to other personnel, environmental concerns became less salient in hospital nursing. At the present time, however, concern

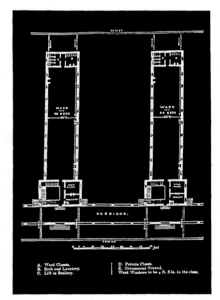

◆ **FIGURE 4–5** The advent of antibiotics and construction material that enabled the erection of high-rise hospitals inaugurated the demise of the open, airy, cross-ventilated wards and pavilion hospitals that Florence Nightingale advocated. (From *The Hospital: A Social and Architectural History* by J.D. Thompson and G. Golden, Yale University Press, 1975.)

with the physical environment is resurging among nurses caring for the elderly, especially in long-term care settings, and among those working in neonatal intensive care units. Both the institutionalized frail elderly and the high-risk neonates epitomize the importance of the environmental docility hypothesis, originally put forth by gerontologists, which postulates that as the ability to control one's environment decreases, the impact of that environment increases (Lawton, 1974).

These brief bits of history serve as a reminder that "what goes around comes around." Although emphasis will vary depending on the patient population and philosophy of the institution, the concept of using the total environment as the major agent of healing is gaining renewed interest. Thus, the concepts that Nightingale put forth so strongly are receiving renewed attention. Her emphasis on the need for visibility of patients via the open ward has given way, however, at least in the United States, to construction of patient rooms that afford more privacy. But there will probably always be a tension between design factors that favor ease of practice by healthcare workers and those that favor patients' desires for security, privacy, and space.

Design and Behavior/Outcomes

Can patient behaviors be directly affected by design? Yes, certain ones can. Patterns of interaction with others can be changed by design features as shown by studies in psychiatric units and long-term care facilities (e.g., Holahan and Saeger, 1973; Sommer, 1969). As suggested, feelings of privacy and security can be affected, as can orientation and satisfaction with setting. Using design to accomplish therapeutic outcomes, however, is best considered as a means to support effective processes of care. Such processes also are dependent on knowledgeable staff working in a supportive social and organizational environment.

A distinction needs to be made between designs that are intended to meet the needs of patients in general and designs that are intended to support processes and functions for specific groups of patients. There is a growing sensitivity to the general needs of patients and visitors. Examples of this are the studies Carpman and colleagues did as part of the planning for the new University of Michigan hospital and their subsequent manual, *Design That Cares* (1986). Interesting implications for design arose when the opinions and perspectives of two groups of infrequently queried users—patients and visitors—were taken into account. Too often, the opinions and perspectives of staff are disproportionately represented in studies of potential users' opinions.

The work by Carpman has not, however, been followed by a post-occupancy evaluation (POE) of the hospital. Systematic POE's are infrequent relative to most new healthcare institutions as a whole, although informal evaluations by users are frequent and often continuous. More often in the literature are reports of unit redesign and its effect on patients and staff. These have been mostly psychiatric units, probably because of the early impetus of Osmond's seminal work on function as the basis of psychiatric ward design (1957).

A problem with design that is based on the needs of large groups of patients and their families is that they then may become prescribed for as a homogeneous group. For example, many modifications of environments to suit the needs of elderly persons are long overdue; but there are variations within that group, and there may be a danger of prescribing for them as though all older persons had the same needs. The only way to handle such variance is to incorporate substantial flexibility in the design.

Another problem is that even if opinions of the major users of a facility are sought, only the patients who are able to respond to the questions will be represented in the results. Little is known about changes in perceptions of the environment for those who are physically ill, or mentally or emotionally impaired. There is a need to "get into the patient's world," but this is a process that requires skilled and sensitive observation and interaction over time. Realistically, the best that can be done in most instances is at least to have persons who are involved in planning spend time in actual situations in the role of the patient. This seems a somewhat old and hackneyed recommendation, but still one of substantial and continuing merit.

Another implication is that it is easier to design for special populations who are together in one place than in diverse settings. The patient diversity on general medical/surgical nursing units makes these units more difficult to plan for than, for example, a coronary care unit. At the same time, large numbers of very small units, each designed for a special subgroup of patients, can be overly expensive when there is a fluctuating census and the need to staff units at safety levels even when there are few patients. Again, flexibility must be built into the design.

How does one differentiate between design that is simply pleasing to users and design that supports therapeutic goals? The difference in many instances may be slight, since pleasant surroundings may be conducive to lessening stress and creating a positive response. However, design that supports therapeutic goals must take into account the functional requisites of patients, as these are influenced by illness or disability. Four contemporary examples include: head-injured patients, emotionally disturbed children, adults in intensive care units, and infants in neonatal intensive care units.

Head-Injured Patients

The first example comes from a nurse experienced in both the acute care and rehabilitative care of head-injured patients (Johnson, 1990, 1991). She described what the physical and social environment should optimally be for these patients in inpatient settings. The major goals are three: (1) maintenance of patient safety in the least restrictive environment possible; (2) eliminating sources of confusion that increase agitation; and (3) fostering social reintegration. Stated as outcomes, these goals would be reworded such that patients would: (1) experience their hospitalization with a minimum of external control and with no untoward events or accidents; (2) have experienced few or no episodes of heightened agitation; and, (3) have made progress toward social reintegration by the time of home discharge.

Depending upon the severity of the injury, there may be cognitive, perceptual, and sensory deficits and, in the early stages, prolonged lack of consciousness. At later stages, agitation occurs as the patient becomes confused in response to external stimuli. Safety must be provided by manipulating the environment, by attending to the sources of stimulation, and by establishing structured schedules. The goal is to decrease sources of overstimulation and confusion that can increase agitation and potential aggression.

Thus, design implications include the following:

1. The nursing unit for these patients should be located within a quiet area of the hospital where through traffic by hospital staff and visitors is minimal.

2. Furniture in the rooms should be easily movable, as safety concerns can mean substituting for the usual bed a special bed in which the mattress is on the floor and surrounded by padded walls three to four feet in height. Such an arrangement provides a barrier to visual and auditory stimuli while still permitting the patient freedom of movement and reducing the need for physical restraints and the risk of injury due to falling out of bed. Use of restraints tends to potentiate agitation by increasing the feeling of powerlessness and lack of control—thus increasing the behavior the restraints were meant to control.

3. Wallcoverings, if used, need to contain designs easily interpretable by the patient. Plain walls in colors that do not arouse anxiety or cause overstimulation are best. Artwork can be confusing to the person with perceptual deficits and probably should not be in the room. High and harsh illumination should be avoided; dimmer switches will be helpful, and normal patterns of light and dark will provide cues as to time of day. Other orienting information such as clocks and calendars should be provided and, whenever possible, items of personal relevance to the patients such as photographs or favorite items.

4. Noise must be kept at a minimum; overhead paging and use of the intercom are sources of confusion because there is no identified source of the voice. Use of pocket pagers is best, but at least a unit mechanism to lower the volume of overhead paging and announcements should be available. Alarms on technological equipment can be modulated.

5. When patients become ambulatory, there need to be alarms or other mechanisms at exits, as patients with heightened physical activity accompanying agitation may not be aware of unit boundaries. Unit designs must permit observation of patient rooms and unit exits. There should be space either on the unit or in individual rooms for various therapy services in order to lessen the confusion related to taking the patient off the unit for such services.

6. Relative to the social reintegration outcomes, unit design should provide space in which social interaction with nursing staff, family members, and other patients is encouraged. Usually this will occur in a rehabilitation unit within the hospital or in a specialized facility. Many of these settings include a large multipurpose lounge area. Such a large space with several purposes but no demarcations can be overpowering and create anxiety; breaking it up into identifiable areas with clear functions is necessary. Planners could, for example, provide a clearly identified area for having coffee, soft drinks, and snacks; an area for table games, jigsaw puzzles, or the like; or a reading area. There should, in other words, be cues to appropriate behaviors created by room dividers, placement of furniture, area rugs, or different wallcoverings. There should be a place for retreat and privacy—the patient's own room furnishes this; but in-between areas also are desirable—such as alcoves or small lounges where patients can interact with only one or several persons and not be confused or agitated by activities in the larger setting.

Emotionally Disturbed Children

The second example comes from a report by Cotton and Geraty (1984) in which they detail how the physical environment of an inpatient children's psychiatric unit was planned to support therapeutic goals. The children in this case were from four to 12 years of age. Five treatment goals were used to guide design features. One goal as stated was: "to provide spaces that represent a continuum of external controls that can be adapted to the needs of individual patients and groups of patients as they fluctuate in their capacity to use internal controls." Rephrased as therapeutic outcome, the wording would be: "for patients to gain the ability to use internal controls over behavior as opposed to reliance on external controls."

The outcome sounds straightforward, but design implications are formidable. There is always a dilemma posed when conveying a safe environment versus a supportive one. Locks, bars, and shatterproof glass are elements of external control and safety but they create distinctively institutional, uninviting surroundings. At the same time, these visual images of protection can be comforting to out-of-control children. In the redesign, the issue of locks was treated by providing the unit with one open-door exit and entrance, but having locks used within the unit on drawers with knives, cabinets with paint supplies, the refrigerator, and the like.

Two quiet rooms were used so that extremely disturbed children would not be subjected to mechanical restraints or overuse of psychotropic medication. Restraint and protection were provided that still afforded relative freedom. For safety, there was vandalproof lighting, carpeting solidly glued under nailed wooden baseboards, no visible pipes or rods, a plexiglas panel in front of the window, and tamper-proof vents for air conditioning, heat, and air exchange. At the same time, nonpunitiveness and coziness were implied by each room being small, with the use of carpeting and warm colors. The window looked out on a pleasant scene; there were no bars; and there was a carpeted window bench. Importantly, the rooms were assigned multiple purposes in order to avoid the single association with bad, out-of-control behavior. Each room was used by staff for interviews with new personnel, performance evaluations, and paperwork. The rooms also were used by children for tutoring, therapy sessions, reading, or napping.

The quiet rooms were adjacent to the kitchen and living room to facilitate fast removal of a disruptive child. The kitchen and living room, where children spent the most time, were farthest from the open end of the unit. Staff space and the children's bedrooms were near the open end of the unit. Other design elements, including types of furniture, were described in the report.

Intensive Care Units/Adults

The third example describes how a fine treatment goal was not well supported by physical designs of patient units in early years, but how changes have occurred from recognition of that fact. The example is that of the intensive care unit (ICU) where the major desired outcome for patients was, and still is, the restoration of stable physiologic status as quickly as possible. Operationally, this was translated as requiring a place designed for staff that would afford them maximum opportunity to give intensive, continuous care aided by high-technology devices. Early intensive care units, however, were invariably created from existing space within a hospital.

Usually that became one large rectangular room with beds arranged around the periphery and the nurse station in the center or at one end, where visibility of all patients was possible 24 hours a day. The merits of ICUs were readily apparent in the form of lessened mortality statistics; the negative aspects were described as unfortunate, but necessary, in light of the greater good. These negative aspects included disruption, by constant overhead bright illumination, of internal biologic rhythms because of lack of a day/night cycle; lack of privacy for patients—privacy curtains were available but not always used, and of course they only afforded visual privacy, not aural, or olfactory. There also was constant noise from machines and various devices, and from staff members themselves. The high decibel level in ICUs has been documented in several studies, but it would take only a quick tour of an early ICU to gain an appreciation of the intense sensory input to which seriously ill patients were exposed 24 hours a day. Parenthetically, coronary care units (CCUs) generally were set up to avoid such extremes of input and to afford the quiet and peace deemed essential for heart patients.

Given the desired outcome for patients in ICUs as the restoration of stable physiologic status as quickly as possible, it became evident that the addition of external stressors in the setting was extremely illogical.

How could external stressors in a necessarily complex environment teeming with technology, nurses, and physicians be reduced? First, it was apparent that patients did not have to be in an open ward for staff to keep direct surveillance over them to detect changes in their condition. Circular or semicircular unit designs with private rooms in which there were glass windows fronting the corridor and between rooms gave the same opportunity for visibility. Sliding curtains on the windows could provide the necessary flexibility between high visibility and desired privacy. Further, the ability to control light, odor, noise, and temperature on an individual basis was immeasurably enhanced by this design, to say nothing of infection control. Particular technologies used only for selected patients also could be incorporated more effectively in single rooms than in open wards. A design incorporating desirable features is shown in Figure 4–6.

Even private rooms, however, do not entirely take care of noise in the ICU. Although carpeting is probably unrealistic for corridors and rooms because of the need to move equipment readily, at least the nurses' station and the physicians' charting and transcribing areas can be carpeted.

Some of the design principles cited relative to designing for care of head-injured patients apply to patients in the ICUs and on general units, since hospitals rapidly are becoming large intensive care units with smaller intensive-intensive care units. One such principle is not introducing elements that can be confusing and subject to misinterpretation by any seriously ill person, such as abstract art, floral or figured drapes, and the like.

Noise abatement procedures in addition to use of acoustic materials on ceilings include close evaluation of new products and equipment to check their noise level. Refusal to buy certain products because they emit too much noise can send an effective message to manufacturers. Padding under printers, telephones, and addressograph machines; nonmetal chart holders and racks; and felt strips on file drawers will all help (Williams, 1989).

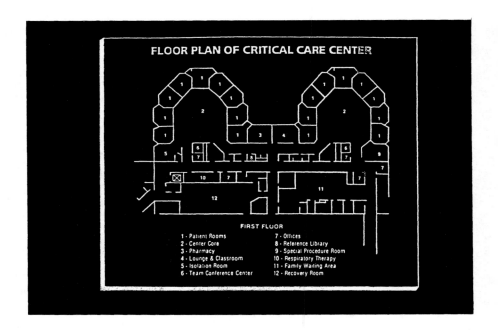

◆ **FIGURE 4–6** Circular or semicircular unit designs provide flexibility and easy access to patients in an adult intensive care unit. (Reprinted with permission from Mosby–Year Book, Inc.)

FLOOR PLAN OF CRITICAL CARE CENTER

FIRST FLOOR

1 - Patient Rooms
2 - Center Core
3 - Pharmacy
4 - Lounge & Classroom
5 - Isolation Room
6 - Team Conference Center
7 - Offices
8 - Reference Library
9 - Special Procedure Room
10 - Respiratory Therapy
11 - Family Waiting Area
12 - Recovery Room

Intensive Care Units/Babies

The final example also is that of an intensive care unit, but one in which the patients are high-risk premature babies—the neonatal intensive care unit (NICU). Outcomes similar to those of adult ICUs have been achieved in these NICUs, that is, reduced mortality and morbidity. However, some of the same problems apply, particularly that of sensory overload. The potential effects of the unit's environment are even greater for premature babies than for adults because of the underdevelopment of their sensory, motor, and neurological systems and because of their precarious physiological stability.

The major environmental hazards to which they are exposed are temperature changes, high illumination, noise, and frequent handling. The hazard of temperature change perhaps has been the best-recognized over time, and considerable attention has been given to protection of the infants through well-constructed incubators. However, it is well documented that exposure of incubators to direct sunlight may result in infant overheating. And, there now is evidence that placement of incubators near exterior windows in NICUs in cool climates can affect the temperature gradient between the interior incubator air and the exterior incubator walls with the potential of greater heat loss for the infant. The implication is that windows, if they are included in the NICU unit design, should be of insulated glass or that thermal drapes should be used (Thomas, 1990).

Lighting in most NICUs, as in early adult ICUs, is continuous and at a high level. The high level is defended on grounds that observation of the infant must be unimpaired. However, a study published in 1985 (Glass et al.) showed that low birth-weight infants exposed to continuous high-level lighting had a higher incidence of eye damage (retinopathy) than those receiving lower lighting levels. There also is continuing concern about the effect of this type of lighting on the sleep/wake cycle and on biological rhythms.

High noise levels in NICUs have been well documented, with the noise coming from infants' crying, the incubator itself and equipment used with it, conversations among staff, use of radios, opening and closing incubator doors, and impulse sounds from banging of other doors, drawers, and equipment. Internal oxygenation of the infants has been shown to decrease under noisy conditions; sleep is interfered with; and there is concern that the immature structure of the infant's ear may make it even more sensitive to noise damage and hence hearing loss (Catlett and Holditch-Davis, 1990).

The problem of frequent handling is a difficult one. Yet observers have documented that infants may be disturbed for medical and nursing procedures as often as five times per hour (Duxbury et al., 1984). This has serious potential for interrupting sleep/wake cycles as well as other physiologic effects from the procedures themselves.

Becker and her colleagues at the University of Wisconsin and a community hospital in Madison have carried out studies directed at minimizing environmental stresses, such as light and noise, and optimizing support for the infant's growth and development through special handling and scheduling techniques (Becker, Grunwald, Moorman, and Stuhr, 1991; Grunwald and Becker, 1991). The interventions were implemented through a broad and intensive staff education program. The outcomes showed decreased morbidity for infants in the study group compared to the control group, decreased days on a ventilator, better behavioral organization, and a hospital stay that was two weeks shorter (Becker et al., 1991).

Recommendations

In sum, the two major characteristics of design for therapeutic outcomes are: (1) that it take into account the functional requirements of patients as these are influenced by illness or disability, and (2) that it support processes of care and treatment aimed at specific desired outcomes. The challenge is a large one and requires a multidisciplinary effort.

Nurses and physicians should be included on design teams, whether in the planning of new facilities or the redesign of older ones. Physicians will be able to articulate the treatment goals, as will experienced nurses who, in addition, have a "handle" on the day-to-day activities that can be more effectively carried out by or for patients with the support of good design.

Nurses and physicians must be part of any team that endeavors to design for therapeutic outcomes, but do not expect all of them to have the same understanding of the built environment as a design professional. Rather, their input is an essential complement to the design professional's skills and of critical importance in articulating the requisites of specific patient groups.

Because of cost considerations and because there are many users within the hospital, there will of necessity be some trade-offs; but concentration on what the therapeutic outcomes should be for different groups of patients will go a long way toward achieving truly functional designs.

References

Becker, P. T., Grunwald, P.C., Moorman, J., and Stuhr, S. 1991. Outcomes of Developmentally Supportive Nursing Care for Very Low Birth Weight Infants. *Nursing Research* 40: 150–55.

Canter, D., and Canter, S. (eds.). 1979. *Designing for Therapeutic Environment: A Review of Research.* New York: Wiley.

Carpman, J.R., Grant, M.A., and Simmons, D.A. 1986. *Design that Cares.* Chicago: American Hospital Publishing.

Catlett, A.T., and Holdtich-Davis, D. 1990. Environmental Stimulation of the Acutely Ill Premature Infant: Physiological Effects and Nursing Implications. *Neonatal Network* 8(6): 19–21.

Cotton, N.S., and Geraty, R.G. 1984. Therapeutic Space Design: Planning an Inpatient Children's Unit. *American Journal of Orthopsychiatry* 54: 624–36.

Duxbury, M.L., Henly, S.J., Broz, L.J., Armstrong, G.D., and Wachdorf, C.M. 1984. Caregiver Disruptions and Sleep of High-Risk Infants. *Heart and Lung* 13: 141–47.

Glass P., Avery, G.B., Subramanian, K.N.S, Keys, M.P., Sostek, A.M., and Frindly, D.S. 1985. Effect of Bright Light in the Hospital Nursery on the Incidence of Retinopathy of Prematurity. *New England Journal of Medicine* 313: 401–4.

Grunwald, P.C., and Becker, P.T. 1991. Developmental enhancement: Implementing a program for the NICU. *Neonatal Network* 9(6): 29–30, 39–45.

Holahan, C.J., and Saegert, S. 1973. Behavioral and attitudinal effects of large-scale variation in the physical environment of psychiatric wards. *Journal of Abnormal Psychology* 82: 454–62.

Johnson, L. (1990). Proposed Change: Creating a Social Space in the Rehabilitation Unit Day Room. Unpublished manuscript. University of Wisconsin School of Nursing, Madison.

————. 1991. *The Physical Environment for Head-Injured Patients.* Unpublished manuscript. University of Wisconsin School of Nursing, Madison.

Kirkbride, T. 1880. *On the Construction, Organization, and General Arrangements of Hospitals for the Insane, with Some Remarks on Insanity and Its Treatment,* 2nd ed. Philadelphia: Lippincott.

Lawton, M.P. 1974. The Human Being and the Institutional Building. In J. Lang, C. Burnette, W. Moleski, and D. Vachon (eds.), *Designing for Human Behavior: Architecture and the Behavioral Sciences.* Stroudsberg, PA: Dowden, Hutchinson & Ross.

Nightingale, F. 1859. *Notes on Nursing.* London: Harrison and Sons.

————. 1859. *Notes on Hospitals,* 2nd ed. London: Longmans, Green, and Co.

Osmond, H. 1957. Function as the Basis of Psychiatric Ward Design. *Mental Hospitals* 8: 23–29.

Rogers, P.J. 1972. Design for Patient Care. *International Nursing Review* 19: 267–82.

Rothman, D.J. 1971. *The Discovery of the Asylum: Social Order and Disorder in the New Republic.* Boston: Little, Brown, and Co.

Sommer, R. 1969. *Personal Space: The Behavioral Basis of Design.* Englewood Cliffs, NJ: Prentice Hall.

Thomas, K.A. 1990. Design issues in the NICU: Thermal Effects of Windows. *Neonatal Network* 9(4): 23–26.

Thompson, J.D., and Goldin, G. 1975. *The Hospital: A Social and Architectural History.* New Haven: Yale University Press.

Williams, M.A. 1989. Physical Environment of the Intensive Care Unit and Elderly Patients. *Critical Care Nursing Quarterly* 12(1): 52–60.

Margaret A. Williams is a professor emeritus at the University of Wisconsin-Madison School of Nursing. She has an extensive background in both nursing practice and education. As an educator, Williams has taught a course for many years for graduate nursing students on physical and social environments for patients. A fellow in the American Academy of Nursing, her research has been widely published.

◆ ◆ ◆

PSYCHONEURO-IMMUNOLOGY

Fourth Symposium on Healthcare Design, Boston, MA, 1991

Millicent Gappell, IFDA

Psychoneuroimmunology (PNI). Another disease? No, it is the art and science of creating environments that prevent illness, speed healing, and promote well-being.

The emerging science of PNI concerns itself with the correlation between stress and health. A large body of replicable experimental and clinical data has proven the connection between biological responses and human responses to sensory stimuli. The data clearly demonstrates that the mind, brain, and nervous system can be directly influenced, either positively or negatively, by sensual elements in the environment.

For the biological regulatory mechanisms to work properly, continuous variations in the amounts of sensory stimulation are necessary to sustain their power to function. The condition of permanent monotony induces pathological disturbances.

British psychologist M.D. Vernon has written, "Thus we must conclude that normal consciousness, perception, and thought can be maintained only in a constantly changing environment. When there is no change, a state of sensory deprivation occurs; the capacity of adults to concentrate deteriorates, attention fluctuates and lapses, and normal perception fades. In infants who have not developed a full understanding of their environment, the whole personality may be affected and readjustment to a normal environment may be difficult."

Yet, the drab interiors that many healthcare facilities present to patients, families, and staff are monotonous, visually trying, and emotionally stressful, especially to people already under stress.

Our physical and emotional well-being are influenced by six major environmental factors: light, color, sound, aroma, texture, and space. These have such an enormous physiological and psychological impact on the individual that a well-designed medical facility properly applying these factors can be considered good medicine in itself. The following are some guidelines utilizing the principles of PNI for more humanistic interiors.

Light

Until recently, the lighting design of a space was only to insure a source for visual functioning, since the ability to see and function efficiently depends on the quantity and quality of the illumination.

Today, designers must be aware of the health benefits of lighting—the field of photobiology. The human system evolved under the influence of the sunlight spectrum to which particular light-sensitive and light-modulated organ systems are specifically adapted. Light, coming into the pineal gland through the retina of the eye, influences endocrine control, timing of our biological clocks, entrainment of circadian (sleep/wake) cycles, sexual growth and development, regulation of stress and fatigue, and suppression of melatonin—a central nervous system depressant used for treatment of Seasonal Affective Disorder (SAD).

Sunlight is vital to the absorption of calcium and phosphorus from the diet for the normal mineralization of bone (see Figure C–1). In infants and children, it is essential for growth of strong bone structure and for full development of immunological defenses against disease. Phototherapy has replaced blood transfusions for neonatal jaundice.

Full-spectrum light provides prophylactic control of viral and staph infections and produces significant improvements in physical working capacity by decreasing heart and pulse rate, lowering systolic blood pressure, and increasing oxygen uptake.

Richard J. Wurtman, M.D., a neuroscientist at the Massachusetts Institute of Technology, states: "It seems clear that light is the most important environmental input, after food, in controlling body function."

Many interiors of facilities are lit by fluorescents. Unfortunately, conventional cool-white fluorescent light at standard indoor levels is interpreted by the human pineal gland as darkness. Studies comparing standard fluorescents and full-spectrum tubes support the importance of full-spectrum lighting, showing that the broad spectrum tube produced a significantly less pronounced reaction of the stress hormones ACTH and Cortisol. Therefore, where fluorescents are used, lights approximating the spectra of daylight should be the choice.

Biologically correct lighting in a building would have the light coming from windows, atria, skylights, and clerestories. Windows are relevant to visual, thermal, and psychological aspects of comfort. Windows with a view provide the daily variation in light, as well as the touch of nature associated with relaxation and restorative powers that encourage faster healing. In an ICU they have been shown to prevent the sensory deprivation that is a cause of ICU psychosis. Using daylight effectively also conserves energy.

Color

It has been demonstrated that color strongly influences human emotions and physiology. Red stimulates the sympathetic nervous system, increases brain wave activity, and sends more blood to the muscles, thus accelerating heart rate, blood pressure, and respiration. Blue triggers the parasympathetic nervous system and is credited with a tranquilizing effect. Color also affects perception. Warm colors seem to advance and cool colors to recede. With the use of cool colors, time is underestimated, weights seem lighter, objects seem smaller, and rooms appear larger. The opposite is true for warm tones. Thermal comfort is also affected by color; people feel cooler in cool-toned rooms and warmer in warm-toned rooms, although the actual temperature may be the same.

Color perception is affected by age. Infants see and respond to sharp con-

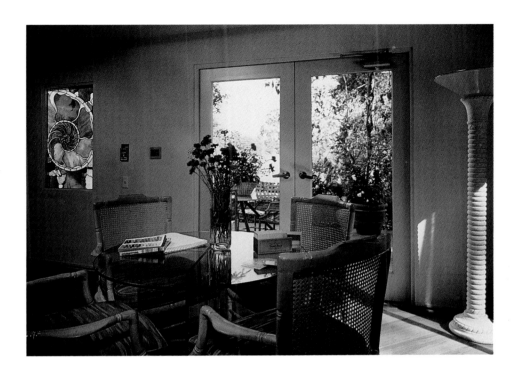

◆ **FIGURE C-1** Sunlight is vital to the absorption of calcium and phosphorus from the diet for the normal mineralization of bone. Shown is the living room of the Chris Brownlie Hospice in Los Angeles, CA. (*Interior design:* Millicent Gappell. *Photo:* Michael Arden.)

◆ **FIGURE C-2** Choosing a color palette depends on the light sources, geographical location, size and shape of the space, type of activity that is being performed in it, and the users' ages. Shown is the living room of the Chris Brownlie Hospice in Los Angeles, CA. (*Interior design:* Millicent Gappell. *Photo:* Michael Arden.)

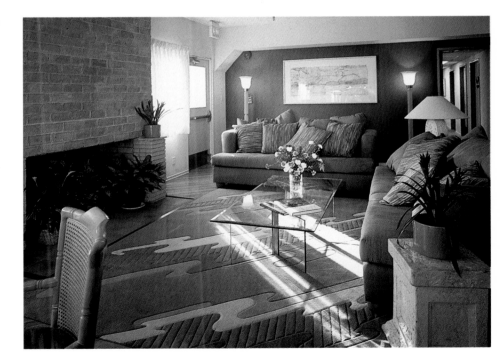

◆ **FIGURE C-3** Bowls of sachet, floral arrangements, and plants can provide pleasant fragrance in the healthcare facility. Ordinary houseplants have proven effective in removing toxic pollutants from the air inside homes and office buildings. Shown is a patient room at the Chris Brownlie Hospice in Los Angeles, CA. (*Interior design:* Millicent Gappell. *Photo:* Michael Arden.)

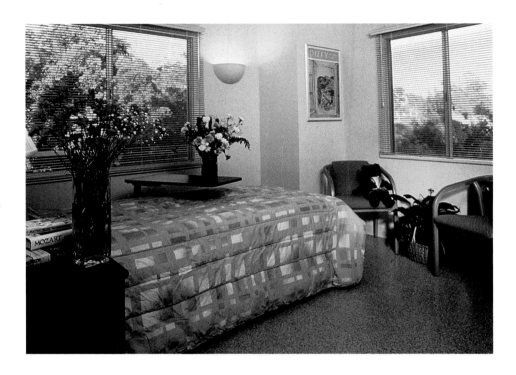

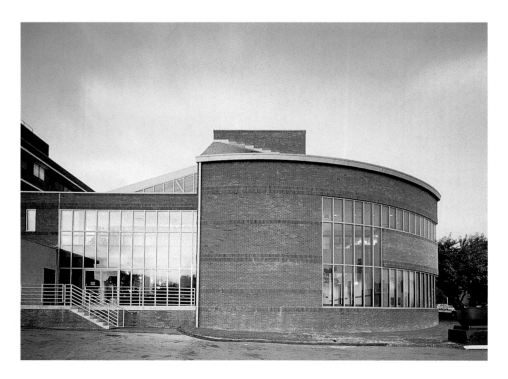

◆ **FIGURE C-4** The curved glass portion of the building was important to reference the context, give the building "no front doors," and lead visually to the front door. (*Project:* Dorothy Bennett Cancer Center at Stamford Hospital, Stamford, CT. *Architecture/interior design:* The Geddis Partnership. *Photo:* Dan Cornish.)

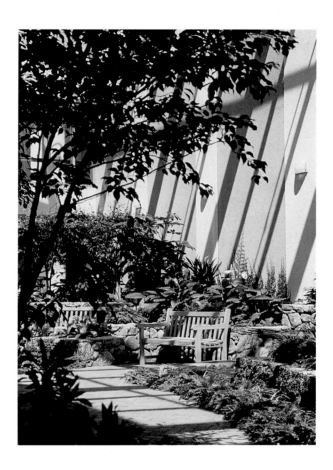

◆ **FIGURES C-5 and C-6** The interior garden and atrium became the geographic, symbolic, and philosophical heart of the center. (*Project:* Dorothy Bennett Cancer Center at Stamford Hospital, Stamford, CT. *Architecture/interior design:* The Geddis Partnership. *Photo:* Dan Cornish.)

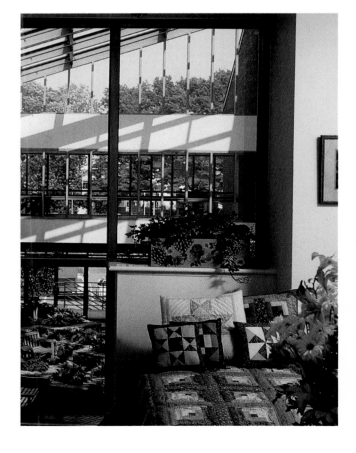

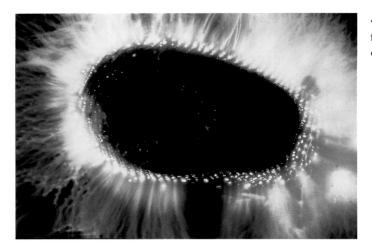

◆ **FIGURE C-7** Kirlian photograph shows colors generated from electromagnetic energy emanating from a living organism. (*Photo:* Dr. Mikol S. Davis.)

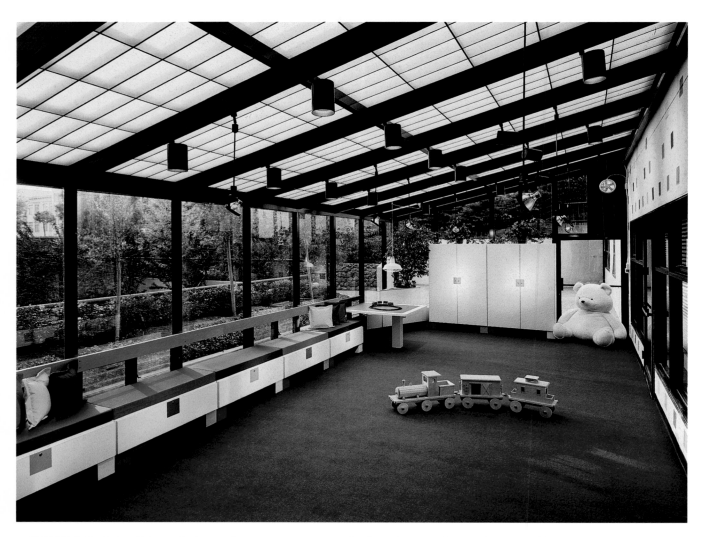

◆ **FIGURE C-8** Color, light, and views of nature are important healing elements for children, as well as adults. (*Project:* Pediatric solarium, Children's Hospital, San Francisco, CA. *Interior design:* Tony Torrice, ASID. *Photo:* Mike Spinelli. Reprinted from *In My Room: Designing for and with Children.*)

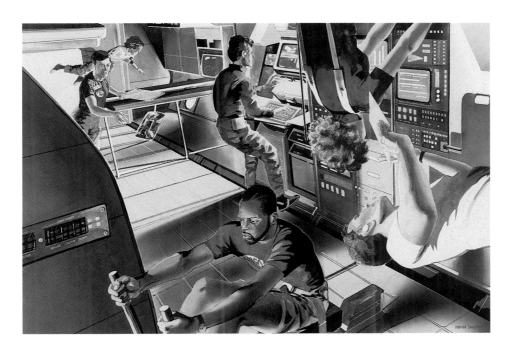

◆ **FIGURE C-9** Research is being done on which colors are appropriate for use in outer space. A rendering of the inside of a habitat module on the space station Freedom uses blue, an appropriate color for outer space because it represents the eyes, ears, and nose and the release of strain and tension. (Space Art by Harold Smelcer. Courtesy of NASA.)

◆ **FIGURE C-10** The design was meant to engender a feeling of openness and honesty in the building for patients and families. It was also meant to stimulate the sense of sight with views and color. (*Project:* Lucile Salter Packard Children's Hospital, Palo Alto, CA. *Architecture/interior design:* Anshen + Allen. *Photo:* Jane Lidz.)

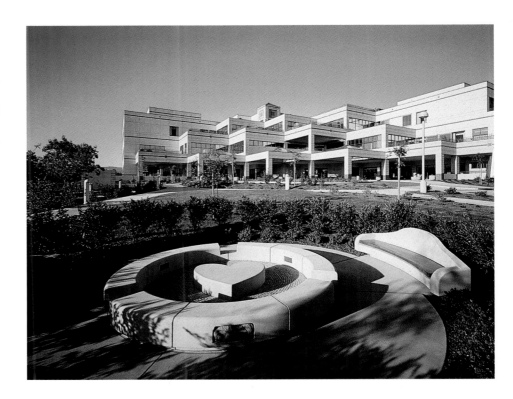

◆ **FIGURE C-11** The wings were extended out in a welcoming way and a small-scale terraced entrance was comprised of a fragmented arrangement of canopies, playrooms, and gardens, intended to be like transparent toy blocks. (*Project:* Lucile Salter Packard Children's Hospital, Palo Alto, CA. *Architecture/interior design:* Anshen + Allen. *Photo:* Jane Lidz.)

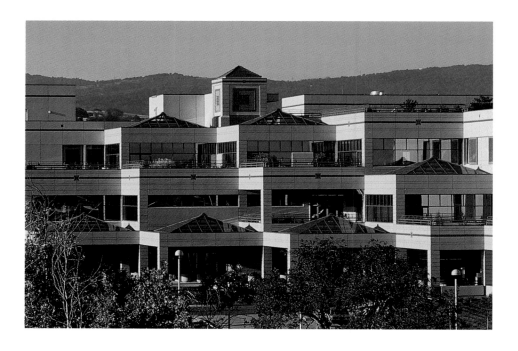

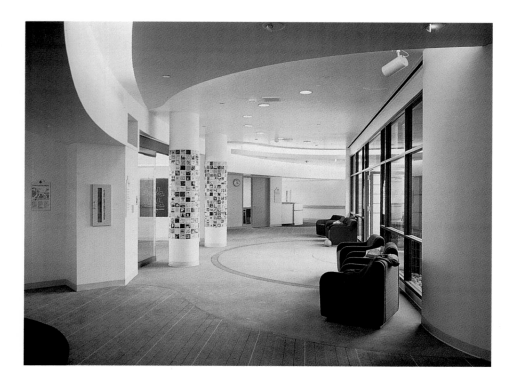

◆ **FIGURE C-12** Sinuous forms of the landscape penetrate the building and give shape to walls, columns, ceilings, furniture, art-work, and interior finishes. The round shape is poetic, calming, sheltering, and fun. (*Project:* Lucile Salter Packard Children's Hospital, Palo Alto, CA. *Architecture/interior design:* Anshen + Allen. *Photo:* Chas McGrath.)

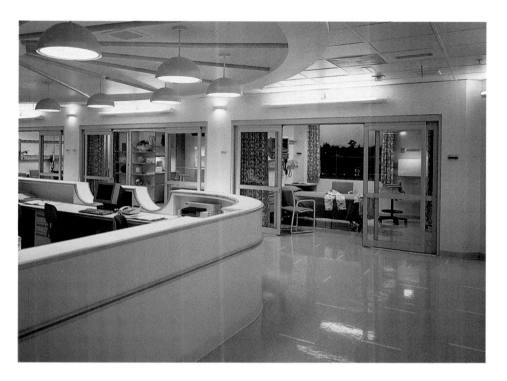

◆ **FIGURE C-13** A warm, neutral color palette of beige tones was chosen so that the environment would not look dated and in order to maximize the visual impact of artwork and elements that children would bring into the environment. Strong colors were used in less permanent, more easily changeable elements, such as upholstery and cubicle curtains. (*Project:* Lucile Salter Packard Children's Hospital, Palo Alto, CA. *Architecture/interior design:* Anshen + Allen. *Photo:* Chas McGrath.)

◆ **FIGURE C-14** A patient room in the Lucile Salter Packard Chidren's Hospital. (*Project:* Lucile Salter Packard Children's Hospital, Palo Alto, CA. *Architecture/interior design:* Anshen + Allen. *Photo:* Chas McGrath.)

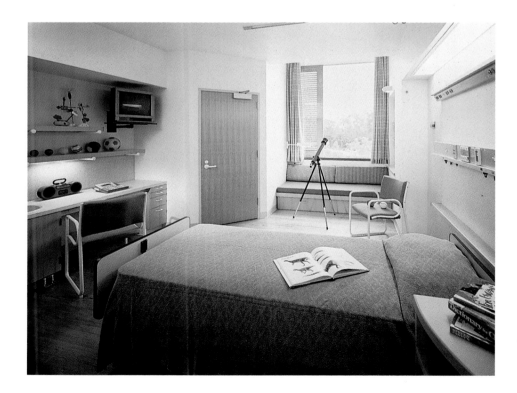

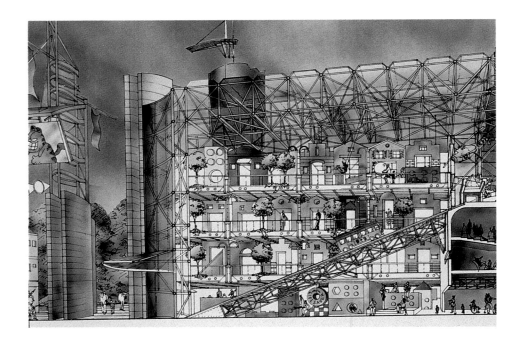

◆ **FIGURE C-15** The firm's challenge was to create physical environments within STARBRIGHT that were as exciting as an "E" ticket ride at Disneyland. (*Project:* STARBRIGHT Pavilion, Los Angeles. *Design:* Kaplan McLaughlan Diaz and Medical Planning Associates.)

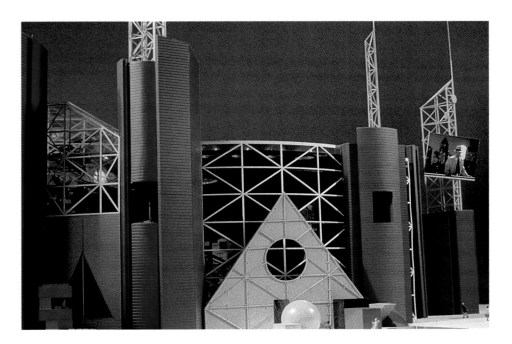

◆ **FIGURE C-16** The exterior design of the STARBRIGHT Pavilion is intended to attract the attention of children but, equally, the respect of adolescents by providing an artistic combination of generic Lego and Tinkertoy-like forms as both structural and decorative features. (*Project:* STARBRIGHT Pavilion, Los Angeles. *Design:* Kaplan McLaughlan Diaz and Medical Planning Associates.)

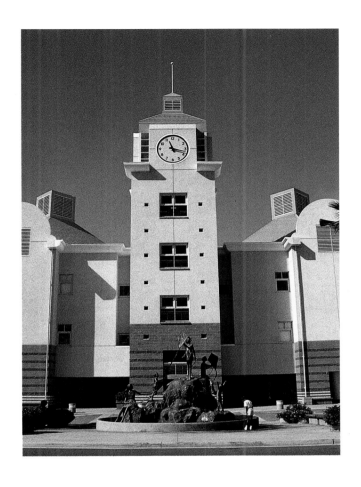

◆ **FIGURE C-17** *Left*. The desire was to create a new, easily recognizable landmark — to take advantage of the heritage and the flora and fauna of San Diego. (*Project:* San Diego Children's Hospital and Health Center Addition. *Architecture/interior design:* NBBJ Architects. *Sculpture:* "Inspiration" by Dennis Smith. *Photo:* Courtesy of the Aesthetics Collection, art consultants for the project.)

◆ **FIGURE C-18** *Below*. Seasonal change is the concept that influences the interiors and the architecture, through the use of color, lighting, and the "openness" of nature. (*Project:* Main reception, San Diego Children's Hospital and Health Center Addition. *Architecture/interior design:* NBBJ Architects. *Photo:* David Hewitt and Anne Garrison.)

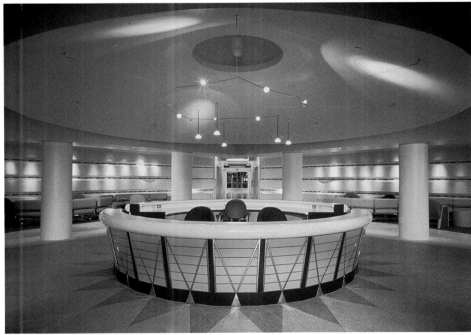

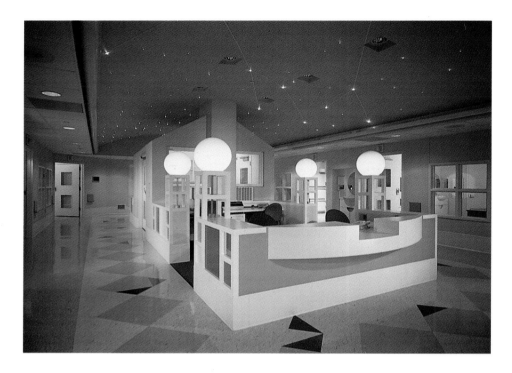

◆ **FIGURE C-19** Imagine the surprise and wonder when a child looks out the window of his room at night and sees the stars shining over the nurses' "home." (*Project:* Nurse station, San Diego Children's Hospital and Health Center Addition. *Architecture/interior design:* NBBJ Architects. *Photo:* David Hewitt and Anne Garrison.)

◆ **FIGURE C-20** Control is provided through the choice of art, lighting, temperature, noise, privacy, and meals. Choice is essential to healing. (*Project:* Patient room, San Diego Children's Hospital and Health Center Addition. *Architecture/interior design:* NBBJ Architects. *Photo:* David Hewitt and Anne Garrison.)

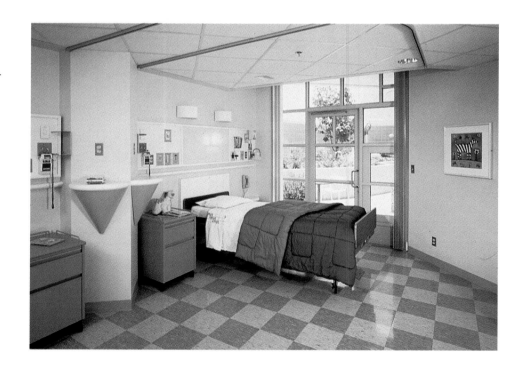

◆ **FIGURE C-21** The inappropriateness of Western-standard hospitals that had brought forth glass skyscrapers in the Saudi desert reinforced the goal to design this hospital in a way that was culturally responsive — while providing all the required technology of a state-of-the-art medical center. (*Project:* Main entrance portal, Aga Khan University Hospital and Medical School, Karachi, Pakistan. *Architecture:* Payette Associates. *Photo:* Paul Warchol.)

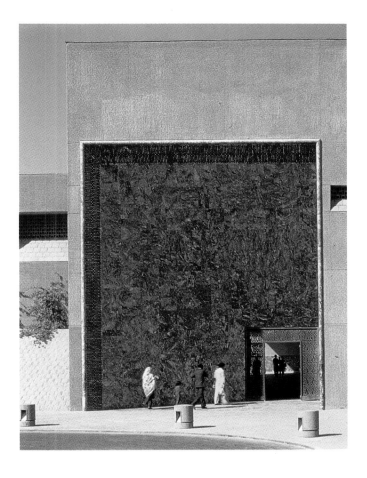

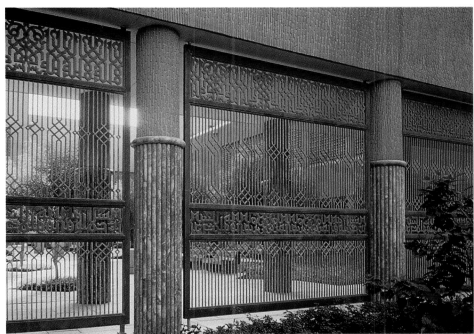

◆ **FIGURE C-22** Payette's design concept captures the spirit of the people who were and are expected to use it. (*Project:* View into courtyard through decorative screen, Aga Khan University Hospital and Medical School, Karachi, Pakistan. *Architecture:* Payette Associates. *Photo:* Paul Warchol.)

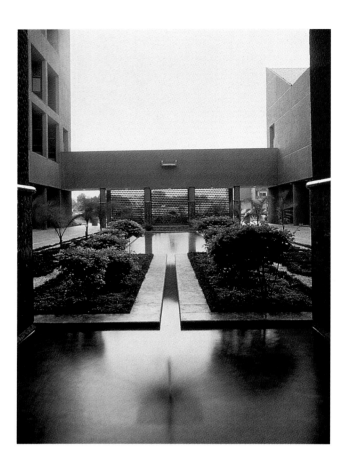

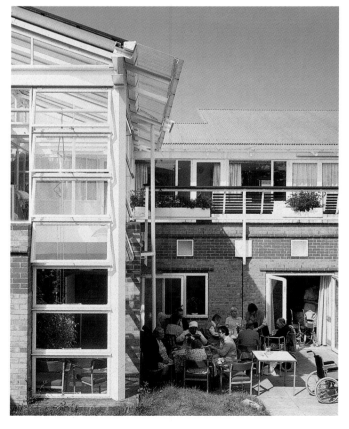

◆ **FIGURE C-23** In Islamic countries, many examples of landscaping are based on the concept of Sasanian courtyards, called "pardis," which is the root word of "paradise." (*Project:* Reflecting pools in courtyard, Aga Khan University Hospital and Medical School, Karachi, Pakistan. *Architecture:* Payette Associates. *Photo:* Paul Warchol.)

◆ **FIGURE C-24** The upper conservatory is particularly enjoyed for the protected exposure to the garden that lets the patient be in nature (life) but inside (shelter), as well. (*Project:* Lambeth Community Care Center, England. *Architecture:* Edward Cullinan Architects. *Photo:* Martin Charles.)

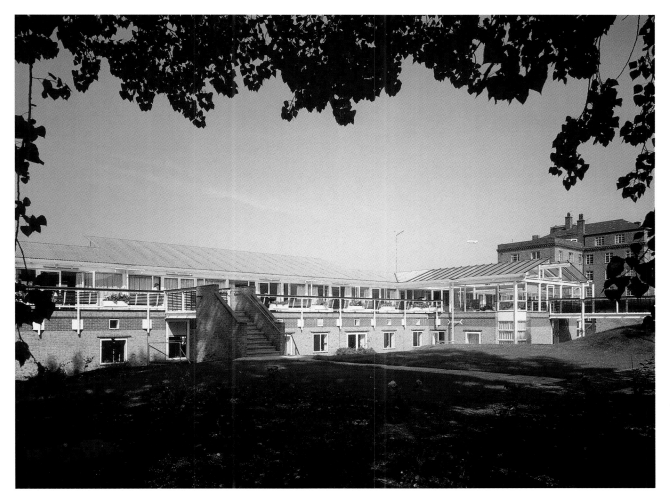

◆ **FIGURE C-25** Generally, the building itself, including the garden and the canteen, were seen as a condition for achieving good-quality care in the center. People praised...the use...of natural light (and) the accessible and homelike physical structure of the building. (*Project:* Lambeth Community Care Center, England. *Architecture:* Edward Cullinan Architects. *Photo:* Martin Charles.)

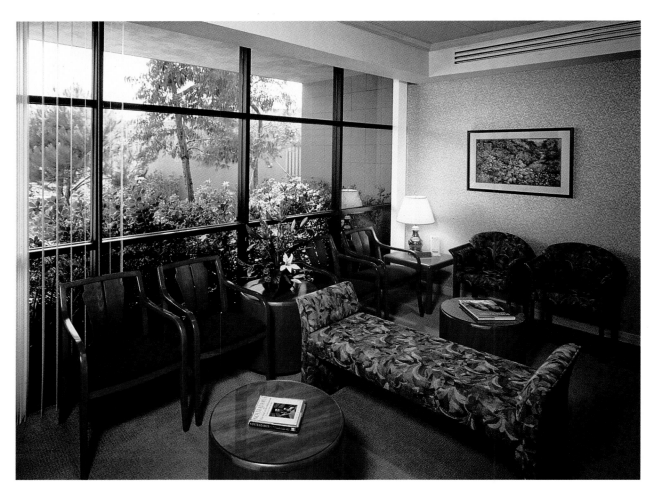

◆ **FIGURE C-26** This example of a physician's waiting room, takes advantage of a view of nature, which research has shown to have many stress-reducing benefits. (*Project:* Family practitioner's office. *Interior design:* Jain Malkin, Inc. *Photo:* Steve McClelland.)

◆ **FIGURE C-27** In an obstetrician's or gynecologist's office, there should be seating that is comfortable and easy to get out of for pregnant women. (*Project:* OB-GYN office. *Interior design:* Jain Malkin, Inc. *Photo:* Steve McClelland.)

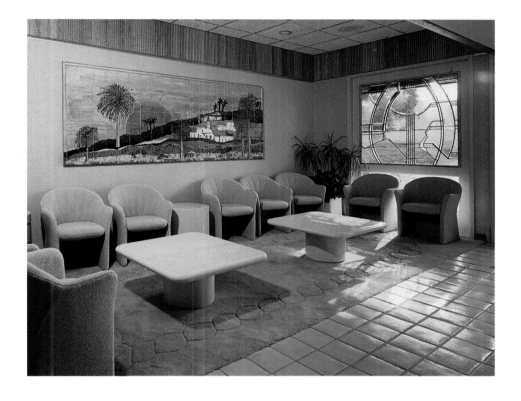

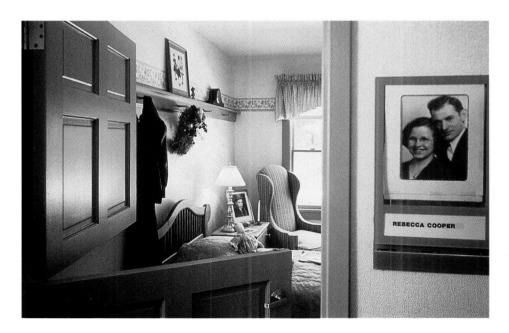

◆ **FIGURE C-28** Enforced routines, structured staff/resident interaction, and institutional models of security and observation were avoided in this residence for Alzheimer patients. The familiar, homelike atmosphere of the bedrooms and shared spaces is believed to elicit more appropriate behavior by the residents. (*Project:* Woodside Place, Oakmont, PA. *Architecture/interior design:* Perkins Eastman Partners. *Photo:* Robert P. Ruschak.)

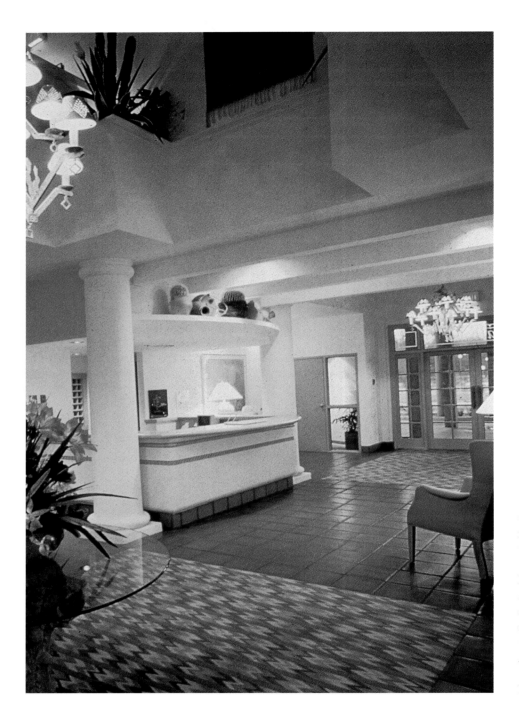

◆ **FIGURE C-29** The building forms and materials in this facility are indigenous to the Southwest, where it is located. Exterior corridors, balconies, and a courtyard pool area encourage residents to enjoy the mild climate. (*Project:* La Posada at Park Center, Green Valley, AZ. *Architecture:* Engelbrecht & Griffin. *Photo:* Assassi Productions.)

trasts and hard edges—at first black and white and then bright, highly saturated primary and secondary colors. As infants develop, they respond to more subtle shades, and by the teenage years their responses have matured. In geriatric patients, the yellowing of the lens of the eye should be considered. Color perception in the blue ranges is lost first. A greater difference in gray values is important, therefore, since binocular vision and depth perception are diminished.

Color perception is affected by the tint or value of the hue and by the adjacent colors, patterns, and texture. Color choices should be guided by geographic location, each of which has different light qualities, natural color palettes, and regional preferences. What is appropriate in the Arizona desert is not appropriate in the Canadian north woods or in foggy San Francisco.

Choice of a color palette, then, among other things, depends upon the light sources, geographic location, size and share of the space, type of activity that is being performed in it, and the users' ages (see Figure C–2). Studies show that a lack of stimulation impairs the functioning of the brain's cortex, causing an increase in heart and breathing rates. A visual environment utilizing a variety of colors and shades is one way of providing needed interest and stimulation for a more productive space.

Acoustics

The most common adverse effect of noise is loss of hearing. But noise does more. Auditory trauma, besides producing generalized stress reaction, produces physiological changes in blood capillary structure, impeding the flow of red blood cells and constricting the vascular channels. This can cause high blood pressure, heart disease, and ulcers.

Noise as a stressor causes irritation and frustration, aggravates anger, and reduces pain thresholds. Not only does it impair hearing acuity, noise has even been proven to affect adversely visual perception and cause diminished learning capacity. For the staff, noise decreases productivity and increases absenteeism.

Babies exposed to a noisy environment are slower to imitate adult behavior, persist in infantile habits longer, and have delayed verbal development and delayed exploratory activity. Infant learning lags in general because it is too noisy to think.

"Calling noise a nuisance is like calling smog an inconvenience," says William H. Stewart, former U.S. Surgeon General. "Noise must be considered a hazard to the health of people everywhere."

The acoustic environment can be improved by the selection of interior surfaces and furnishings that do not reflect or amplify sound waves. Walls and ceilings that are irregularly recessed are effective in scattering sound waves. Although surfaces and furnishings can have varying sound-absorbing qualities, an area with adequate amounts of carpeting, fabric, wood, acoustic tiles, and sound panels can provide a quieter environment.

The positive side of sound is music. It is possible to effect physiological change, for example, control heart rate and lower blood pressure, by coordinating music to the rhythms of the body. Music can also be a conditioned stimulus for relaxation and pain reduction and a distraction from discomfort. The audioanalgesic mechanism includes endorphins produced by the thrill response that occurs when listening to music. Music, being nonverbal, evokes responses on an emotional level, thereby working as a mood changer, and creates synthesis of the other senses. A music library is essential.

Aroma

Scent may be called the silent persuader, influencing mind, body, and health. Smell, the oldest and deepest of the senses, is also the most evocative, stimulating the brain to recall complete memories. Smell impulses travel a faster, more direct route to the brain than visual or auditory impulses, going directly to the limbic system, the seat of emotions. Smell and emotions are very closely intertwined.

Odors get their meaning through conditioning. However, there are certain odors, like rotting garbage, that are inherently unpleasant and can produce nausea. Any smell that is too strong will be disagreeable. Unpleasant smells (e.g., ammonia) increase breathing and heart rates. Conversely, pleasant smells (e.g., spiced apple and light florals) are stress reducing.

Bowls of sachet, floral arrangements, and plants can provide pleasant fragrance in a healthcare facility (see Figure C–3). And there is an added benefit to plants: some can clean the indoor air. Current research indicates that ordinary houseplants have proven effective in removing toxic pollutants from the air inside homes and office buildings. Common plants such as philodendrons, golden pothos, spider plants, peach lilies, and English ivy can effectively clean indoor air by absorbing toxins—such as formaldehyde, benzene, and trichloroethylene, the three most common indoor pollutants—through microbes on leaves, roots, and in the soil. As well as cleaning the indoor air, real plants provide design interest and a needed touch of nature.

Tactile

The skin is the largest of human sense organs, yet touch is the most neglected of the senses. Air quality and thermal comfort of an environment are perceived through skin. One's accuracy of movement is dependent upon the sense of touch. Learning, alertness, and vitality are enhanced through tactile sensations.

Bodily comfort is insured by properly chosen furnishings—soft bedding and fabrics, rounded corners, and ergonomically designed furniture. Inability to move or operate furnishings can produce stress and anxiety in the patient and contribute to the patient's sense of helplessness and dependence, while creating an extra burden for the staff.

Placing controls for nurse call, lighting, telephone, television, and radio within easy reach of a patient enhances self-reliance and increases patient safety. In multibed rooms, each patient should have equal access to controls of such items as windows and television. An environment scaled for young children enhances their sense of independence.

The tactility of the space may be enriched by interesting surface treatments, a variety of fabrics and finishes, and differing scale in furnishings to provide an environment that is both comfortable and comforting.

Space

The space we create controls us, and the way the physical space of service settings is arranged can strongly enhance or inhibit the program of care. Individuals require added privacy and an assurance of ample space of their own at moments of tension and social change. Therefore, it is essential to have space that is private, even if it is just a drawer that locks.

Floor design affects patient satisfaction. For example, a radial floor design with the rooms arranged around the nurse station provides the highest patient stress reduction because the proximity to the nursing staff supports feelings of security and well-being.

Progressive care settings, which are characterized by sensitively designed interiors, furnished more like hotel rooms or homes, encourage faster recovery. These spaces have lounges, dining rooms, and pantries that patients are encouraged to use. In such settings, patients are more active, more social, have less feeling of being confined and institutionalized, and consequently feel better and recover faster.

By incorporating the principles of PNI into a facility's interior design, positive physiological responses can be maximized among patients, resulting in shorter stays and higher earnings for the hospital. And the environment that produces positive responses in patients creates the same reaction in the nursing staff. A PNI-designed facility can help reduce nurse burnout, minimize stress, and assist in employee retention.

This new approach to design can change the way space is used by providing sensorially stimulating environments that enhance well-being. PNI-based interiors can provide a blueprint for the design of memorable surroundings that enrich the human spirit and humanize the "inhospitable hospital."

References

Alexander, C., et al. 1977. *A Pattern Language.* London: Oxford University Press.

Birren, F. 1978. *Color and Human Response.* New York: Van Nostrand Reinhold Co.

Bonny, H.L. 1986. *Music and Healing.* Seattle, WA: American Holistic Medical Association.

Doty, R. Olfactory Communication in Humans. *Chemical Senses* 6(4): 351–74.

Goldstein, A. Thrills in Response to Music and Other Stimuli. *Physiological Psychology* 8(1): 126–29.

Goldstein, K. June 1942. Some Experimental Observations on the Influence of Color on the Function of the Organism. *Occupational Therapy and Rehabilitation.*

Halpern, S., and Savary, L. 1985. *Sound Health.* Glenview, IL: Harper & Row.

Hollwich, F. 1979. *The Influence of Ocular Light Perception on Metabolism in Man and in Animal.* Springer-Verlag: New York, Heidelberg, Berlin.

Hughes, P.C. 1983. Natural Light and the Psychobiological System of Man. *CIE Pub. 562.*

Jokl, M.V. June 1984. The Psychological Effects on Man of Air Movement and the Colour of His Surroundings. *Applied Ergonomics*: 119–25.

Lewy, A.J., et al. 1980. Light Suppresses Melatonin Secretion in Humans. *Science* 210: 1267–69.

Maas, J.B., et al. 1974. Effects of Spectral Difference in Illumination on Fatigue. *Journal of Applied Psychology* 59: 524–26.

Maier, H.W. Fall 1992. The Space We Create Controls Us. *Residential Group Care and Treatment* 1(1): 51–59.

Minckley, B. 1968. A Study of Noise and Its Relationship to Patient Discomfort in the Recovery Room. *Nursing Research* 17: 247–50.

Montagu, A. 1973. *Touching: The Human Significance of the Skin.* New York: Columbia University Press.

Ogle, J. 1985. Exploring Scent Therapy. *New York Times*, November 17.

Olds, A.R. 1985. Nature as Healer, Readings in Psychosyntheses. Ontario Institute for Studies in Education.

Plack, J.J., and Schick, J. 1974. The Effects of Color on Human Behavior. *Journal of the Association for Study in Perception:* 4–16.

Rider, M. 1985. Entrainment Mechanisms Are Involved in Pain Reduction, Muscle Relaxation, and Music-Mediated Imagery. *Journal of Music Therapy* 22(4): 183–92.

Smith, R.C. February 1986. Light and Health, a Broad Overview. *Lighting Design + Application.*

Solomon, G.F. (in press) Psychoneuroimmunology: Interactions Between Central Nervous System and Immune System. *Journal of Neuroscience Research.*

Ulrich, R.S. 1984. View Through a Window May Influence Recovery from Surgery. *Science* 224: 420–21.

Van Toller, S., and Dodd, G. 1988. *Perfumery, the Psychology and Biology of Fragrance.* London, New York: Chapman and Hall.

Wolverton, B.C., Johnson, A., Bounds, K. 1985. Interior Landscape Plants for Indoor Air Pollution Abatement. *NASA Office of Commercial Programs—Final Report.*

Wurtman, R.J. 1975. The Effects of Light on Man and Other Mammals. *Annual Review of Physiology* 37: 467–83.

Millicent Gappell, IFDA, is a certified interior designer located in Los Angeles, California. A pioneer in the field of psychoneuroimmunology (PNI), she is a broadcast media authority on the positive effect that the environment plays in health. Gappell also teaches accredited courses about PNI to healthcare professionals, designers, and architects.

◆ ◆ ◆

CREATING A TOTAL HEALING ENVIRONMENT

Fifth Symposium on Healthcare Design, San Diego, CA, 1992

Patrick E. Linton

I am not a designer, architect, consultant, or paid professional speaker. I am a hospital CEO. I enjoy small-world community hospitals, because I can develop a closer relationship with the people and the community.

I am also very interested in spirituality, both on a personal level and in its role in the healing experience and process.

What I have to offer is three things. The first is a conceptual model from a CEO's perspective of what a total healing environment might encompass. Then, as someone who is attempting to create a total healing environment, I can offer my experiences. Perhaps most importantly, I hope I can inspire design and healthcare professionals to realize the importance of the mind, heart, and spirit in a very personal way when they talk about creating healing environments.

There is much debate right now in Washington, D. C., about healthcare reform. When I hear those discussions and look at the models that various politicians and committees are proposing, I observe that the focus is on reforming the financial delivery mechanisms of healthcare. However, reforming the healthcare product will require discussions among design professionals, owners, administrators, staff, physicians, communities, patients, and families—at conferences, in hospitals, offices, lounges, and hallways.

When we reform the healthcare product, we should focus on tapping the greatest low-cost healthcare resources: the mind, heart, and spirit of the individual patient. I am not comfortable with the term "patient," but in our society, that is the phrase we use. So I will use it, even though I think it is a very disempowering term. I actually prefer to use the term "healer" when I refer to patients.

There are tremendously powerful healing potentials within each human being. When we are talking about designing and organizing healing environments, what we are really trying to do is find effective ways to engage those inner healing potentials within each human being.

What Is Healing?

The term "healing" is used quite a bit by design and healthcare professionals. What actually is healing? Is there a common definition of what healing represents? I'm not sure there is one; I'm not sure one is needed. But it is important for each of us to consider what healing means to us personally. Each of us may have a definition of healing that is very individual.

When I began thinking about healing and creating healing environments three or four years ago, some of the questions that I considered were:

• What is healing?
• Is healing the same as curing? Is healing caring?
• Is healing an event or is healing a never-ending process?
• Where does healing come from?
• Does it come from outside the human being or does healing come from within the person?

- What is it that heals? Is it our bodies, our minds, our emotions, our relationships, our attitudes, our perspectives, our spirit?
- What is a hospital?
- Is a hospital a place for curing? Is it also a place for healing?
- Is a hospital a building? Is it equipment and technology? Is it people?
- Who are the healers? Are the healers the doctors, nurses, housekeepers, and administrators, or are the patients themselves the healers?

Again, I do not pretend to have all the answers to these questions. Yet, from my perspective as a CEO, here are some of the things I have concluded:

- Healing is bigger, deeper, and more far reaching than curing, but both are closely related.
- Healing usually involves more than just the physical vehicle, as it also touches upon the mental, emotional, and spiritual aspects of what it means to be a human being.
- Healing comes from sources within and outside of the patient, but primarily from within.
- Hospitals need to expand beyond the medical model of curing to newly developed models of healing that recognize and consciously work with the mind/body/spirit connections researchers are beginning to understand.
- Healing is not just something that happens magically or spontaneously. It is something that can be consciously pursued and influenced by the person who is being healed.
- We are all in the process of healing all of the time. The only distinction between caregiver and care receiver is one of acuity; both have the potential to heal from the experience.
- Humankind's eternal quest seems to be the search for itself, its God, peace of mind, and peace of heart. Healing seems to occur when people get back on the path in this particular quest.
- Healing seems to be a continuing process of connection, or perhaps reconnection, that people bring into their lives.

When I think about healing, I think of surgery. What does not seem to fit into the definition of healing I have just described is that the surgery itself is often seen as the healing procedure. What does seem to fit is that we also talk about the need to heal as a result of surgery. That seems to be how society has embraced the term "healing" when referring to a very traumatic or invasive physical procedure. We actually have to heal from the very curing treatment that we have allowed ourselves to go through.

But the concept of connection, or healing reconnection, can also be applied to relationships or ideas we become connected to that expand our consciousness of things we were not connected to previously. Within our families and social relationships, we connect to our individual histories and heritages. Connections to nature are very powerful healing connections. Connections to deeper parts of ourselves in the continuing process of self-discovery are part of the healing journey.

Yavapai Regional Medical Center

Yavapai Regional Medical Center (YRMC) is in Prescott, Arizona, which is about 90 miles north of Phoenix yet south of Flagstaff. Even though Prescott's "rugged West" origins are ranching and mining, it has a distinct midwest landscape. The town has a Victorian "courthouse square" feel to it.

When I was hired in 1988, YRMC had already begun the process of constructing a 110,000 square foot patient tower. YRMC was a bit of a turnaround situation, which was why I was attracted to it. It was not until 1991 that we began to set a future course for the hospital. We were in a crisis mode, trying to get ready to move into this new building. In retrospect, in light of our vision of the total healing environment, I would have designed many things differently. But we did not have the vision before we went into the design phase.

I saw my role as the leader of this hospital as one of working with individuals to come up with a vision for the organization. The vision that we came up with at YRMC of creating a total healing environment was this:

> We are trying to create an environment in which the people of the hospital work in partnership with patients and their families, seeking peace of mind and peace of heart, as well as physical cures and comforts. The reason is that we are beginning to understand the indivisible relationship that exists between body, mind, and spirit.

There are some key words and concepts here. The first is the concept of partnership with the patient and the family. As Don McKahan indicated in his presentation, often not just the person who happens to be residing temporarily in a hospital bed, but also the family is going through a healing process. This vision underscores the importance of individual responsibility. I wonder how much we really heal people, or if we are simply assisting the person in managing his or her own healing process.

Another important concept to consider when working with holistic and mind/body approaches is semantics, because sometimes groups in our society respond to certain terms and concepts in a negative way. For example, in Prescott, the clergy from the area wanted to meet with me to hear about the kinds of things I was working on with the hospital. We had a wonderful discussion. They were concerned, however, about the phrasing of the vision. Originally, I talked about the relationship between the body, mind, and the human spirit, thinking that "human spirit" might be a phrase that would appeal to large numbers of people. But some people in the clergy told me that spirit is not human; spirit is divine in origin. When I asked them what terminology they preferred, they debated back and forth. What we came up with as a group was simply the term "spirit."

North Hawaii Community Hospital

In 1992, I left YRMC to head the North Hawaii Community Hospital, which has not yet been built. This truly is a wonderful adventure that I have been fortunate and blessed to participate in.

The northern part of the Big Island of Hawaii is grossly underserved in

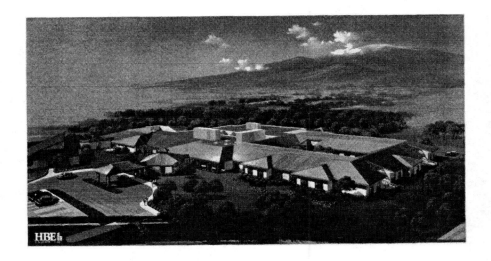

terms of access to acute care and other types of healthcare services. The community, for the past five or six years, has been working hard to come up with the money and the support needed to start its own new hospital. Community leaders want it to be a very special kind of hospital, so they asked if I would come out and work with them to develop a hospital based on the concept of a total healing environment. In very simple terms, I now have $25 million at my disposal, a supportive board and community, a generally supportive medical staff, and a piece of ground to work with.

Mauna Kea is one of the five volcanoes that form the island of Hawaii. Working on the island is really unique, because the island is relatively young. It is 800,000 years old, formed by a tremendous, creative energy of nature. There is one volcano on the south end of Hawaii that has been continuously erupting for 10 years. So the island is changing and recreating itself, even as I speak. That creative power can be inspirational.

Cinder cones on the island look like hills. Native Hawaiian culture says that the cones are very powerful in their healing impact. One on our site is called Buster Brown. We were thinking about putting the hospital on top of Buster Brown but decided it would be hard to access.

Background on Healing

The concept that the mind, body, and spirit are somehow connected in the healing process certainly is not new. In fact, it goes back centuries. Hippocrates was the one who said, "I would much rather know more about the person who has the disease than the disease that the person has."

One hundred years or so ago, Louis Pasteur and a contemporary had an ongoing debate about what was the more important factor in healing. Was it to eradicate the foreign agent from the body? Or was it to improve the health of the host tissue, within which the foreign body or the foreign agent might be lodged? That debate went on for more than a year. On his deathbed, Louis Pasteur's contemporary, who had taken the side that eradication of the foreign agent was more important, finally gave in and admitted that the health of the host tissue is a much more important factor in dealing with disease.

Over the past decades, particularly since World War II, we have seen tremendous advances and improvements in medical technology and science. We have shifted almost too far in that direction. I certainly would not want to go backward, nor would I want to halt the advancements in medical technology. But somehow we need to bring components other than technology and science back into balance.

When we talk about creating healing environments, we are not thinking of substituting these environments for medical technology and science. We are trying to balance those things with the natural healing potentials that reside within the human being. In the vision of a total healing environment the external interventions of medical science can be balanced with the internal potentials of the patient. Ultimately, what we want to do is to create an environment that will be powerful in invoking the inner healing resources of the patient in order to enhance the effectiveness of the physician's outer healing resources.

Psychoneuroimmunology

In forming my thoughts and models, I have studied some of the research coming out of the field of psychoneuroimmunology. The first studies using the scientific model in this area probably were done in the 1930s. Psychoneuroimmunology refers to the study of the relationship between the mind and the immune system. Actually, it is the relationship between the mind and the brain, nervous system, endocrine system, and the immune system. As research continues in this particular area, scientists are finding that all of the body's systems are constantly interacting and influencing each other. The human being, even at a physical or psychological level, is a very holistic, interdynamic entity.

In the field of psychoneuroimmunology, it has been known for some time that negative emotions, particularly those that are chronically held and suppressed, can have negative physical impact. Emotions such as rage, depression, hate, fear, and frustration may actually manifest as a physical disease.

In addition, we are beginning to appreciate that the opposite may also be true—that positive emotions openly and creatively expressed may actually have positive impacts on health. In Hawaii, there is a term "aloha." It means hello and good-bye, but it also means love. So when we talk about the aloha in the room, we mean the aloha that is coming from people. I do not know why we cannot begin to talk about the use of love in hospitals. Let us talk about it openly and warmly and accept the role of love, joy, and peace in our lives, as well as in our hospitals.

The research in the area of psychoneuroimmunology breaks down into two levels. One is the research being done at the micro or cellular level. Researchers using microscopes are beginning to see how these body systems are interrelated in a biochemical way. They are beginning to see how the brain and the nervous system are able to produce neurotransmitter cells. Almost like a lock and key, certain receptor cells are constructed to be the receptor cells for certain neurotransmitters. When that healing connection is made, the immune system begins to react.

Researchers are also finding out that the same process works in reverse.

The immune system also produces neurotransmitters, which are sent out through the body. The brain has receptor cells that pick up these neurotransmitters. When the brain is engaged, it becomes a pharmacopoeia. The most wonderful drugstore that exists is in the human brain. Somehow the brain and the nervous system know how to produce the right amount of chemical and get it in the right dosage to the right part of the body.

The macro, or behavioral, level of research is discovering that, in the psyche of the human being, emotions, thoughts, beliefs, and values have an impact on what is happening at the biochemical level. For people in depressed states, the connection at the cellular level is physically impaired and vice versa. We are going to see much more in the years ahead in this particular area.

Here are some of the findings that have come out of the study of psychoneuroimmunology:

- A study done at the University of California in San Francisco found cancer patients whose attitudes were active instead of passive exhibited much better immune function and slower tumor growth in their cancers.
- Another study of cancer patients done at Johns Hopkins in Baltimore showed that there might be a link between the progression of the disease and emotional suppression of chronically held emotion.
- In an experimental group of elderly patients with cancer diagnosis, those who engaged in relaxation training three times a week had much increased natural killer and T-cell activity in their immune systems compared with the control group.
- Another study of cancer patients found that those in the experimental group who were using not only relaxation, but also positive and guided imagery techniques experienced increased stimulation of lymphocytes, antibody production, interluken two cell activity, natural killer cell activity, etc., in their immune systems.
- A study done at Ohio State did not focus so much on the patient, but on the caregivers for a group of Alzheimer's patients. In the experimental group, those caregivers who were involved in support groups were found to have significantly higher percentages of natural killer cells in their immune systems.
- A major series of studies done at the University of Southern California, Los Angeles (UCLA) separated patients into four different disease categories: ulcer disease, hypertension, diabetes, and breast cancer. Within each of these four diagnostic categories, there was a control group that really was going through standard treatment and protocols, as well as an experimental group. With the experimental group, researchers gave subjects a brief 20-minute education and information session on how to be a more involved patient. They explained how to become more active and involved in the healing experience, how to talk to physicians or nurses and ask them questions. Researchers found that in each of these disease categories, in each of the experimental groups, those who were more active in participation with their doctors had improved health status. That tells me something about what we should be doing in hospitals in terms of teaching and coaching patients how to become more involved in what is happening with their treatment.
- In various studies that have been repeated multiple times, researchers

found that the psychological state of happiness was actually a better predictor of future coronary problems than any other clinical variable. Cholesterol, smoking, diet, etc., were not as accurate predictors as the psychological state of happiness. The second most accurate variable in predicting was job satisfaction.

- In another study, people who are in high-demand and low-autonomy positions have two to three times the risk of heart problems. When we talk about empowering management techniques and approaches, it is not just to get increased productivity or to motivate an organization. It is because sharing responsibility helps people's health.
- People who help others tend to feel healthier, and in one study of 2,700 male volunteers over a 10-year period, the volunteers had death rates two-and-a-half times lower than expected.

Total Healing Environment Model

The center of the Western healing model is still high quality medicine. There are different types of healing systems throughout the world; no one system contains all the answers, but perhaps it is time to begin sharing and go beyond the limits of one particular system. Nevertheless, in talking about creating a total healing environment, we need to be practical. In Western culture, the primary focus and model that we are working with is allopathic or osteopathic medicine.

Yet, when creating a healing environment, it doesn't matter what the core of the model is. I can create a healing environment around a naturopathic, ayruvedic, or Chinese herbal medicine approach. It doesn't matter, either, whether we are working with physicians or chiropractors. When working toward a more holistic approach and creating that kind of an environment, we are naturally going to see health professionals become more collaborative and open to other healing approaches.

To develop the conceptual model for the total healing environment, I created a matrix by intersecting two overlapping continuums. (see Figure 4–8.) The vertical continuum begins at the top, with the environment that is external to the human being and moves down the continuum to the environment that is within the human being. In quantum physics, as one gets to the subatomic level, it is very difficult to see where the boundary of a human being stops and the boundary of his or her environment begins. In effect, I am not sure where my hand stops and the podium begins at a subatomic level. So I truly see this as a continuum.

Similarly, along the horizontal continuum, we are talking about the elements of the environment on the left side of the matrix that are physical in nature. On the right side of the continuum, we are talking about the elements in the environment that are psychospiritual in nature.

The intersection of these two continuums thus results in a model for our total healing environment that is comprised of four quadrants.

1. *First quadrant.* This contains the physical environment that is external to the patient, or human being: elements such as color, views, equipment, appearance of staff, lighting, and other sensory stimuli that design professionals deal with.

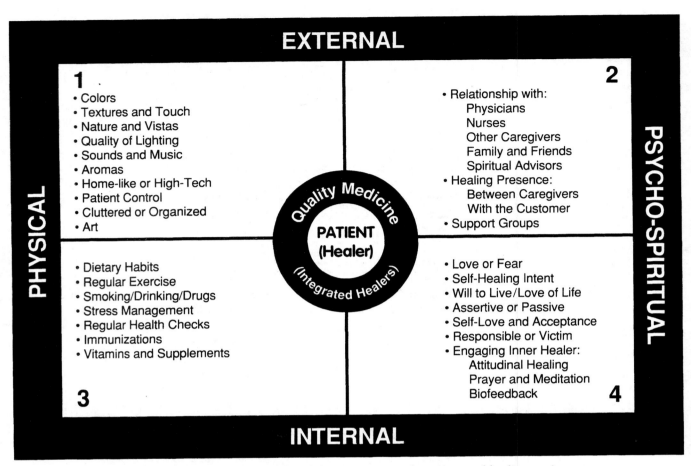

EXTERNAL

1
- Colors
- Textures and Touch
- Nature and Vistas
- Quality of Lighting
- Sounds and Music
- Aromas
- Home-like or High-Tech
- Patient Control
- Cluttered or Organized
- Art

PHYSICAL

Quality Medicine
**PATIENT
(Healer)**
(Integrated Healers)

- Dietary Habits
- Regular Exercise
- Smoking/Drinking/Drugs
- Stress Management
- Regular Health Checks
- Immunizations
- Vitamins and Supplements

3

2
- Relationship with:
  Physicians
  Nurses
  Other Caregivers
  Family and Friends
  Spiritual Advisors
- Healing Presence:
  Between Caregivers
  With the Customer
- Support Groups

PSYCHO-SPIRITUAL

- Love or Fear
- Self-Healing Intent
- Will to Live/Love of Life
- Assertive or Passive
- Self-Love and Acceptance
- Responsible or Victim
- Engaging Inner Healer:
  Attitudinal Healing
  Prayer and Meditation
  Biofeedback

4

INTERNAL

◆ **FIGURE 4–8** The model shows four quadrants with variables that contribute to a total healing environment.

2. *Second quadrant.* This contains the elements in the external environment that are psychospiritual in nature. These include relationships with physicians and nurses, the reputation of a hospital, caring of staff, conversations in public areas, and the help of relatives. How can we analyze what is happening in our organizations to improve the healing impact of things happening in this particular quadrant?

The key phrase in this particular quadrant is "the healing impact of relationships." Perhaps the most powerful relationship in the healing experience is the relationship that human beings have with themselves. In terms of external relationships, one of the most powerful relationships is the relationship with the physician. The power is beginning to shift, however, as patients become more active, informed, educated, and desirous of becoming involved with and directing their own care. Society is beginning to take back some of the power it has given physicians over the years. Unfortunately, we had disempowered ourselves, in many respects, as human beings, and we had created a very dependency-oriented model in healthcare. We are still very much dependent on physicians and their knowledge and very much dependent on other healthcare professionals—having given that power to them.

In a hospital, nurses are the group of people with whom patients spend the most time. Unfortunately, bureaucracies, regulations, and joint commission standards require that nurses do more paperwork, and this has taken them away from patients. We are trying to find ways for nurses to spend more time developing healing relationships with patients and families.

When I talk to nurses, they all say, "Don't forget the housekeepers." Next to the nurses, the housekeepers may spend the most time with the patient in the hospital. How many have ever thought about the housekeeper as a healer? Perhaps housekeepers could be trained to create a therapeutic presence when they are in a room; to embrace openly and love and accept the human being in the bed near them without even having to say a word. If they can engage in conversation, it might help in the healing experience even more.

How many remember guest relations training that came into vogue as hospitals went into major competitive environments in the 1970s and 1980s? I became very sad at that time, because all of a sudden I saw the business acumen increase, which is wonderful; but it became the entire focus of what we were trying to do in hospitals. Everything we were doing was geared to increasing market share and improving the bottom line financially. Somehow I saw the heart of the healer, that very precious commodity, being squeezed and buried underneath layers of politics and bureaucracy and under a business orientation that did not care much about what was happening on the heart side. In this new paradigm, we are going to see the heart reemerge.

3. *Third quadrant.* This is the physical environment within the human being, or patient. It includes the patient's physical condition, existence of other diseases, condition of other body systems, and the patient's diet. We are seeing tremendous strides being made in diet, exercise, lifestyle changes, etc. I am so pleased to see that, because we know that if people are in generally good physical states when something goes wrong with one body system, generally the healing experience is much more positive.

4. *Fourth quadrant.* This is perhaps the most powerful quadrant in this healing environment. It deals with what is happening within the mind, psyche, and spirit of the individual patient, or human being. This includes issues such as the patient's outlook on life, psychological state, will to live, willingness to take responsibility, acceptance of self, view of disease, and trust in treatment. It is where the greatest untapped potential lies. Everything that we are doing in the other quadrants has an impact on what happens here.

This brings up the question of what patients contribute to their own healing experience? We have heard for many years about the concept of the will to live. If patients have that, their chances of recovery seem to be improved. We are also discovering that having that will might be a matter of choice, not just a natural phenomenon.

If we were to look at a frequency distribution curve of our patients and do a psychographic profile, we would see that probably 15 to 20 percent do not want to take responsibility for their mental and emotional state. They are in the hospital to get the pill, have the surgery done, and go back to their lives.

At the other end of this distribution curve, there are probably 15 to 20 percent of patients who do not need to be coached or educated, because they are going to demand to know what is happening to them. They are going to study and research their disease, select the treatment they want, select which physician to work with, and demand of the nurse, "Why wasn't my medication given at 2 P.M. like the doctor ordered?" These are our so-called problem patients. Problem patients, we know through studies, get better faster. Why? Because through self-initiation they are engaging the healing parts of themselves.

The 60 percent in the middle are the people, who, to some degree or another, want to become more involved. They want to know how they can become more engaged and be a contributor in their healing process. It is up to us to help coach them, advise them, help bring them to the approach that is right for them. We do not have the right to force our will upon another human being. We do not have a right to take our personal philosophies, belief systems, or religions and "lay" them on someone else. We have to give patients a variety of options in a healing environment so that they can select for themselves what will engage their mind, emotions, and spirit.

Studies have been done with patients who meditate, use relaxation training, breathing, visualizations—all that I call the "softer therapies." Patients select those therapies themselves, work with them, and become active participants in their own care.

A task force on psychoneuroimmunology at UCLA has worked with patients for a number of years, putting them into a quiet environment, working with breathing and guided imagery to get them into a relaxed state. Researchers got patients to visualize their heart pumping blood through the shoulders, down the arms, and into their hands. Then they got patients to visualize that blood flow increasing in volume and speed. Using biofeedback techniques, researchers demonstrated to over 95 percent of the patients that they were able to raise the skin temperatures of their palms usually 10 to 15 degrees Fahrenheit.

The message is not that by increasing the blood flow to their hands, patients can cure their disease. But patients come to realize that they can influence what is happening to them.

Implementation Tracks

I have created a "Greek healing temple" diagram to illustrate possible implementation tracks. The key is creating the total healing environment. There are five implementation tracks that we must move through to achieve the vision.

1. *Self-mastery.* Individual employees within the hospital must be given opportunities to work on their own healing, personal growth, and development.

2. *Culture development.* Developing a positive organizational culture involves looking at the team concept, which is not a rigid concept. We are not working just with the X-ray or laboratory team, but with a very fluid concept of team. So one might be with his or her departmental team in the morning and be part of a cross-functional team in the afternoon. One might be the team leader in his or her morning session and a team member in the afternoon.

It is important to work from the inside out in transforming hospitals—before the physical environment is designed or programs developed. The people, attitudes, values, and spirit of the organization itself has to shift in order to accommodate these new paradigms. Leaders who can be effective in leading groups of people in this direction are needed in the culture development area.

3. *Quality of service.* Good technical and clinical quality is first and foundational. Staff has to be getting the right pill to the right patient in the right dosage, using the right route at the right time. If we are not doing this, we have no business going on to some of these other things. Service excellence is important, although standards of quality will be measured differently in the future—perhaps based on more holistic approaches.

4. *Community relations.* The healing environment within a hospital does not exist in isolation. Hospitals have to determine how their healing environment (as an organization) is going to fit within the larger community that it serves.

5. *Business and financial development.* The financial aspects of this paradigm shift are not a barrier. Instead, these might be the control mechanisms that society uses to tell us when and how fast it wants to move into this next paradigm of what healthcare is going to be. To know when society is ready, just look to see if the money is flowing in one's direction. If the money is not flowing to support this paradigm shift, it probably means society is not quite ready for it.

In Hawaii we have been blessed. The community has embraced these concepts. In 1991, in the entire United States, there were 55 gifts to hospitals and healthcare organizations of one million dollars or more. Our hospital has seven such gifts so far. It is a 50-bed hospital. The Big Island of Hawaii might be unique in terms of the potential for philanthropy, but this tells me that people are ready for holistic healing and the money is beginning to shift in the direction of supporting it.

Implications for Healing Design

I would like to close with some suggestions for design professionals who wish to help create total healing environments:

- Understand how the external, physical environment (quadrant 1) relates to the other quadrants to form a total healing environment. What are the impacts?
- Know how the features and qualities of the physical environment empower patients and help to invoke their own inner healing potentials.
- Understand how to design healing spaces that balance the need to be functional in support of medical diagnosis and treatment, the need to empower people in support of the healing model, and the need to be cost effective.
- Consider how to work with clients to create healing design experiences and processes. The actual process of creation can be very healing in itself for all those involved. Embrace the concept of designer as healer.
- Become living, breathing personifications and examples of the concepts

and values of healing. Actively work on healing and expansion of life as a way of living and being.

In ancient Hawaiian healing traditions, much of the healing focused around the "kahuna" (medical doctor). At North Hawaii Community Hospital, we also have our kahuna. The wisdom that emanates and radiates from this kahuna has this last message:

> Life force, or "mana," constantly flows through us and manifests physically, mentally, and emotionally. We clog or block the flow of mana with our fears, our doubts, and limited self-concepts that originate from our egos. When we are filled with fears, doubts, or limitations, we lose our balance and our harmony with life, which is called "pono," and a state of disease can result. Healing is the ongoing process of seeking and maintaining pono through peace, love, faith, and expanding consciousness. When we maintain pono, we remain open to the experience of life, regardless of its form, and we realize the state of beingness and connectedness with ourselves and all of life, which is "lokahi."

Patrick E. Linton is CEO of North Hawaii Community Hospital, a community organization that is creating a new 50-bed acute care hospital serving the residents of the northwest portion of the Big Island of Hawaii. He was hired in 1992 to develop this hospital following the ideas and concepts he has developed under the heading "Creating a Total Healing Environment." Prior to coming to NHCH, Linton served as CEO of Yvapai Regional Medical Center in Prescott, Arizona, which, under his leadership, was given the 21st Century Innovators Award in Healthcare from The Healthcare Forum and 3M Companies.

◆ ◆ ◆

DEFINING AND CONVEYING DESIGN VALUE

Fifth Symposium on Healthcare Design, San Diego, CA, 1992

Barbara L. Geddis, AIA

A discussion of the value and worth of design in this "new generation" of healthcare interests me profoundly. The search for the proper medium, the best language, and the most appropriate tone necessary to inspire an institutional client to seek higher aspirations is an exhilarating and sometimes frustrating odyssey—one I pursue every day in my practice. Thus, what I offer other professionals today is a highly personal set of beliefs and acquired strategies that have often formalized this search. At the heart of the odyssey is the very old question of how to persuade others in a gentle, but convincing, way that design and excellence in design can and should make a tangible and palpable difference in people's lives. This is a driving and all-inclusive goal in my firm's work in architecture, planning, and interiors. But this may not be a goal shared explicitly by the majority of healthcare clients.

Conveying and instilling the need for value demands that value be defined in a manner that is readily understandable to the layperson. Neither program narratives nor budget parameters can truly define the level of quality sought by the sponsor.

What is the value of good design?

Value is the extra, added magical quality that makes a place memorable, remarkable, serene, or simply comfortable for those who readily spend time there every day.

Geoffrey Scott in *The Architecture of Humanism/A Study in the History of Taste* (Charles Scribner's Sons, New York, 1969) wrote:

> Values (whether in life or art) are obviously not all compatible at their most intense points. Delicate grace and massive strength, calm and adventure, dignity and humor, can only coexist by large concessions on both sides. Great architecture, like great character, has been achieved not by a too inclusive grasp at all values, but by a supreme realization of a few. In art, as in life, the chief problem is a right choice in sacrifices.

In a healthcare, or specialized residential setting, it is still impossible to prove any of the following: that life is extended by a pleasant environment; that high technology is made more effective in a lovely space; that more revenue will flow into an institution just because it is hospitable; and that patients will heal and recover more quickly in a place emphasizing dignity and intimacy. But in my heart, I do believe that all of these possibilities exist and that belief fuels my firm's design approach. Let's face it, many users (consumers, visitors, short- and long-term residents) of an institution do not want to be there and have little choice in the matter. And if they have made the selection themselves, this decision was rarely based primarily on the physical environment. Yet at the same time, they are the primary beneficiaries of whatever quality designers have been able to create. They are our real clients, and they are often confined to a small physical "universe." How, then, can value offer attributes of freedom to confinement?

I would like to continue with a few additional quotes that emphasize my theme today—defining and conveying design value.

"Everything takes form, even infinity," said Bachelard in 1958.

Design value is not a subjective judgment. One can define and must continually try to define the softer and more elusive intentions of design to a client in an objective way. Furthermore, it is essential to do so in the healthcare sector, where there are so many other powerful competing criteria.

"Architecture depends on Order, Arrangement, Eurythmy, Symmetry, Propriety, and Economy," said Vitrivius in the first century B.C. His description remains crystal clear and striking. His language and vocabulary may be antique, but the concept of value is assumed in every one of his ground rules from the outset.

Finally, a quote from Andrew Saint deals with architects' responsibility to lead and inspire: "[Architects] must raise to the level of ideal those aspects of architecture whose worth is plainly perceptible to everyone."

I am going to present a case study of a recently opened project, The Carl and Dorothy Bennett Cancer Center at the Stamford Hospital in Stamford, Connecticut (see Figure C–4), that began programming in January 1991, received its temporary certificate of occupancy 11 months later in December 1991, and was finally dedicated in April 1992. It is a comprehensive outpatient cancer center for ambulatory patients and their families. This fast-track project had its site, budget, and footprint size previously defined by others (six years before my firm got involved), as well as a long-awaited opening day. Yet at the same time no advance definition of design intention or stylistic goals had ever been discussed.

Case Study Comparison

What are the means by which design value can be conveyed at various stages in the process, and how did it happen step-by-step in this case study?

1. *Precontract:* How does one convey in an interview or proposal process that one's work has a high level of design and therefore, value?

In this case, two dozen architects were evaluated and reduced to a half dozen. The remaining six were then asked to do a "concept" for the building—some built models and did renderings; most did plans. My firm did none of the above. Instead, we wrote a piece on design philosophy, approach, and considerations in designing for cancer patients and their families.

The moral of the story is that giving away "free design" at an interview does not help design professionals' status as value-leaders.

2. *Programming:* How does one address design goals in a process that stresses square footage and functionality?

In this case study, we participated fully and actively in the programming process, though we were not the programmers of record; we volunteered as the "sketchers" of proximities and clusters. We quickly found that plan sketching with this client was immensely useful for immediate playback of program testing.

To illustrate the moral of the story, the old programmer in me often borrows from Shakespeare: "The play's the thing in which you catch the conscience of the king." Inside the programming process, key clues to a design path may be found only in wide-ranging discussions with the users (but not in the square footage listings). In this case, it was a discussion of an elusive concept we called "the third entity." That was our code term for all of the non–department-owned spaces (outside of radiation therapy and medical oncology) for patients, families, and the public: counseling room, nutrition classes, all the waiting spaces. We continually asked, who is our client for "the third entity" and who is available to interview? One of the administrative vice-presidents volunteered to serve as the "owner" of the pivotal spaces.

3. *Schematic design:* How does design value become a criterion for weighing alternative design approaches?

Design goals have to be documented early in schematic design. In this case, we held a goal-setting meeting with executive administrators, and asked varied questions about intentions, goals, and dreams. By no means was this client group comfortable with the questions. But eventually, a series of published design goals became the summary of this meeting. We referred to these again and again throughout the project—when key choices about design arose. We also used them in the forward to our architect specifications. (And I also used them as the basis for our first two postoccupancy sessions, which were held in the past two months.)

In this presidential year when the words "new generation" and "change"

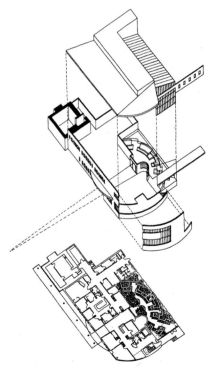

◆ **FIGURE 4–9** Axonometric and ground floor plan shows the building's unique design. (*Project:* Dorothy Bennett Cancer Center at Stamford Hospital, Stamford, CT. *Architecture/interior design:* The Geddis Partnership.)

keep coming up and when the economy is sluggish at best, many find it hard to talk about style and design, of form beyond function. However, the moral of the story is that almost every client can be drawn out on these issues. Almost everyone in a service sector at some time in their career had, and has, noble service intentions. We have to find these intentions and reinforce them. Sometimes we accompany these written goals with historic pictorial images to suggest mood or ambiance. In this case we used words. We could not find a comparable building type that was the right metaphor.

4. *Design development:* How does one keep "value" in making the many microdecisions to refine design as cost becomes a major factor? Design development is the least understood phase of design, in which microdetails should be reprogrammed and the design begins to crystallize. At some point, the design's inherent character is strong enough so that decisions are easy and obvious to a layperson.

In this case, we had a fast-track project in which we had no proper design development phase at all, since construction start was continually pushing us on. Nonetheless, we had three or four heavy-duty "value" engineering meetings with the preselected contractor on many key design issues, such as:

- Why did we need such an expensive roofscape?
- Why did we need such an elaborate canopy drop-off?
- Why did we need glass on the curved portion of the building and continuous lintels rather than punched windows?
- Why did the interior garden have to be roofed at all? Wouldn't an open courtyard work just as well?
- Why did our parapets have to be so high and decorative in the linear accelerator area?
- Why did we have to have a brick cavity wall and not brick on stud wall construction?
- Why did our operable and fixed windows have to look alike and have zero sight lines?
- What did any of this have to do with cancer treatment?

What was of value to the client? The roofscape did matter, but it didn't have to be copper or standing seam metal. It was then detailed as high-profile shingles.

Given the published goals, the dialogue was eased but not easy. Nevertheless, the client was generally onboard and decided the following:

- The canopy did matter. It had to look substantial (not fabric). There was precedent at the hospital, but more importantly, cancer patients are often dropped off by others who then park elsewhere and have to find their way back. However, we could not use Aleucobond, the seamless metal we preferred.
- The curved glass did matter. The client agreed that this referenced the context, gave the building "no back doors," and led visually to the front door. By the way, the building sits in a sea of parking and is approached from three different sides.
- The interior garden and atrium did matter profoundly. After being initially criticized for pulling the building southward and reducing parking spaces, the garden grew to become the geographic, symbolic, and philosophical heart of the center (see Figures C–5 and C–6). All major circulation paths and axes relate to it.

There were some areas lacking consensus:

- The parapet height did not matter to the client. We were unable to convince them that lining soldier courses on the blank facade of the heavily shielded linear accelerator would successfully camouflage its massive wall.
- The brick cavity wall was a judgment of value left to our recommendation. We said we could not recommend a wall system criticized by the National Masonry Institute, so the cavity wall was built and we are watching it as its second winter approaches.
- The client did not initially understand our theory of windows (i. e., that fixed and operable should look the same), until we had actual samples on site to look over. Then they understood the "value" right away. But to keep the zero lot line, at the last minute we had to change from casement to pivot for cost reasons.

5. *Construction documents and administration:* How can one properly maintain a watchful eye on those targeted areas important to "value" and detail? How can one continue to make choices as shop drawings appear, as change orders arise, and alternate means and methods are suggested: flooring on the main floor, ceramic tile or VCT or pavers or carpet, pavers in the garden versus baumanite?

Once the architect and the owner have agreed on the design goals and the architect has struggled to realize these goals in the drawings and specifications, it is time to carry out and enhance these goals in the construction process.

Construction contracting methodologies vary tremendously in today's market. From construction management to lump sum open bidding to design/build, there are as many ways as there are contractors—every day there is a new wrinkle. Because of this myriad of possibilities, each with its own pitfalls, the architect plays the most important role in preserving design goals during construction.

Although different strategies may be employed to maintain and enhance the design goals under different contracting methodologies, there are a few principles that should apply in any scenario:

- The contractor/construction manager/subcontractor must know what the owners' and architects' design goals are from the start. These should be clearly articulated in the negotiation process and, if possible, incorporated into the documents or agreements. The contractor should be encouraged to offer suggestions on how better to achieve these goals.
- Choices are constantly required during construction. The architect must consistently and tirelessly evaluate these choices for the owner in light of the design goals. This is an ongoing process in solving such things as: evaluating substitutions, reviewing value engineering proposals, and adding discretionary "upgrades."
- The architect should be flexible in the construction process to allow the shifting of value from one part of the project to another. Often it is clear after the bids come in that "a little less of this would buy a lot more of that." The architect is in the best position to recognize and facilitate this type of value shifting so that the project's design goals may be better achieved. It often takes extra effort to overcome the criteria of owners

and contractors in order to achieve this type of flexibility. Important trades are made.
- The most significant way architects can maintain and enhance the design value of their projects during construction is to *stay involved*. Leaving decisions and choices in the hands of such people as owners, contractors, construction managers, and owner representatives is to remove the single most important voice in defending the project's design values.

6. *Postconstruction:* How does one keep communication open with clients who work and live in the spaces, and track how the important and "valuable" components of the concept and space are performing and enduring? We have already conducted the first two sessions of our year-one postoccupancy sessions, using a 12-point checklist that has been immensely useful. This list was inspired by the work in elderly housing of Sandra Howells 15 years ago.
- Sufficiency
- Accessibility
- Maintenance and maintainability
- Safety
- Security
- Adaptability
- Interactivity
- Aesthetics
- Personalization
- Operability
- Functional quality
- Other issues/action items

Conclusion

It is easy for a client to want the best of design, the best details and finishes, and the most inclusive program. But, ultimately, it is not that easy if all of these qualities cost a lot more than they expect. It is easy to want value, including good value in design (as in consumer products); but as in all other products and services, there must be a consensus on what constitutes a fair cost for better value.

At the same time, there has to be agreement between the client and the design professional on what is worth protecting. In the case I have described, there was a documented, up-front agreement on intentions. There were guidelines and a framework for discussions. There were early-phase site models for board and fund-raising presentations. There was a language for discussing the soft areas, the non–bottom-line areas, the "third entity" I mentioned earlier. In the months in which the center has been open, interesting enough, a "third entity" program director has been hired to run interdisciplinary programs. Volunteers have been actively involved in reception— a flower is often given to any incoming patient or visitor, as well as fresh fruit and cookies. There is talk of a tea cart in the garden. There is discussion of the fact that the patients would like the phones to be answered as Bennett Center, not Bennett Cancer Center, a subtle but important difference.

It is the design professional's responsibility to offer an intellectual and practical dialogue on higher values, to define them with and for clients, to track them throughout a project, and to be the first and last one on the project still referring back to those higher aspirations.

Unfortunately, there is very little room in this highly public process for Zeuslike thunderbolts. Gaining a client's trust and respect, especially in this highly regulated and multiheaded sector, is a process requiring faith, stamina, love, humor, imagination, and craftsmanship. I hope that this case study of a hospital-based ambulatory cancer center has recorded how some of the key milestones in defining, defending, and conveying design values were reached. The real recipients of whatever success we achieved are the cancer patients who visit this place 40 to 50 times over a few months, half of whom will not survive, half of whom will.

When we began the predesign phase, I met with a young woman as she was undergoing intravenous chemotherapy. She was sitting with a bandanna on her head in the existing long-term room with her husband and children, who were watching a movie on television. One of the clients said, "Here's the architect, tell her what you want." She pointed toward the window (a view of a brick wall) and said, "Give us something beautiful to look at and to focus on." I think we have, and I hope all who see it agree.

Barbara L. Geddis is principal of The Geddis Partnership, in Stamford, Connecticut. During the past 19 years, she has served as principal architect, master planner, and programmer for more than 200 projects in the United States, including a wide variety of nonprofit and private institutions, healthcare facilities, long-term care facilities, and college campuses.

◆

◆

◆

◆

◆ Chapter

FIVE

DESIGN TECHNOLOGIES

COLOR FOR HEALING

*First Symposium on
Healthcare Design,
Carlsbad, CA, 1988*

Antonio F. Torrice, ASID, IFDA

This discussion will be in four parts. The first part will be a quick "tour" of my background, designed to share the ideas and the plans that formed my education and, consequently, my career style. Mine is an unorthodox approach to healthcare design, justified by the fact that I believe we all have in our background the information and the tools needed to work as interior designers. The second part will provide the vocabulary necessary for approaching color in the healing setting. The third part will highlight some projects that illustrate what is happening in today's healthcare environments, point out areas in which we have yet to solve problems, and underscore the great potential of color as a design tool. Finally, I will mention some reading materials and design tools that can help us create more helpful well-being spaces.

Background

I was academically trained at Villanova University in Pennsylvania, where I majored in special education and child development. I can honestly tell you that, at that time, I never thought my education would be used for cleaning out closets to create puppet theaters and decorating bedrooms for children!

As I look back, I realize what tremendous training and opportunity I had to enable me to put together the worlds of child development, psychology, and interior design. These are actually very sympathetic partners. During an internship that was part of my training at Villanova University, I lived with 57 brain-damaged children in a foundation called Devereaux. Devereaux is a private, nonprofit organization that deals with behavioral problems in children of different ages. The unit, or school, I worked in was just north of Philadelphia, where children between the ages of 6 and 11 lived with an excellent staff. Older children lived in cottages away from the main house to learn to socialize with small groups of their peers.

Among my many jobs at Devereaux was to encourage children to talk about their feelings. Some of these children had been legally placed in Devereaux by the courts to protect them from parents who were abusive or counterproductive to the child's well-being. So these were angry children, damaged children, children who had a hard time talking about their fears and feelings. But they would talk very freely about things they didn't like. For example, "Why is the clock up there? I can't see the clock up there. That must be for you; that's not for me." Or, "I hate that color bedspread. That is the worst color bedspread I have ever seen." Or, "Where do my shoes go? He's got a place for his shoes. Where do my shoes go?" They would talk about their personal space, their immediate environment, the room that was their room or not their room. These were the things they volunteered freely. As a young psychologist, I began to make mental and real notes about these children and their environment. But I never thought I'd be designing rooms for them in a few years.

During that time, I also taught Montessori, worked with children two to five years of age, and read many books about the California methods of teaching—Montessori, special education, and free schools. Then I read a book by Sally Raspberry, who taught in an apple orchard somewhere near

San Francisco, and I decided I wanted to meet her. In 1973 I joined my colleagues in the "covered wagons" that moved to the West and met them all in San Francisco in the unemployment line! There were too many of us for too few jobs. To make a living, I did whatever kind of work came about—a waiter in a restaurant, a busboy, and finally a stockboy for a store called Design Research.

Design Research began in Boston's Harvard Square, bringing to America the Scandinavian design concept "form follows function." Not only were the store's coffee mugs beautiful and colorful, but they also stacked very neatly and were dishwasher proof. This design concept was also applied to fabrics with bold, bright colors and to modular furniture that stacked, evolved, and converted into other things.

My job as a stockboy at Design Research was helping the display lady move her ladder around and unbox things for her. On occasion, she would ask me to display mugs in certain places. Later, she noticed that sales would go up wherever I placed the red mugs and that they sold faster than the blue mugs. Why did this happen? I told her that I knew about color therapy and occasionally used that knowledge in creating displays. I knew that people were drawn to certain colors, but I wondered if this applied to the items in the store. I tried arranging the silk blouses a certain way and it increased sales. "How about pots and pans?" I wondered. Rearranging the pots and pans display also increased sales. Within three years I was named national codirector of display for all nine Design Research stores, which included designing and displaying merchandise for each store using color as a seasonal selling tool. I did all this for $3.25 per hour. Freelancing was decidedly the answer!

In 1975, I went into downtown San Francisco and began to go into shops I was attracted to. I proposed to each store's management that I would rearrange their display windows for no fee if I received a 10 percent commission for all goods sold out of the window. They agreed, and I did very well that Christmas! It didn't matter what kind of store it was—the Nature Company, Roots Shoes, or Just Desserts. It didn't matter what kind of merchandise it sold—pots and pans on Mondays, silk blouses on Tuesdays, jewelry on Wednesdays. People were drawn to color and light. It brought them into the stores and, I hoped, would inspire them to make a purchase.

One of the stores I began working for was Lenore Linens. Located in San Francisco for many years, they sold bed, bath, and table linens to the design trade. I had created a very successful showroom for them. When a decorator's show house committee toured the city looking for new designers and sponsors, they saw the showroom and asked the shop owner if he would like to participate in the show house. He would. I would. We did! So on a Sunday afternoon in early January 1979, I went from being a display artist to a decorator.

To begin the project, I went to the show house where I found many trained designers bidding to design 35 rooms. I picked my favorite room and, in 25 words or less, described what I wanted to do with it. I picked a second choice room and a third choice room in case my favorite was given to someone else. Then I went home to wait by the phone. Sure enough, the phone rang. I was told that I had received not one, but all three rooms. The shop owner was delighted. I told him that I was going to do what I do the very best: design a room for children. I also told him I wanted to use his six-year-old daughter, Allison, as my client. The shop owner was unsure about whether children and decorators' show houses went together or whether anyone would spend money to decorate children's rooms, but he agreed to let me try it.

I went back home and pulled out all of my psychology tools—eye-hand coordination games and colored cards—then went to the show house with Allison. I sat down in the three-room suite with her and said, "Allison, if you could live in this room, what would it look like?" What ensued was a wonderful project called "Suite Allison." The remarkable experience for both Allison and me was the fact that it was her room and the people who saw it realized that her input was evident everywhere.

One of the wonderful things about decorator show houses is that consumer magazines use them to focus on design talent. *Better Homes and Gardens* saw my work and asked me to become a designer of children's rooms for several of its publications. It was an exciting adventure to work with props and sets and build wonderful rooms for children that evolved around their needs, through their eyes, through their perception. As a result, many, many letters addressed to me poured into the magazine's office. Interesting enough, for every ten letters received, six were from handicapped children's parents. They asked questions like, "Do blind children perceive color? My child is blind." I was back where I began, returning once again to psychology in a rather unique, new way—designing spaces for special children.

In 1979, I created a company called Just Between Friends to work with these special children. The company consisted of 37 wonderful people, who built rooms for and with children. Since then the business has grown to include building rooms for adults with handicaps, senior citizens, and now, quite to my delight, the homeless around the country.

These special-need groups have been overlooked. It's amazing to me that 23,000 interior designers alone make their living as part of the American Society of Interior Designers (ASID). Yet their clientele includes only five percent of the U.S. population. Where is the remaining 95 percent? Where are those who not only want us, but need us—the children, the handicapped, those in healthcare facilities?

Then, a bolt of lightning came out of the sky and changed everything I had been trying to accomplish. I had been knocking on the doors of hospitals, day-care centers, and senior citizen centers offering my design services. Unfortunately, my knock fell on deaf ears. Then in 1985, ASID singled out my work to receive their "Oscar," the Human Environment Award. From that moment on, everything changed. Hospitals called me back. And once again, I entered a field that opened up tremendous potential for those who are needy—the field of healthcare pediatric design.

Rooms for Special Needs: The Three 'Cs'

The following examples depict the results of my efforts and the results of the work of many people around the country. I am very pleased to discuss them as part of an ongoing effort to communicate the great tool that color can be in our lives.

In building rooms for people with special needs, I consider three "Cs": choice, color, and convertibility. It's very important that choice come first. When I build rooms for those with special needs, especially children, parents often ask me to build the room that they never had. Mom wants a canopy bed with a Laura Ashley bedspread and matching wallpaper. Dad wants basketball wallpaper and a racing-car bed. A noble thought, to say the least, but often not what the child wants. In fact, when children are upset by the room mom and dad create for them, they may tear it apart to show how upset they are. Ever wonder why a child's room is never neat? Perhaps it's because it's not the child's room—it's mom's or dad's room.

When I create a child's room, I play a very simple game. I open up a large brown paper bag or get a piece of white art paper and lay it flat on the floor. Using only a black or brown crayon or marker, I simply draw a bird's-eye view of the room on the paper—a floor plan.

At this point, I have already met with the child's parents and made a list of things that they and the little one and I have agreed will go in the room including areas for sleep, study, storage, laundry, toys, and sleep-over friends. Item by item, I go through the list and ask the little one, eye-to-eye, questions like, "Where do you sleep in this room? In the corner? By the window? Next to the door?" Wherever the child points to on the paper, I write down the word for that activity. I put a word in every place in the room; so every place has a word.

During a second interview, I ask more detailed questions such as, "Describe that sleep area to me. Is it high? Is it low? Oh, it's a bunk bed. Who sleeps on top? Who sleeps on the bottom?" I'm working with form and shape now. As the questions evolve, so does the master plan of what the child perceives as his or her personal space.

This also is true for adults. We all have our own creature needs, particularly people in hospitals. Those same needs exist as you move into treatment centers—the need for comfort, the need for curling into a fetal position, the need for texture, color, light, and fresh air. In fact, we build better zoos for animals than we do healthcare facilities for the sick. We give zoo animals fresh air; we give them water; and we give them a natural habitat. We don't even do that for our senior citizens.

I then take these sketches home and prepare a portfolio for the child's parents. Each portfolio cover is a different color, the colors of the spectrum: red, orange, yellow, green, blue, and violet. As an example, I have brought a young boy's portfolio that I'd like to describe to you. Inside the portfolio is a blow-by-blow description of the boy's room. There are areas for music, dance, art, tea parties. There is a description of what happens in each area, how it works, and where problems might arise. There are research reports on color and light and their scientific background. There are also brochures and mail-order catalogs so the parents can purchase merchandise that might very well outfit the room if, in fact, the parents want to create the room themselves. There are paint chips chosen by the little one in the color interview, some color cards, and of course the most important element: the sketches.

There are two identical sets of sketches in each portfolio. Mom and dad get their own set on which they can make changes, notes, and additions. The little one gets a set, too. It's our contract, a paper relationship that takes their ideas and makes them real. The sketches are like coloring book drawings—they are bold, black and white pictures of the child's room that turn a dream into reality.

Let's take my friend Michael, for instance. When Michael was three-and-a-half, his parents invited us to work with him. Michael had a hearing problem and a speech problem, and he rarely talked. He had become very shy. Michael's mother was pregnant with her second child and feared that when the child was born, Michael might feel pushed out of the family circle.

When Michael and I first met, he began designing his own room nonverbally, describing in a crayon drawing how his room was to be laid out. He striped the walls from the bottom to the top in gradations of width. He created a desk area that was a formation of adjustable ladders. He turned his closet into a puppet theater. Now why would a boy who doesn't talk want a puppet theater in his room? Because it was the only place where he would talk. He would get inside the closet and tell me where he wanted his desk and his chair. This was his place to be heard and not seen.

On the other side of Michael's room, he expanded the stripes into a rounded arch to sleep under—an arch that resembled the soft, round ribbons of a rainbow. There were soft bathmats on the floor and some living things in the room as well. These items are "signatures," ideas that make this room Michael's room. They cost no more to purchase, but they create ten times the positive effect.

Color as Light

The second "C" I use is color, and I will explore what that is. I am not going to talk about the "summer, fall, winter, spring" theory. I am not going to talk about the "mauving of America." These are pigment theories. Red paint and yellow paint put together bond; the molecules mix and become a third color—in this case, orange.

There's another way that color works in our lives that is much different: color as light. Red light and yellow light put together do not create orange light. They each move, as sound does, in wavelengths—one color at one speed, another color at another speed—to create the visible spectrum. We know this is true from our friend Sir Isaac Newton. He taught us that if you take a prism and beam white light at it, the prism will bend the light, fanning it out into red, orange, yellow, green, blue, indigo, and violet colors—the invisible spectrum.

We know that the body receives light in two ways. One is through the retina of the eye. Artificial or natural light bounces off the back of the eye and, through a series of reactions, to the brain to give us color cues. We know that color appears different to people who are blind, who have cataracts, who wear contact lenses, eyeglasses, or sunglasses. We know that color appears different when the light coming into the eye is altered, and that light affects human physiology as well as psychology.

Another way color affects us is how our skin receives light. Our skin works very much the same way a prism does. When light hits our skin, the light bends. As it bends, it fans out into the visible spectrum of red, orange, yellow, green, blue, and violet.

Some research suggests that light wavelengths pass through tissue matter and are absorbed into sympathetic tissue matter throughout the body. This information was first made known to me in a book I read as an intern by a gentleman named Semyon Kirlian. In the 1930s, Kirlian and his wife, Valentina, were electronic technicians in Moscow. They were often asked to repair equipment used in electrical therapy. While repairing this equipment, Kirlian was fascinated by the way that electrical therapy worked: An electrode would be placed on the flesh of the patient, a switch would be thrown, and a spark would go off. That spark intrigued Kirlian. Because his hobby was photography, he took a photographic plate with him one time when he was asked to make repairs. He held it very carefully under the electrode, put his hand on the switch, and threw the switch. In the process, however, he burned his hand. That burn changed the focal point of his entire career. What he had done was photograph his hand at the moment it was absorbing electricity. What appeared on the photographic plate were colors emanating from his fingertips. He became excited about what he saw and began photographing many other phenomena.

The colors captured in Kirlian photographs (See Figure C–7) *are* exciting! The tip of an index finger just pricked by a needle and photographed appears pink around the damaged tissue matter and blue-white around the healthy tissue matter. Blue-white appears around the cold part of kitten's paw cooled by an ice cube. A photograph of a solid gold earring shows where the finger of the photographer first touched it: The area is pink with turquoise around it.

Perhaps one of the most world-renowned photographs, taken in Southern California by Dr. Thelma Moss, is called "Phantom Leaf." It shows the leaf of a geranium plant photographed while electricity was passing through it. The image appears to have a "corona discharge," a white ring of electromagnetic energy, on the rim. Dr. Moss also photographed the same leaf after cutting off the leaf tip. The image of the entire leaf appeared in the photograph; but the missing piece appeared pink, as do the missing limbs of victims who have lost an arm or a leg.

What is being captured in Kirlian photographs? To be honest, we don't know. The Kirlian equipment is too primitive, and what is known about it is pretty much confined to Europe. Europeans have been way ahead of us on this matter.

In 1967, the Pentagon began using the Kirlian method to photograph Vietnam soldiers before and after battle. The same method was used on the Washington Redskins football team before a big game to help identify stress.

The information that resulted from each test was inconclusive. What did trigger my interest, however, were the results of the same research used on those who were handicapped. When light is absorbed into the body of a healthy person, it appears in Kirlian photographs as the following colors:

- Red appears around the hip area, the base of the spine, and the sexual organs. Red is the most highly energizing color because it increases the heart rate and the respiration rate and encourages motor activity.
- Orange appears in the liver and spleen area and near the circulatory system. All body fluids, plus the lymph system and the nervous system, are affected. Orange has a very tonic effect.
- Yellow appears in the areas of the heart, lungs, and respiratory system.
- Green appears in the throat area, the area where vocal skills originate.
- Blue appears around the eyes, ears, and nose—the sensory areas of sight, sound, and smell.
- Purple appears around the cerebral cortex, the top of the head, the brain, representing nonverbal activity and the thought process.

In Kirlian photographs of healthy individuals, the spectrum appears to run up the spine from the bottom to the top, in that order. But when the method is used to photograph handicapped individuals, light does not seem able to enter an area where a disease or dysfunction is located. In a person who has liver cancer, no orange appears in the Kirlian photograph of that patient. In a person who has a speech problem, no green appears in the Kirlian photograph of that patient. In a person who is deaf or blind, no blue appears. I felt this observation merited further exploration.

The Color Card Game

After studying Kirlian photography, I developed a "game" to help design rooms for my special children. I created six colored cards—red, orange, yellow, green, blue, and violet—on glossy paper that reflected light. Then I simply asked the children to choose a card. I did not ask them what color was their favorite, connoting a right or wrong answer. I did not ask them what color they wanted their bedroom painted—again, connoting a right or wrong answer. I simply asked them to choose a card. In every situation involving handicapped children, they chose the color card that corresponded to their damaged body part. The deaf child chose a blue card. The child with a speech problem chose a green card.

This game helped me to design Michael's room. Michael had a speech problem. He had stopped talking. He had withdrawn. He chose a green card (throat area) and an orange card (circulation). I then gave him a green and an orange crayon and the black and white room sketch and asked him to place these colors wherever he wanted. Whether on the bedspread, carpet, or walls, wherever he put the color was fine. When he was finished coloring with those two crayons, I took them away and gave him the balance of the crayon box minus those two crayons to finish the sketch. Even at three-and-a-half years of age, Michael had graduated the stripes in the walls in shades of orange from light at the bottom to dark at the top. This is a "signature." He had ignored the area rugs, each of which I thought he would make a different color, and colored the entire floor green. The combination of his not talking and his wanting to crawl around on the floor, plus the fact that green was his favorite color, plainly meant green wall-to-wall carpeting. When Michael was finished with the green and orange crayons, his mother asked him to decide what colors would go in the rest of the room. He very spontaneously grabbed a color other than orange or green; he chose the "nonverbal" purple to color his entire closet.

Color and light are powerful tools that can open us up physiologically and psychologically. Michael is now 11 years old. He writes beautiful poetry. He speaks proper, fully projected English and has an IQ of 116. He could have been considered a retarded child. Of course, his parents' love, his diet, and the school system in which he was placed were factors in his development. But so was the room where he spent the first seven years of his life.

Color Choice and "Volume"

There are other colors besides the primaries. Black is the absence of all light—therefore the absence of all color in light. It is not a recommended color for a living environment, but it's very good for creating a dramatic effect in museums and theaters and for highly stylized spaces as seen in magazines. White is the opposite; it's the presence of all light—therefore, the presence of all color in light. If a designer is afraid to use a color for some reason, white is the safest choice—particularly if there are lots of people sharing the space and the designer is afraid of overwhelming them on one level or another. The earth tones—browns, grays, and animal colors such as fawn, squirrel, and dove—do what they purport to do: They ground people. They level people off. They don't elevate; they don't slow people down. That's why these colors are often used in offices; they keep people away from the water fountain and coffee machine. I suggest that a little pink and yellow might increase productivity in the workplace.

Choosing color is like choosing a radio station. For example, rock-and-roll music might be red, classical music might be blue, and something in the middle, like country and western, might be green. The intensity of the color might represent the loudness of the music. Even though I may choose rock-and-roll, it may not be very loud. So it is with color. When a child picks a color, I go to the paint store and pick up 10 to 15 shades of that color. Then the child can tell me how "loud" the color "volume" should be.

A Personal Kirlian Photograph

Because I became so interested in Kirlian photography, I wanted to photograph my own body under different conditions. I asked a doctor who had the apparatus if I could use it for my research. I went to his office and sat in front of an open window. There was no filtered light in the room, only the light of the sun on my face. Then I wrapped my head in different color cellophanes so that only those colors would come into my eyes. For instance, I wrapped red cellophane around my head so only red light entered my eyes. Then I photographed my finger on the apparatus. The image showed a red corona discharge around the tip of my finger; this meant that a high wavelength of light was evidently running through my body on the red end of the spectrum. The joint in my finger showed a blue-white corona discharge; in a healthy person whose spectral colors are balanced and properly absorbed, the color shown would be white.

Then I took off the red gel and wrapped a green gel around my head. Less than 30 seconds passed between photographs. Yet in the second picture of my finger, the color blue was more predominant in the corona discharge and the color red was less so. My heart rate also slowed down, as did my respiration rate. The green gel was calming me down.

I quickly took the green gel off and wrapped the blue gel around my head, thinking that blue might be the best color for me. In fact, it was. There was an almost completely white corona discharge around my finger in the photo. I had evidently balanced my "body prism."

Natural Light Simulation

When we are surrounded by natural outdoor light, there's an equal balance of each of the colors of the spectrum in our bodies. Under fluorescent light, this balance is tremendously distorted. A cool-white fluorescence gives off a preponderance of yellow and orange color as it bounces throughout the environment, distorting the colors we perceive under natural light. A warm-white fluorescence is even more distorting; in fact, yellow and orange go right off the chart.

Today, there are many full-spectrum light bulbs on the market. They seem to come closest to simulating the effects of natural light. We can make tremendous changes in people's environments by using technology that re-creates nature.

An object will appear different under different sources of artificial light. Under a full-spectrum light bulb, a vase will appear the way we expect to see it in sunlight. But under a fluorescent light, the vase will appear a little more yellow, as will carpets, wall coverings, furnishings, and window treatments in healthcare (and other) spaces.

Whenever reading research on color, one should always ask one important question: Under what quality of light was the research done? There's been talk about the "pink cell" and how it affected violent prisoners. Under different qualities of light, however, the responses of those prisoners changed. Always ask the question, how are color and light related in this research?

Sexually Determined Color Preference

I find no sexual differentiation between the color choices of boys and girls. Boys don't pick certain colors and girls pick other colors. We do know that when babies are born, they see contrast: black, white, and gray. They very quickly memorize the placement of the eyes, nose, and mouth on a face as dots or dark spots in a neutral field. It's that memorization that reminds babies who they are looking at.

Within a few days, babies see their first color—the color red. It stands to reason that if you put a boy into a blue nursery and a girl into a pink nursery, the girl will see pink long before the boy sees blue. She will reach out for the color, more quickly developing eye-hand coordination.

Color Intensity

There are no sexually determined color preferences; but there are developmental preferences that we, as human animals, must keep in mind when specifying colors. I find that the more severe a person's handicap, the louder the "volume" of that person's color choice. A very profoundly deaf child will choose a very intense color; a mildly hearing-impaired child will choose a soft version of that same color. For instance, Michael's room is a very "loud" orange because he had a very dramatic need for it. Orange is also one of his favorite colors to wear.

Scott is another young friend for whom color volume was important. Scott was just 12 years old when he became the subject of my second decorator show house project. After interviewing 37 boys and girls, I chose Scott because he was very special. He had been profoundly deaf since birth. His parents very early wanted him to learn more than sign language; they also wanted him to learn to read lips.

I began working with Scott by bringing him into the room I had chosen to design and asking him what the room would look like if he lived there. The room ended up being blue—deep blue. The color blue represents the eyes, ears, and nose—eyes that watch lips in order to communicate when ears can't hear words. Scott's room has many surfaces that help multiply the effect of the blue color he chose. The walls he faces as he works allow natural light to come into his body through reflection and windows. Color was also used as an organizational tool on the stacking, storage furniture that surrounds the room; blue tells him where his clothes are, yellow his toys, green his school supplies.

Color in the Healthcare Environment

Today we are focusing on the healthcare design professional. Great things have been happening in the past two years, and great things are yet to be done. The call to arms is here. There are some people and associations I would like to acknowledge, whose efforts as role models in the industry are remarkable. They include the Association for the Care of Children's Health, Hansen Lind Meyer, Anshen + Allen, The Ritchie Organization, Ellerbe Becket, Thompson Design Associates, Texas Scottish Rite Hospital, Leo A. Daley, NASA, Langdom Wilson Mumper, the HMC Architects, and Living & Learning Environments. These are truly some of the best in the country.

Anshen + Allen created the "art cart"—a cart containing nicely framed pictures of Bruce Springsteen, Madonna, kittens, whales, puppies, and Monet reproductions. The cart can be rolled into a hospital room so that children can choose two or three prints to put on the wall near the bed to give them the feeling of being "in my room."

In the Children's Hospital in Philadelphia, you will see a nest, or pod, on each floor that allows children to leave the wing without leaving the floor. They are well-lighted, colorful play spaces with wonderful views from up high. In the interior lobby of the hospital, children can enjoy themselves surrounded by water fountains, animals, birds, fish, and interesting sculpture.

In some of the projects from the Kaiser Group of California, the complexion of reception areas is changing. These are the first areas in a ward a child sees. Note how the colors are more muted, softer, and more enveloping; they are not aggressive or abrasive. They seem to say, "Come on in and get comfortable." Today's reception areas are becoming more hospitable, as they should be in a hospital. They're becoming more like lobbies in hotels, with colors that are calming and nurturing.

Hospital hallways where there are no windows now have good lighting. There are color contrasts of light against dark. Nothing is worse for a senior citizen than trying to find a railing that is the same color as the wall; they can't see it, just as they can't see a bedspread that matches the carpet when they try to sit on the bed.

It has never been more true that "from whence you came, you shall return" than in designing environments for children and seniors. Treatment rooms should be soft and color reflective. Their colors should complement skin tones—warm, nurturing flesh tones. Not bloody tones or aggressive tones, but soft, enveloping tones.

The work of Mary Jean Thompson of Nevada brings a homelike atmosphere to medical facilities through the use of texture and color. In one example, the eye focuses on blue when one is feeling blue, on pink when one is feeling "in the pink," and on yellow when one is afraid. In addition her use of wood, natural textures, light, and greenery helps bring the outdoors inside.

The Memorial Hospital of Rhode Island uses a lot of color and light interplay and is palatial looking. Splashes and bold statements of color allow people to transcend the hospital environment, leaving behind sadness and sickness and bringing them into a place that is uplifting and encouraging. Hallways and reflective surfaces also bring in light where sunlight cannot be found.

Floor color is another way that color can be used in new and imaginative ways. Red may lead to one area of the hospital, yellow to another, blue to another, and green to still another. Each color, because it is placed low on the floor where children can see it, visually directs them to where they want to go.

Wall murals and art are very important in supplying color to very specific healthcare environments. And color should be used on the ceiling, as well, so the end-user, the patient, can see it on the way to surgery or in the recovery room. This improves greatly over bright fluorescent lights that shine in a patient's eyes.

In the numerous centers across the country that treat children with drug and alcohol dependencies, children are surrounded by earth tones. These colors calm them and bring them back to earth.

Color is beginning to be recognized for its importance in pediatric ward playrooms. In Children's Hospital of San Francisco, there is a playroom with areas of red, orange, yellow, green, blue, and violet. Each area encourages a different activity—red for motor skills, orange for eye-hand coordination, yellow for the chest area, green for voice/communication, blue for the eyes, ears, and nose, and purple for fantasy play. Also included in the playroom is a miniature kitchen that resembles a home kitchen. It even has a real refrigerator and a stove with handles that move. Added to this playroom is a solarium that won the 1987 Halo Lighting Award (see Figure C–8).

Color and the Space Program

Outer space is the future of design. In outer space, research is now being done on color. The results are going to affect the way we use color in design on earth (see Figure C–9). What man sees in outer space is actually negative space—nothing. It's black, and the eye must constantly strain to find something to focus on; this creates great eye fatigue and muscle tension. This gives us some healthcare design clues. Rather than allow someone to sit in front of computer screens of a single color, how can we help prevent fatigue and tension with color and light?

Our key contact with outer space is the space shuttle, which is an enormous design challenge for professionals in the healthcare field and every other profession. In outer space, we need to be concerned about the shuttle passing by the sun every 90 minutes. This means people in the shuttle experience 16 sunrises and 16 sunsets every day. Research done in space will help us find answers to the problem of how to provide patients with a sense of time when they have no point of reference. The interior of these shuttles must become hospitable for the 20, 60, or 90 days they are in space. What happens to man in such an environment? Are Kubrick, Spielberg, and Lucas all correct in presenting outer space in black, chrome, and gray? Or should the green of trees or the blue of water and sky go into outer space with man? We must decide this. We are discovering that the effects of color on man in these facilities are very remarkable.

If one were to see a natural shot of our last space mission taken by NASA, you would note that the interior of the capsule is predominantly blue. Blue is a most appropriate color, representing the eyes, ears, and nose, and the release of strain and tension.

In an artist's rendering of Project Galileo, each of the modules holds two to four people in a space about the size of a trailer or railroad car. The modules are supplied by power from solar disks that collect light from the sun and store it. Like an apple from a tree, the disks are plucked from a storage station, shuttled to the space station, and plugged in.

Before I close, I would like to recommend several books. They include *Health and Light* and *Light, Radiation, and You* by Dr. John Ott—books that discuss the reaction of the human body to smoke detectors, digital watches, lead pencils, and other everyday items that prevent absorption of light—and *Color and Light in Man-made Environments* by Drs. Frank and Rudolf Mahnke, which discusses color selection for hospital wards, pediatric centers, and nursing homes.

The late Antonio F. Torrice, ASID, IFDA, was a designer/author/lecturer who devoted his career to serving as an advocate for children, the physically challenged, and the homeless. The co-author of In My Room: Designing for and with Children *(Ballantine Books, 1989), he was honored in President George Bush's "Points of Light" program.*

◆ ◆ ◆

BEYOND SILENCE: MUSIC AS ENVIRONMENTAL DESIGN

Fifth Symposium on Healthcare Design, San Diego, CA, 1992

Susan Mazer
Dallas Smith

Note from the Authors: When one considers the experience of healthcare consumers as they utilize the facilities in which healthcare is delivered, the questions that need to be addressed are ones pertaining directly to the reality of the experience, in contrast to the intentions or objectives stated by the institutions. The waiting areas (patient and family holding areas, including patient rooms) represent the place where accumulated tension and anxiety define patient care. Thus, this presentation was set up to introduce this issue by allowing the participants to have an analogous experience. This was done through a performance of 180 seconds of anticipatory silence without prior notice.

Other portions of this presentation that were experiential and do not translate easily into written form have been replaced with an overview of their intention.

Smith: (after 180 seconds of silence) The first piece we performed was titled "Healthcare Waiting Areas: 1993." How did the silence make you feel? In nature, there is no such thing as a pure vacuum. In healthcare facility waiting areas, as well, there is no such thing as pure silence. During those

180 seconds of "silence," there were still sounds in this room: the door in the back opening and closing, waiters rattling dishes, the noise of the ventilation system, and the sound of people breathing. You were wondering, perhaps, what was going on? Did *I* do something wrong? When are *they* going to tell me what to do? Do *they* know what they are doing?

This is how most people may experience time spent waiting in a healthcare facility. However, in this case, there were only 180 seconds—three minutes—of uncertainty. How much longer must one wait for information or an explanation in a medical crisis? What kind of environment must a waiting area be to be comforting? The discomfort of uncertain silence, of not knowing what our rights are, of not knowing whether we can even ask, often continues throughout the healthcare experience. With the addition of beepers, buzzers, overhead paging, computer printers; the sounds of suffering, laughing, crying, inappropriate conversation; and the 24-hour rock station on the radio at the nurse station, the sounds of the environment are often much worse than "silence."

There are any number of elements in the sound environment that can violate the best physical design.

In this presentation, we are going to continue the conversation about creating healing environments. Our focus is the aural environment. All of us have just experienced silence for 180 seconds. It was a rather innocent silence, because we are not here because we are in pain, suffering any trauma, or under the influence of medication—all of which can distort time and make minutes seem like hours.

We see the environment functioning as the context for the delivery of healthcare services. All too often, that environment runs counter to the purpose of healthcare; counter to the intention of the services that are being delivered by various specialists and highly trained individuals. *Whose environment is it?* Who is ultimately accountable for the quality of this space and its impact? *If the environment is not healing,* what is it? Once the facility is built and the patients, families, and staff have arrived, the responsibility for the quality, both visible and nonvisible, may easily be put on the designer. Often, we have heard the comment, "Well, that is just how hospitals sound. There is nothing that can be done." In regard to the sound environment, perhaps unlike other physical components, each individual, each event, each conversation, each cry of pain, becomes part of the space.

It may be true that nothing can be done about some elements required in the hospital. However, there is much that can be done to affect the totality of the environment. The total healing environment cannot be realized by isolated individuals. There must be an institutionwide shift of consciousness so that the people who are in the facilities every day keep the healing environment in place.

Mazer: When we present workshops on music as environmental design, questions concerning the economic justification for this program do arise. What is clear is that the sound environment is a fact; it exists whether or not we deal with it intentionally. Thus, a price is being paid for the unintentional, perhaps untended sound environment, in the form of institutionally generated stress, pain, anxiety, and accompanying symptoms. Institutionally generated symptoms are seldom addressed. However, we know that human beings experience stress, fear, and anxiety, especially in situations where they have limited control. The increased stress can affect the recovery process. Silence in an institution is an illusion; it is relative to various other sounds; and it is not neutral or absolute. Silence has its own quality and can be shifted. In the middle of the night when the lights are out and patients are alone, the aural design of the institution is still working. Our goal is to address the sound environment from the human experience of being a caregiver and also a patient.

More Than Just Opinion

The auditory reflex gives us information about when a sound occurs, what that sound is, and where it is located. Once we recognize the sound, we then bring meaning to it. In fact, a neurological synthesis occurs in which the brain puts together what we see with what we hear. When we are only hearing, without the sense of sight, our hearing ability is intensified. Thus, the impact of the sound and our efforts to bring meaning to it are mutually increased.

Music—organized sound—has meaning beyond itself. We, as individuals, connect who we are, what has happened to us, what is currently happening to us, and how we feel with music that is playing. Music is cultural, historical, and personal. It has been a major indicator of social and political mores for as long as it has been recorded. Thus, opinions about music are opinions about who we are in relation to our past and present.

When people talk about music, the conversations that usually result are centered around opinions. People say, "I like country and western music." Or, "This is the song we played on our first date." Or they say, "This is the song I remember my mother playing for me." Music produces strong opinions that are based on past experiences. It creates boundaries and defines generations. Music is a statement of cultural identity and represents both the parts of our history that we would like to access and the parts we would like to forget.

What can be done in healthcare facilities to access those opinions and histories to create another type of experience? As Dallas mentioned, we found that when we first approached healthcare facilities about improving their environmental sounds, we heard the words, "But, this is what a hospital sounds like." Administrators told us, "Your music could be too loud. How could you perform live music, especially with the amount of equipment you require?" So we decided we had to do an intervention in the institution. If we were going to transform the healthcare environment, we had to get the staff to believe and know that it could be different—to move from a stand of "impossibility" to one of "possibility."

We developed a music-in-residence program for Washoe Medical Center in Reno, Nevada, to serve as an environmental intervention. We organized it so that we were positioned on a particular unit for up to eight hours. It was the most difficult engagement that we ever booked ourselves into—long hours, with insufficient lighting and staging. We did not know what was going to happen. We had to convince the nursing staff through this "experiment" that the environment could be different due to music.

In oncology, we had logistical problems in locating an appropriate place to perform due to the physical equipment and the sound level. The nurses, wanting this to work, made many voluntary concessions regarding the volume and placement. I was very concerned that when we started to play, the music would be an unwelcome distraction. The nurses not only did not complain, but they made whatever adjustments they needed to in order for our "experiment" to work in this unit.

After we had played for about four hours, the nurses reported that patients who had been on morphine every hour and a half had not asked for medication in more than three hours. They also noticed that some of the patients who were having chemotherapy treatments had requested to be hooked up to the IVs and wheeled out to the hall to listen to the music. At about 7 P.M., after we had been there for six hours, Dallas gave, on request, one of the most astonishing renditions of "Misty" I have ever heard him play.

The nurse manager said that she noticed her staff was far less stressed than usual. Staff members then started talking among themselves and realized that the environment could be different. Thus, in order to bring music into a healthcare facility, environmental design has to be redefined for staff members so they realize they need something different, and know it to be possible. In addition to the oncology unit, this program was offered in rehab, dialysis, admitting, neurology, med-surg, and emergency. In all situations, the staff and patients experienced a significant change in how they and their unit functioned.

The workshop we have developed, "Music: A Life-Altering Decision," is an eight-hour CEU-accredited program for nurses and CME-accredited program for physicians as an experiential workshop. It includes empirical information about the research that has been done on the relationship between music and medicine. Our goal is to give the staff an opportunity to identify environmental components that are changeable, the impact those elements have on both staff stress and patient outcomes, and the possible strategies for the ongoing creation of a healing environment. Although our main focus is the aural component, we address all variables. The workshop deals with opinion and personal history, because all participants have opinions that function strongly in how they relate to where they are and what is happening to them.

We have learned that if the staff and administration do not understand the issue of aural space and its impact on patient care, the use of music is very limited and the negative impact of the existing sound environment is ignored. We have also found that, in terms of the elements of design, the sound environment is a living, organic, dynamic component. It is changing from moment to moment.

I am sure that if we went back and looked at how each of you processed the three minutes of silence with which we began this presentation, we would see some interesting things. During the "performance" we did specific things, such as getting ready to play our instruments and then not playing, fussing with music, and so on. Such silence, without explanation, is occurring when the patient has few felt rights to ask questions, and at a time when he or she has intensified anxiety by virtue of his or her reason for being in a hospital. Such a silence is not neutral. The confusion, tension, frustration, and any other feelings that you felt are similar to the feelings experienced by patients and families when they enter waiting areas or the emergency room. They are greeted by a receptionist, and they wait, and wait, and receive little information.

We emphasize to hospitals that waiting time needs to be a proactive time for caregivers and patients. They are either going to be better or worse off for having to wait. They will seldom be the same after four hours of waiting, compared with when they first came in.

Smith: If there is a visual environment that is displeasing, one can close one's eyes. However, it is very difficult to shut out the sound environment. In fact, closing one's eyes can make one even more sensitive to the sound environment.

Mazer: One of the issues we deal with in terms of healthcare design is time management, but not in terms of administrative productivity and all that has been associated with it. We speak now of all the minutes and hours during which a patient lies in the hospital while the protocol is working. More hours pass with the patient being unattended than attended. The experience of time is negotiable. It is perceived and experienced differently, depending on who we are, what type of environment we are in, and the types of relationships that are exhibited around us. Given the opportunity and capacity to alter time as experienced by the inpatient, we become responsible for that part of patient care.

A Sampling of Research

For some of our work, we have had to review the research on music and medicine. At one point, we thought about putting our music aside and doing research ourselves. But it would have been research that told people what they already intuitively know. We did not believe this was our mission. Then we had the good fortune to speak with Dr. Clifford Madsen, a noted music therapist at Florida State University in Tallahassee, Florida. It became clear that the Center for Music Research and similar organizations and individuals are doing substantial research in the field of music as it relates to medicine. The issue of implementation, however, remains the challenge.

Through Dr. Madsen, we were able to access a meta-analysis, prepared by Dr. Jayne Standley, also of Florida State University. She reviewed the major research on music and medicine and compiled a summation of 30 relevant studies, selected from 80 documented studies. Studies were reviewed and eliminated for the meta-analysis based on certain criteria, including the credibility of the clinical setting. Studies utilizing artificially induced pain or anxiety were not included.

The research implied several conclusions: (1) women respond to music with somewhat greater effect than men; (2) it was also noted that the Effect Size was greater (Since a great deal of research has been done in labor and delivery, this obviously influenced this conclusion. Because childbirth is limited to women, that statistic will probably remain out of proportion. As mentioned, the number of female participants in the study definitely affected the results of that study.); (3) music has greater measurable effect when there is some pain present; (4) music has been shown to enhance the impact of an analgesic and is also better than just the analgesic or anxiolytic by itself. Obviously, greater or lesser degrees of wellness are harder to measure than moving from conditions of pain and anxiety to a neutral state. The use of music as a protocol, as opposed to entertainment, is measured in the same way as any other protocol—that is, when a change in the condition is evidenced or reported; and (5) the most conservative measure of music's effect is the patient self-report, followed by physiological measures and observational measures.

I know few patients who will say that they feel worse than they actually do, but many will not say how bad they feel. This is especially true when the method of dealing with pain involves more pain, or when pain can indicate the procedure that most frightens the patient. A dramatic measure of music's effect was obtained in a study of noradrenaline levels, secreted when anxiety is experienced, as measured in pre- and posttests. Results were more dramatic when live music was presented by a trained music therapist. I do not know what kind of recorded music was listened to, and I do not know who the music therapist was. The study indicated that live music has more impact than recorded music. That may be debated and depends on the quality of either. Fortunately, modern technology has finally allowed recorded music to be bigger than life.

The delivery systems used in these experiments are not adequately described in any of the research. The reports say that researchers used a cassette player or headphones. There is no indication of when records (LPs) were used and no indication of the quality of the performances or who performed the music. So, when we look at the research, it is clinically heavy and musically light. The music is not dealt with in enough detail.

In terms of physiological measures, music has been found to affect the respiratory rate, amount of medication for pain, and anxiety levels. Length of labor and childbirth was shown to be dramatically affected by music (Figure 5–1). In fact, one study over 24 hours of 50 women in labor showed that John Philip Sousa marches definitely had a positive effect.

In terms of research to be generated and programs to be offered, the results must be manifested in healthcare objectives: in improved rate of recovery, decreased length of stay, and reduced stress as exhibited by staff and families. What healthcare designers hold themselves accountable for must be transferred into therapeutic objectives.

Smith: These statistics were compiled over many years of studies. In fact, the discipline of music therapy has been in existence for 50 years or so. Uniformly, the results indicate that the use of music in conjunction with other treatments yields better results than the absence of music. Despite the weaknesses on the music side of the studies, we are amazed that the results of these studies have not been applied. They have not permeated the medical industry at large. In fact, staff music therapists are relatively rare. When they are present, they are often looked down upon, equated with pet therapists, physical therapists, and the like, all of whom rank below doctors, nurses, and nurse's aides.

Defining Music Therapy

I would like to distinguish our work from traditional music therapy. The therapy model offers a one-to-one patient/therapist relationship. In this kind of music therapy, music is used as an administered protocol for a measured amount of time. We do not treat patients. We treat the space in which patients are placed. Our approach is to use environmental design that will affect the institution at large, which holds the patients, staff, administrators, families, visitors, and so forth. If that design is incorporated into the overall plan, our work should create positions for music therapists to help keep that environment in place.

However, as I said earlier, one person alone cannot make this change. The responsibility for the healing environment cannot be put solely on the shoulders of the designer, music therapist, or any other specialist, because every

◆ **FIGURE 5–1** Using control and music groups of 100 women each, researchers found statistically significant differences between the two, demonstrating a remarkable stress-reducing effect of music. In particular, if military music is chosen, trumpets and drums contribute to the desired effect, creating some kind of inner discipline. (*Chart design:* Glenn Ruga.)

EFFECT OF MUSIC ON BLOOD PRESSURE LEVELS DURING CHILDBIRTH LABOR OVER A 24-HOUR DAY

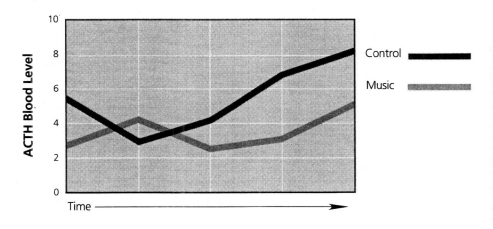

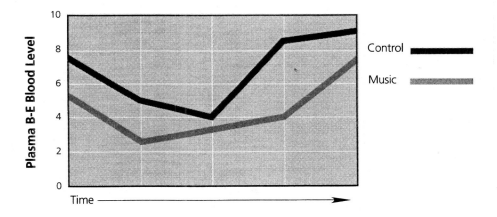

Source: B. Halpaap, R. Spintge, R.Droh, W. Kummert, W. Koewgel, "Anxiolytic Music in Obstetrics," in *Music in Medicine*, eds. Ralph Spintge and Roland Droh (Grenzach: Editiones Roche, 1985), pp. 145-54.

individual staff member is responsible for keeping that environment in place 24 hours a day.

Churches have done a great job of creating environments. When people walk into a church, even if no one is there, they know what is appropriate and what is not. We would like to see that same respect generated upon entering healthcare institutions. Unfortunately, often when music is added, it is done in such a way that the waiting room feels like a shopping mall, an elevator, or "happy hour" at the bar. There are places for these types of music in our lives, but such music is not appropriate for healthcare environments because of the denial implied and, thus, the negative environmental impact.

A suggested listening list that identifies music that "heals" (implying that music not listed does not heal) has been requested by many individuals and institutions. Unfortunately, it is not that simple. Just as doctors cannot deliver the "magic pill" that cures all, musicians, regardless of their intention, cannot deliver the "magic song" that will heal everyone all the time. We seek to empower the healthcare professional to be sensitive to all levels of musical impact—which include ethnic, cultural, personal, and spiritual elements—and to become astute at encouraging the ongoing redesign of a space that may seem static. What will work for an 85-year-old Alzheimer's patient may not work for a 17-year-old paraplegic. On the other hand, we have seen a demonstration of a sound environment that is appropriate for both these individuals.

The healing environment must be created from moment to moment through the skills of a knowledgeable staff as they interact with the patients, visitors, and one another. The ideal sound environment may vary from patient to patient, from one time of day to another, and from one unit to another.

Mazer: In terms of how to create a healing sound environment, at this point, we could probably document more of what does not work than what does. However, all of our experiences and the evidence coming from research indicate that some things certainly help more than others.

Healing Healthcare Systems is the newest addition to our healthcare projects. It is 24-hour audio/video programming for in-room patient television. We have found, both in live performance and in the results of offering this programming, that when a tool is offered to assist in those issues that medication cannot address, it is easily accepted and used. We have found, as musicians, that if we are appropriate to and honoring of our audience, if we know what we are delivering, and if we do it with great intention, the audience will become open to the music as a positive experience. Thus, it is possible to move beyond conflicting personal tastes.

We consider the needs of the patient to be primary, our objective being to facilitate the recovery process. If adding music and visual images to the space inspires a patient to request his or her own music, we consider that to be a positive step in the patient's participation in his or her own recovery. When patients start asking their families to bring in something else, this request generates a conversation that is positive and proactive in designing the environment in ways that personalize the room.

A study was referenced by Dr. Standley regarding the use of music in neonatal intensive care. The music therapist measured the decibel level of the respirators and the incubators in the intensive care unit. It was about 75 decibels, which is louder than a freight train and not quite as loud as a boiler room (Figure 5–2). A lullaby tape with a woman's voice, ethnically matched to each child, was recorded and played at 80 decibels, so as to mask the sound of the respirator. Researchers found that the experimental group that had the tapes and lullabies left intensive care seven to ten days earlier than the control group of infants who had not received the music therapy.

Another study done with epidural anesthesia, which can be compared to conscious sedation used in gastroenterology procedures, showed that anxiety measured through specific blood analysis was far lower with the use of music. In outpatient procedures, the amount of certain kinds of sedatives required is often partially determined by the emotional (and accompanying physical) state of the patient. Once again, we see that the patient's experience of the environment, prior to and during treatment, translates into the reality of the healthcare experience.

When we discuss this experiment with doctors, we ask them why, if the research is credible and answers all the questions that medicine needs to

◆ **FIGURE 5–2** The decibel level of respirators and incubators in an intensive care unit is about 75 decibels, which is louder than a freight train and not quite as loud as a boiler room. (*Chart design:* Glenn Ruga.)

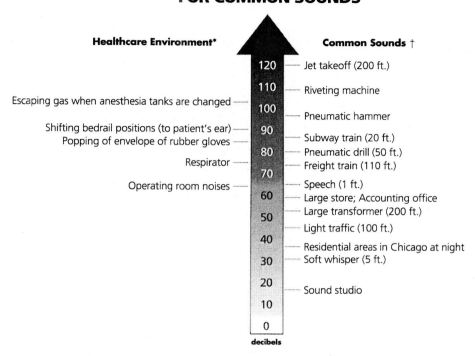

TYPICAL SOUND PRESSURE LEVELS FOR COMMON SOUNDS

Healthcare Environment*

120 — Jet takeoff (200 ft.)
110 — Riveting machine
Escaping gas when anesthesia tanks are changed — 100 — Pneumatic hammer
Shifting bedrail positions (to patient's ear) — 90 — Subway train (20 ft.)
Popping of envelope of rubber gloves — 80 — Pneumatic drill (50 ft.)
Freight train (110 ft.)
Respirator — 70 — Speech (1 ft.)
Operating room noises — 60 — Large store; Accounting office
Large transformer (200 ft.)
50 — Light traffic (100 ft.)
40 — Residential areas in Chicago at night
30 — Soft whisper (5 ft.)
20 — Sound studio
10
0

decibels

Common Sounds †

* The New England Journal of Medicine, Vol. 328, No. 6, pp 434.
† Courtesy of General Radio Company.

know about what works, has it not penetrated the medical community? Cassette tapes, at most, are $10 each. Considering the economics of healthcare, why is it that something so cost effective has not penetrated the medical community? At the same time, we look to designers to be in partnership with us in using this information to convince clients to design the aural space intentionally.

Smith: I might add that all of these statistics from the annals of music therapy came into existence prior to the birth of psychoneuroimmunology, which, in brief, recognizes the impact of the patient's attitude and emotional state on his or her immune system. This is something that we, as musicians, having practiced our art all of our lives, know instinctively. It has taken both time and persistence to get the statistical documentation from enough double-blind studies of medication plus counseling, versus medication alone, to prove that the psychological component can indeed go beyond the limits of medicine alone.

Trust

During this workshop, the participants did an exercise that demonstrated the impact of sound in shifting them from fear into trust in a brief amount of time. The exercise involved partners walking each other around the room, in silence, with one partner blindfolded. While the environment was contained in one space, with a group of individuals known to each other, the addition of music shifted the quality of the space.

This exercise was designed to demonstrate the power of the aural environment as it affects patients when other factors deprive them of control over their own environment. Blindfolded, the issues of color and light are moot. There is, however, an exaggerated sense of hearing as one tries to gain and maintain a sense of the space. Thus, the sounds in the room, the approximate location of physical objects and other people, and the loss of orientation, together, cause a dramatic increase in stress. Participants in the two workshops reported an elevated heartbeat and other physical manifestations of fear.

Mazer: We are obliged to heed the reality of the patient experience when specific sensory deprivation exaggerates the impact of those senses still in operation. In the previous exercise, you played both patient and caregiver. The role vacillates between having control and having no control, having more information and having less information. This is the nonverbal, physically invisible component of healthcare that needs to be addressed. When we look at these things that happen to patients in the best, most brilliantly designed gurneys, wheeled by the most highly trained individuals, how do we deal with the fear that dramatically affects patient outcomes?

Can we, as healthcare and design professionals, hold ourselves accountable for the quality of the space in which we place patients? It is possible to deal intentionally with medical crises in ways that minimize fear. Some of that fear is healthy and normal. It is part of being alive. How do we cut through the silence that is so oppressive and shift to a safe space? Some of you—no matter who was around you during this exercise—did not feel safe when your eyes were closed. As human beings, we loathe being out of control.

How can we build trust into the design of healthcare facilities? Can we do it in a very intentional way? We have done this exercise for many different groups and it has never generated a different result. When the music starts, people report that the tension goes out of the person they are leading around. It can be noted that the music is unfamiliar, new, and that it is different each time we do this particular exercise.

When you consider the use of music as environmental design, it is important to remember that the uncertainty and anxiety you have experienced here is real. Yet, you are healthy and safe, and you have chosen to be here in this room. In a hospital, people are not healthy, they seldom feel safe, and their very presence there is by limited choice.

What Is Appropriate?

Are we to assume that if we provide music for all patients in every therapeutic situation, that they will always be receptive to it? Let us remind ourselves, that patients are not asked what kind of a needle should be used or when an I.V. should be administered. In the use of music as environmental design, it is necessary to consider what music might be appropriate to the recovery process, as opposed to the kind of music that may be preferred in a casual, nonprofessional setting. Patients trust healthcare professionals to deliver what is appropriate and will best serve their recovery. Yet, regarding the use of music in healthcare, a specific kind of relationship is needed between the staff, patients, and the music. It is a different kind of intimacy and trust. When music is appropriately introduced to a patient, our experience has been that the patient becomes willing to try it.

For example, there was a woman who had been in an accident and was in traction in which she was face down, suspended at a 40-degree angle. Patients using this particular apparatus are not able to sleep. It is a very painful position and in addition to the pain generated by the injury, they cannot move. Thus, the medical need for rest is countered by a physical inability to get enough rest. A nurse who had taken our workshop went to this young woman and proposed that she try listening to a specific tape of music on a Sony Walkman for ten minutes. The young woman was understandably irritable and resistant. But upon listening to the music, she was able to sleep for three hours—the most she had slept in days.

There is a point at which we have to trust that it is the relationship that will create the opening. A relationship has to be built, which is why the beginning of this work is the educational process.

Smith: We have had the experience of music crossing generational and ethnic barriers. Certainly, if it is instrumental music, as opposed to vocal music, the music is more likely to have a universal appeal. The minute there is a song with lyrics, it triggers a certain specific, limited meaning. But if I play an Indian flute, one does not have to think of India in order to have a positive experience with the type of music I am playing. Also, we attempt to avoid musical clichés. What we played today has been more improvisational, in order to avoid falling into any particular style.

Mazer: Our work in music and healthcare is about using music as environmental design. We are committed to excellence in all aspects of healthcare delivery. We are committed to the creation of an environment that projects an aesthetic that is appropriate to the recovery process, to the human process. We hope to create a place for music to be experienced in a more powerful way than it may have ever been experienced. We would also like those who are afraid of listening to music they have never heard before to validate our position that music does not have to be familiar to work in a healthcare environment.

Smith: I would like to make a few comments in conclusion before we play one last number. We compare the design of music to the design of the healthy diet. It is possible to design a diet that, though totally healthful, is nonetheless totally unappetizing.

Music is the same way, in that some people seek to contrive healing music. As they remove elements that might not be healing, they end up with a bland style of music that is not appetizing intellectually or aesthetically. We think that variety in music is healthy.

The most important thing we hope we have done today is to encourage you as individuals to use music in the design of your lives and carry it into your professional lives. It is amazing how people will tolerate bad institutional design that they would never put up with privately, at home, in terms of lighting, color, and sound. We know how to make our personal living spaces comfortable, and we feel empowered to do so. It is unfortunate that we can go into public places every day that we would certainly never want to live in, nor spend any time in, much less try to recover and heal in. We control the environment that, in turn, controls us. So, let us feel empowered, as individuals and groups, to bring all the elements together to create a total healing environment.

Susan Mazer and Dallas Smith are composers, performers, producers, and educators based in South Lake Tahoe, Calif. They are the creators and producers of "Healing

Healthcare Systems," 24-hour audio/video programming for in-room patient television. They are members of the board of advisors for the ART of Living Institute and are on the national board of the Association of Healing Health Care Projects.

◆ ◆ ◆

ART FOR HEALTH: EMERGING TRENDS

Fifth Symposium on Healthcare Design, San Diego, CA, 1992

Helen G. Orem

"Can you remember where you were when the paradigm shifted?" This title of an essay by Marilyn Ferguson, published in her April 1991 *Brain/Mind Bulletin*, has stuck with me, and I like to think that I helped give the paradigm a push. That was in the mid-1980s, when, as art director for the Clinical Center at the National Institutes of Health (NIH), I was given responsibility for a new approach to interior design, wayfinding, and art.

There was a reason why the NIH saw the need for an "art director" for the Clinical Center—a position that had not existed previously. The story begins with architecture, and I would like to give some background on the movement toward patient-driven healthcare design.

The dictionary defines "environment" as "the aggregate of surrounding things, conditions, and influences." Well, what is this new element in healthcare delivery systems everyone is so excited about? Let's look at our society over the past 20 or so years to try and find those elements that shape "perception," that is: how, we as Americans, form judgments about our healthcare environments.

Let's look at architecture, sculpture, and public places. Let's consider the hospitality industry, and, briefly, look at retailing. Then, I will ask you to recall your own perception of what might be called "the hospital experience."

As the medical practitioners themselves would say, "To prescribe a cure, we must first understand the disease."

The Built World

Let's begin with a look at the built world—the box, cube, or container that shapes our American cities; the practice of architecture; the public place and its opportunity for a statement of some sort, usually rendered in sculpture, fountains, or gardens.

The age of modernism in architecture is perhaps best typified by Mies van der Rohe in his crisp, rigid Park Avenue Seagram's Building in New York City, built in 1958. It has been referred to as a summary of both the machine age and modernism. Lacking decoration, steel, bronze, travertine, and glass spoke for themselves. Modernism, or "contemporary" design, spread to Chicago and westward (in fact, everywhere), creating the perfect expression of the corporate headquarters within—the center of American technology and commerce.

Modernism brought with it the giants of contemporary architecture—

Skidmore, Owings, and Merrill (SOM), Eero Saarinen, Edward Durrell Stone, Perkins & Will, I.M. Pei, Harry Weese, Kevin Roche, Louis Kahn, and many others. Modernism was the only way to go, and everyone went there—and they seemed to speak with one voice. The voice was concrete, steel, and glass.

Add to this arena what was happening in art and sculpture in public places. Here, the brutalism of steel is seen as a further homage to the machine, as in a work by Louise Nevelson that was placed at a hospital entrance—a work that soon became known as "The Rusted Bedspring."

As an artist, Louise Nevelson considered herself to be an isolated system. She is quoted as saying, "If they blow up the world, that's not my business. My business is to work." And work she does, in a most arresting medium and style. But we have to ask ourselves, "Is it appropriate in healthcare? What message does it convey?"

Perhaps the epitome of this self-assertion of the artist over social values—a hard intellectual approach over intuitive wisdom—was evident in the controversy that raged over the removal of Richard Serra's monumental steel sculpture "Tilted Arc." This work, funded during the construction of the Jacob K. Javits federal office building in downtown Manhattan in 1981, has come to represent the ultimate in uncompromising modernist art dominating its space—a public plaza—as the heroic, belligerent ego of modernity.

By now, most people are aware of the embroiled saga of this work and the result of the public hearing spawned by a petition signed by 1,300 government employees which read in part, "It has dampened our spirits every day. It has turned into a hulk of rusty steel and clearly, at least to us, it doesn't have any appeal. It might have artistic value, but just not here . . . and for those of us at the plaza I would like to say, please do us a favor and take it away."

The government consented, and the rest is history. Serra sued the government for $30 million—$10 million for loss of sales and commission, $10 million for harm to his artistic reputation, and $10 million as punitive damages for the violation of his human rights. The art world defended Serra, because this populist revolt was seen as a challenge to all artists everywhere; but in 1987 the work was removed to storage.

It was a victory for the common man. A statement by the people who used the plaza and who worked in the buildings around it—they were, after all, "the client"—the taxpayers, the users, and their voice had been heard. They were saying, "What about our rights?"

The removal said something about government-funded art in public places and it said something about the wide chasm that separates modernism from the rest of us. But the arc was removed. Was this, perhaps, the first nudge in the paradigm shift?

Reaction Against Modernism

By 1975, the world of architecture was in a full-scale reaction against modernism. Society was breaking down a monolithically white Anglo-Saxon Protestant conception of itself—blacks had come to the lunch counter; women had come out of the kitchen; gays were declaring their rights; the disabled demanded access; and the elderly realized they had needs and rights and a power base. Mainstream America was giving voice to its constituent minorities, just as architecture was emerging as a pluralist discipline with many voices.

Now the movement featured richness and diversity where there used to be sterile functionalism and uniformity. Even time-honored concepts of zoning were challenged, leading to mixed uses, preservation, and the integration of urban functions that had been so carefully segregated by the antiseptic planners of the 1960s.

The new test became vitality and liveliness—two characteristics that contain the word "to live" and not the word "machine."

Postmodernism had arrived, and, with it, the freedom to be creative again: to invent, to rethink the purpose of the building and its interior spaces, as shown in the work of the Farrington Design Group. Its design for Resurgens Orthopaedics in Atlanta, Georgia, was featured in the October 1992 issue of *Contract Design*. As the article explains, "The knee bone's connected to the leg bone and the leg bone's connected to the hip bone," which is demonstrated in the structure of the physical spaces—in the experience of the facility itself. This interior reads "bones, joints, and structure . . . orthopedics . . . sports medicine," and it is Farrington's concept of structural elements as representational forms that become the "art." Like familiar examples from the high baroque, sculpture and architecture have become merged into a common statement. Art is not an add-on. We might call this movement "constructivism."

But never content (and perhaps that's a good thing), architects are now pushing the envelope toward something they call "deconstructivism." Personally, I do not begin to understand it . . . the buildings look as though they are either falling inward or flying apart . . . visual excitement carried to extremes.

Deconstructivism is baroque—the architecture contains within itself the essence of all plastic arts. If the high baroque was "frozen music," then the music was by Johann Sebastian Bach. If we hear subliminal music from deconstructivism, it may be works by John Cage, or it may be cacophony—the collision of a freight train with a gravel truck.

Yet the popularity of deconstructivism in architecture is what counts here. Buildings like the new hotels at Disney World in Orlando, Florida, come to mind. This is free enterprise at work. If the buildings succeed, and there is every indication that they will, the Disney Corporation will be very pleased.

Disney's architecture is not funded by taxpayers' money and is not up for a populist referendum. The market will vote with its credit cards, and this brings up the issue of competition and the second area of inquiry, the hospitality industry.

The Hospitality Industry

We are all familiar with the grand hotels of the 1920s and 1930s—the Plaza and the Waldorf in New York City, the Palmer House in Chicago, and the Mark Hopkins in San Francisco. No matter what the city, there was "the" hotel in town that set the standard for style and elegance. But these were hotels for the rich and famous. The rest of us stayed in roadside motels outside town and only dreamed about the grand hotels we had seen in magazines and movies.

We ate at Howard Johnson's and learned about the power of color and shape—orange and turquoise inside and out, the familiar roof line with a cupola on top visible from the highway, and the same dependable menu from Maine to Florida—long before McDonald's Golden Arches.

Through chain restaurants and later, motels, we came to realize that standardization and quality control could provide a more dependable product than independent mom-and-pop operations, and we took a certain pride, and perhaps relief, in finding a familiar shape and color in a distant town far from home.

But the grand American hotels were—and are today—a study in taste. In fact, in the 1920s and 1930s, Americans saw taste as reconstituted European elegance. Thus, interiors featured colonnades and brocades, gilt-framed mirrors, gleaming mahogany paneling, overstuffed lounge seating, and an aging concierge in a field marshal's uniform—all borrowed from The Grand Tour. America had yet to discover herself.

Beginning perhaps in the 1970s, the hospitality industry came alive again in a boom cycle of expansion and construction that lasted until the recent recession. It has been said that the healthcare industry will dominate the 1990s as hospitality dominated the 1980s.

But what did the hospitality industry build? No more fake European elegance. American architects had discovered a new idiom, soon to be the standard for hotels and office plazas across the country—the atrium.

It began perhaps in Atlanta, with John Portman's Hyatt Regency Hotel. Here, the first atrium lobby with exposed interior elevators set the standard for others to follow. For a few years, the Marriott Marquis in Times Square in New York City gained more in publicity from its daring architecture than any new hotel in town. People wanted to stay there just to ride the elevators and look down into its incredible lobby. They wrote home about it.

An essential element in all high-rise construction, the common elevator, had been transformed into a signature form of entertainment, and the passengers did not look outward at a distracting city view, they looked inward, at the lights, the spaces, the finishes that read "Marriott." They were like a captive audience in a commercial, and they loved it.

As more and more Americans traveled, more and more became familiar with the atrium; and because of its "good vibes," we began to associate an atrium space with a hospitable space—a place where we had fun, or were welcomed, or just enjoyed ourselves, away from the cares of home and office. The atrium had gained in our perception of architectural spaces, and lobbies with low ceilings would seem noisy and crowded thereafter.

The hospitality industry also knows that people want to feel "at home," even in a 30-story high-rise, and that attention to interiors, corridors, and elevator lobbies can remove some of the stigma of hotel living. So we have become accustomed to the use of mass produced reproduction art, color coordinated to the room decor with attention to the colors and textures of the fabrics, bedspread, drapes, and wall finishes. The rooms are generic—designed to offend no one—but not unpleasant.

But it is the main lobbies that impress us, and here's where the artists of today make their statements. If we liked the ornate clock at the Plaza, we also associate with Eric Orr's sculpture in the lobby of the Marriott in San Francisco—five stone and bronze towers down which water flows into a "pool" of polished black pebbles, quiet, with rippling motion and a certain grace.

There are many other examples, but the point is: The hospitality industry is aware of the opportunity an atrium provides for the display of original art—art that makes a statement about the company and the building and its concern for its customers' environment.

And what is the American hotel experience today? From years of traveling, I can say that it has never been better. Intelligent, well-trained people make reservations; alert, helpful personnel are at the entrance—not the officious doorman-with-his-hand-out from the 1950s; there is a courteous staff; computerized checkout on the room TV; and clean rooms—with plenty of towels!

Our perception of staying away from home, of being received and processed and directed, is formed largely by the efficiency, personal attention, and pleasant environment we associate with our hospitality experience, and we will not settle for anything less.

But the quality of our American hospitality industry was not spawned by decree, it was earned by competition. As competition for the healthcare dollar forces our established institutions to take a fresh look at their own mission, they, too, must come to see the patient as a customer—as an individual—who deserves the respect he has come to demand from a competitive free market.

Whether we express this comparison or not, we measure our healthcare experience against the architecture, the interior design, the personnel, and the environments we have come to expect from traveling in American hotels.

But the hospitality industry tells us something more. We are now entering the world of patient hotels associated with healthcare facilities. These are nearby lodging for outpatients and their families, located at, or convenient to the medical center, clinic, or hospital.

As we move in this direction, the opportunity exists to bring the expertise of free market competition to the design and operation of patient hotels—to see that the healing environment, the integrated application of colors, textures, materials, and the arts, begins at check-in, and is continued, strengthened, and reflected in all related patient spaces within the complex, so that the patient experience in the facility is presented with one voice.

Learning from Retailing

What can healthcare arts learn from retailing? Americans grew up with strip shopping centers lining their highways. But there was another form of retailing that developers and planners had forgotten—the "market."

In the 1960s, the noted shopping center developer James Rouse, given an opportunity to play a role in the revitalization of Baltimore's Inner Harbor area, remembered the human values of the marketplace he knew from Baltimore's rich heritage as a market center for dairy products, German and Polish sausages, farm produce, and seafood from the Chesapeake Bay. The market Rouse remembered was not a strip center, but a block-long, high-roofed structure housing a variety of interior stalls leased out to the many different vendors whose products, sights, and smells vied for attention. It was a busy, noisy, exciting place where hand trucks loaded with bushels of softshell crabs pushed through crowds of shoppers from Baltimore's inner city as well as its trendy suburbs. Shopping at Lexington Market was a Baltimore experience.

In what has now become a model for mixed use redevelopment, Rouse's Festival Marketplace at Inner Harbor in Baltimore recreated some of that sense of visual excitement, variety, and delight that characterized the farmers' markets of the 19th century. The concept was so successful that it has been extended to Boston's Quincy Market at Faneuil Hall and New York's South Street Seaport.

Critics decry the "malling of America"—the concentration of goods and

◆ **FIGURE 5–3** The atrium, an architectural feature first popularized by the hospitality industry, is now common to many hospitals. Shown is a model of the Homer Gudelski Inpatient Building at the University of Maryland Medical Center in Baltimore, MD, done by Zeidler Roberts Partnership, Architects.

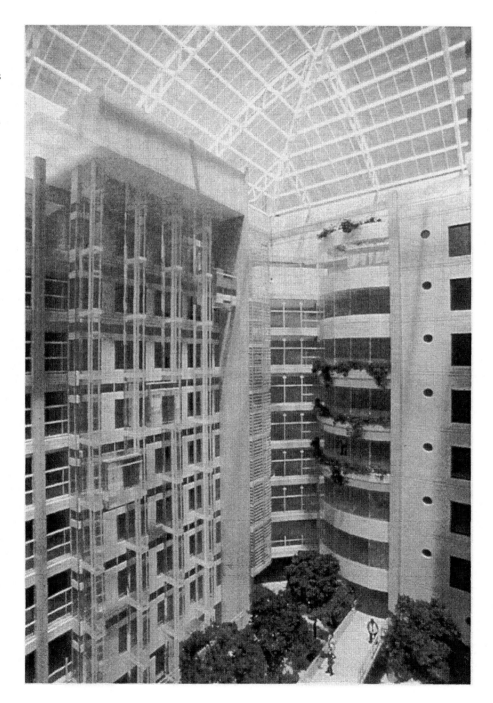

services in ever and ever larger regional shopping malls; but we, as consumers, have responded with enthusiasm. We demand the free parking that malls provide, we have come to expect the very latest in enclosed mall environments—the interior landscaping, waterfalls, piano music, seasonal performances, and visual excitement. We delight in the variety of goods, services, theaters, and restaurants available to us in this festival atmosphere, all under one roof.

What should healthcare planners learn from malls? They should learn that American retailers and the competitive free enterprise system continually strive to bring consumers the ultimate shopping experience through the creative process—through architecture and interior design—and thus, as consumers, we have seen it all.

Our perception of the healthcare experience is molded by our response to shopping malls, and we will make comparisons that lead to judgments about the quality of the healthcare delivery system based on these visual and sensory experiences we bring with us.

Which is not to say that those experiences are all favorable. Healthcare delivery is not retailing. The flashing lights, the color-saturated primaries, the pervasive "mall music" and the aroma from a dozen fast-food outlets are all incompatible with healthcare environments. But some of the best "interiors" are done for America's top retailers, and the images projected in their store spaces tend to establish our own sense, not only of taste, but also of reassurance and acceptance.

Recently there has emerged a trend toward the integration of retailing with healthcare; if we are to add patient hotels, then the design of the medical center of tomorrow will require input from both the hospitality industry and commercial leasing experts.

If the popular uprising against establishment dictated public art nudged the paradigm a little, the hospitality and retail industries of the 1980s were giving it a hard push.

What of the Hospital Experience?

I am sure each of us has had different hospital experiences, but probably the one common impression on which we can all agree is dehumanization. At times, we felt like an experiment in a high school biology lab.

How did this happen? Well first, our medical facilities from pre–World War II days were unprepared for the population boom of the postwar years. To meet the surge in demand, hurriedly designed and built extensions and add-ons were thrown up almost overnight to add capacity. Second, our medical facilities, like our postwar architecture, were a reflection of modernism and its credo.

Perhaps most important, hospitals that reflected these modern and postmodern trends had another element forcing them in a particular direction. They were "doctor driven," and often doctor owned. The physician was the client and the architects responded to the client's demands:

- Bare = clean
- Brightly lit = efficiency
- Paging systems at top volume = communication
- Mysterious shiny equipment = latest technology.

Then, in the 1980s, modern technology created a miracle world of incredible machines and procedures—each new breakthrough more fantastic than the last. Yet no one thought about the "person" inside the patient—of his or her spiritual or emotional well-being—of his or her reaction to the experience.

No one asked, "Is the patient's emotional state a contributing factor in the success of the protocol?" The operation on the biomedical model had succeeded, but the spiritual patient had all but died.

Someone once said about VA hospitals, "If you're not sick when you come in here, just wait a while."

Competition and Consumerism

And then two very healthy, very American, factors emerged: competition for patient dollars and the power of the patient's voice as a consumer—to have a say in the way healthcare would be delivered.

Running concurrently with the decline of modernism was this new-found voice of the patient demanding a more people-friendly healthcare space—in particular, there was a reemergence of art as a component of place.

Also, medical research had begun in the relatively new field of psychoneuroimmunology, the study of the neuronal and hormonal bonds between mind and body and the effect on healing. Dr. Roger Ulrich, speaking at the Third Symposium on Healthcare Design, citing his now well-known documentation on the use of a window to the outside world and its effects on recovery rates, identified a new focus: that healthcare environments should be targeted to patients, visitors, *and staff.*

By now, a new awareness of choices was being expressed, and the first area affected was labor and delivery.

San Francisco architect James Diaz notes the emerging changes in maternity wards—a signal victory for women—and points out that women are the demanding voice in patient-driven hospital systems. A recent survey notes that 75 percent of healthcare demand in the United States is made by women.

While most changes in labor and delivery were of a positive nature, many feel that the movement went too far in "Laura Ashley-ing" the whole process. We women after all, are the ones who know that balloon drapes are dust catchers and do not belong in a room with newborn lungs, no matter how welcoming they might have appeared the day before delivery.

The second area to benefit from the new approach was the neonatal intensive care unit. Manufacturers were supplying products in primary colors that built visual clutter. Noise and harsh overhead lighting is actually harmful to premature infants. Neonatal units being built today are softer, quieter, less jumbled areas of care and security.

A third area of concentration recently has been cancer facilities, typically outpatient clinics. Outpatients come to the clinic for treatment on a regularly scheduled basis. The process of immunology is time consuming. Patients will make many visits to the clinic over this time period and, on each visit, they will spend time undergoing chemotherapy in a reclining chair, facing a wall, looking at . . . what? So the environment of the cancer facility must respond to another factor—sameness. Time is seen to progress when the environment changes, not dramatically, but in response to nature and the cycle of the year. The visual environment in a cancer clinic, therefore, should respond to this need for change, not to be different, but to add interest and variety.

One tested approach has been the changing art show with works by local artists hung in the lobby or corridors, changing every several weeks, and allowing patients, staff, and visitors alike to share the benefit of an art experience. The approach I recommend, is to limit the shows to works that are for sale, works which are priced fairly, and to require that 20 percent of the sales proceeds are returned to the institution as a donation. Thus the artist receives 80 percent of the sales price of any works sold during the show. Since typical commercial galleries charge 40 percent or more to promote an artist through a similar show, artists are encouraged to price their works to sell while they are on display at the facility.

There are no losers in changing art shows. Patients and staff benefit from the visual variety and interest and from the change of scene; the artists benefit from an opportunity to reach a new market; and the mission of the facility is carried back to the local arts community through publicity in the local media.

We have looked at some of the major influences driving healthcare decisions today:

- A new freedom in architecture and the multipurpose atrium
- The hospitality industry—"we know what service means"
- Interior design influenced by retailing—"we've seen it all"
- Competition and consumerism vs. doctor-driven institutions.

Through this review process I have tried to emphasize the concept of perception—how does the market see an institution or facility? What message is it trying to send?

Arts Consultant's Role

I would like to focus now on the role of the healthcare arts consultant or advisor. What, exactly, does the arts consultant do? When the outpatient clinic was built at NIH in the mid-1980s in response to the universal trend toward outpatient care, the architects chose an all-glass box solution to the challenge facing them: to create an 11-story addition to the world's largest brick-faced building. These new clinics were without difference or distinction. Patients were met with confusion, endless areas of technical equipment, and a cold, sterile lobby. This was the federal government's largest biomedical research facility, entertaining visitors from all over the world, and it was saying nothing about itself or its mission at NIH.

In the 1980s, the first problem at the new Clinical Center addition was really twofold: image and wayfinding. As the arts director, I wanted to establish an art presence at the main escalator lobby, and I wanted a piece that met very specific requirements: It should read "healing," but not "doctor"; "local," but not identifiable with any city, town or place; and (I didn't know the term at the time) "politically correct," that is, not representative of any particular race, creed, or culture.

NIH is located in Bethesda, Maryland. The city gets its name from the Old Testament reference to the "Pools of Bethesda," a healing place. It was

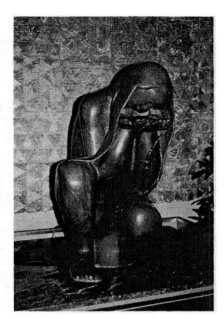

◆ **FIGURE 5–4** "Healing Waters" sculpture fountain by Azriel Zwet was chosen for the lobby of the ACRF Building at the National Institutes of Health in Bethesda, MD, for its human element and water reference. (*Photo:* Orem Associates.)

natural, then, to look for a water element or fountain. But there were lots of those—we see them everywhere—and I wanted something with a human element. The subject of healthcare after all, even biomedical research, involves people .

I finally found it in a work by a local sculptor, Azriel Awet. It is the figure of a woman—without distinguishing features, one who might even be a native American, drinking water from her cupped hands, as she kneels by a pool. The piece was placed on a base, and a recirculating pump keeps a steady trickle of water dripping from her cupped hands. The subtle sound of water is reflected off the large abstract wall piece behind her, commissioned from local artist Gail Watkins.

Named "Healing Waters," her image was adopted by the Clinical Center as the logo for its letterhead and for all announcements it issued regarding activities taking place there under its newly created Arts and Humanities Program. The image has become so closely associated with the Clinical Center over the past six years that, today, small maquettes of the sculpture are given out as awards by the director, in recognition of outstanding achievement.

In arts consulting, we call this a "statement piece"—a strong visual element that says who you are and what you do, without using the written word. A statement piece must be carefully considered since it conveys a stronger, more immediate image than all the printed words a marketing department can write.

Our next step at NIH was to begin building a permanent art collection and, in this venture, I was given the support and encouragement of both the director and several key department heads, each of whom was an active art collector in his or her own right. I looked to the local arts community first, but then expanded my range and began buying from sources outside the metropolitan area. We were fortunate to acquire several examples of American "WPA" art, small-scale proposals submitted for consideration as Post Office murals during Franklin D. Roosevelt's administration. Although our collection is varied, with works representing Latin America, Asia, and Africa, as well as contemporary works, these pastoral scenes contain just the right balance for NIH: They are government sponsored, authentic, and speak to rural America or early Bethesda without being sentimental.

Throughout this process of selecting and acquiring art for the permanent collection, I was faced with the question: What is appropriate subject matter for a healthcare setting?

In art, everyone is an expert, and everyone has his or her own particular tastes. After some give and take, I settled on a solution—a jury. We reviewed slides, or sometimes original works, on a periodic basis, receiving input from an established panel of people in both healthcare and the arts. If a submission was too sweet, or too aggressive or hostile, or even if the color scheme seemed to suggest something unsettling, it was out. But we were careful not to become so bland, or so neutral, that we excluded vitality and strength. One thing we all agreed on—we wanted original art, no reproductions that a patient might have seen somewhere else, and we did not want puppy dogs or kittens—the sort of thing weekend painters love to do—or anything that looked like calendar art, or a get-well card.

We made our position clear in written guidelines. I cannot overemphasize the importance of established criteria for the selection of art in a healthcare environment. It tells what is wanted, and it tells what is not wanted. Arts consultants will be overrun with well meaning volunteers—sometimes people in high places—who wish to give them "just the right thing" in return for a tax deductible receipt at (their) statement of value. Arts consultants have to be able to turn these offers down politely and without alienating the prospective donor. One way to do this is through the jury system or by following written guidelines. Another way to do it is to ask if the donor would be willing to make a similar donation in the form of cash.

In the corridor to the patient rooms, I placed art in a hallway to encourage exercise—walking—accompanied by an "Observant Walker's Guide," describing the art, telling something about the artist, and noting how many postrecovery feet the person has walked, from piece to piece. The art here is not just for the spirit, it is also a medical tool.

The problem of moving people around in a strange environment brings us to the term "signage," which is already obsolete. Today's term is "wayfinding." I started with color coding, based on a handout map or floor plan of the building, and then added recognizable visual elements that don't need words or numbers—art. Perhaps I was influenced by "red right returning" from my days cruising on the Chesapeake Bay, but I firmly believe that a reassuring object, whether it is a red channel marker or a piece of sculpture, is the best aid to "navigation." And so we placed clearly identifiable pieces at important locations, where they would be seen and remembered.

Working with our hospital administrators, I was asked to reconsider the entire approach to pediatric clinic design, and here we made some major discoveries. Pediatrics is another whole subject, beyond the scope of today's discussion, but it is an area in which a healthcare arts consultant can make a significant contribution. To be brief, saturated primaries are out. Cartoon characters are out. Circus is out. Participation is in. Involving the children in participating in their own environment gives them a sense of empowerment—and that is, again, a medical tool.

The Parameters of Healthcare Arts

As a licensed interior designer, I am anxious to become involved in all forms of design from the early concept stage, to remodeling—or even redecorating just one office—or redesigning a more efficient nurse station.

Others may limit their services to the permanent collection, changing art shows, music, wayfinding, and community relations. We are a multitalented profession, but we all share a common objective: to create a better healthcare environment through art. To summarize:

- An arts consultant is involved in the creative process.
- An arts consultant will work in cooperation with architects and interior designers in the formative stages of planning and design for new construction, bringing his or her expertise to the decision-making process.
- An arts consultant can be retained by the client to advise on the development and implementation of arts and humanities programs at an existing institution or facility. Once these systems and programs are in place, the consultant works with staff to demonstrate and advise how the programs can best be placed into operation. Then, standing by as an advisor, the consultant turns over a working package to the client, and

steps aside. The programs, if properly implemented, should be self-directed thereafter.

- An arts consultant can be an in-house staff member with a working knowledge of architecture, interior design, facility maintenance, hospital administration, and the world of art, whose primary responsibility is cultural enrichment, training, implementation, and development—building bridges between medicine and the community.

When I formed my own consulting firm in 1990, there were only a few people out there with my experience and my message, who wanted to limit their practice to healthcare arts exclusively. Many others had come to healthcare arts through the disciplines of architecture, interior design, or hospital administration or through graduate programs in fine arts.

But as I talked with people around the country, I soon realized that there were successful arts programs already in place that had evolved from the same need we felt at NIH in the 1980s. These programs were originated by institutions and architectural firms that had anticipated the demand for a patient-driven environment and had done something about it.

Duke University Hospital, for example, had established a Department of Cultural Services under the direction of Janice Palmer. Palmer's *The Hospital Arts Handbook* should be required reading for anyone entering this field.

The University of Washington Medical Center at Seattle had already created an exciting arts program under the leadership of Lynn Basa. That program continues today, as one of the model programs now in place in the Pacific Northwest.

Planetree, a pioneering healthcare movement dedicated to changing the way patients and guests experience hospitals, was opening new facilities on the West Coast including the Mid-Columbia Medical Center in The Dalles, Oregon, the subject of a forthcoming Bill Moyers PBS Special, *Healing: The Mind-Body Connection*.

Similar programs were underway at Children's National Medical Center in

◆ **FIGURE 5–5** Many hospitals and clinics, such as the Lombardi Cancer Research Medical Center in Washington, DC, are integrating the performing arts into their programs.

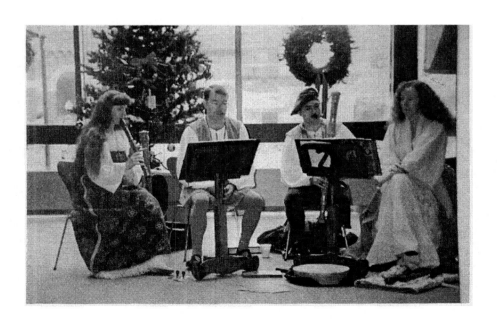

Washington, D.C.; Vanderbilt University Medical Center; Marin General Hospital in California, whose art program is directed by Beverly Dector; Johns Hopkins Medical Center; Bay State Medical Center at Springfield Massachusetts; and university hospitals in Iowa, Virginia, Florida, Wisconsin, Minnesota, Indiana, and Michigan, to name just a few.

One program that has come to my attention recently deserves special note. In Warren, Ohio, (population 56,000) the Trumbull Memorial Hospital (TMH) prides itself on its arts and humanities program developed and administered by Marianne Nissen. TMH runs a comprehensive program including visual and performing arts. The hospital promotes the arts program by publishing pictures and articles in its periodical *Topics* and by producing mail-outs and handout brochures that feature the works of local Ohio artists, as well as works done by patients of the hospital.

Today, representatives from more than 55 different healthcare arts programs in America and England find an avenue for the interchange of ideas in the Society of Healthcare Arts Administrators.

New Paradigm, as Old as the Renaissance

In the 15th Century, Brunelleschi "did" the L'Ospedale degli Innocenti, the Foundling Hospital, for Lorenzo de Medici in Florence, Italy. This combined the fresh air of the early Italian Renaissance with patron-sponsored healthcare and lifting the concept of "hospital" out of the medieval monastery into the realm of political and social responsibility. A grand *patron*, Lorenzo insisted that only the most creative architects and artists of his day be commissioned to create the Foundling Hospital—a place of healing for children. Can we afford to do less?

I would like to conclude with some observations on emerging trends:

1. *Art in architecture.* Today's trends are toward more freedom in architectural expression without slavish adherence to established styles. Hopefully, architects today are designing people-friendly buildings for the client, and not for the AIA awards committee.

We are seeing a greater use of familiar forms and materials and, I think, a return to "nature"—that is, to more organic elements in design, away from geometrical and abstract symbolism and expression.

Other art-in-the-atrium solutions have been presented at these Symposia previously, but one that I am very impressed with is the Hospital for Sick Children in Toronto, Canada, designed by the Zeidler Roberts Partnership. The art includes a series of murals by artist Louis de Niverville, depicting happy days out-of-doors, which brings sunshine and sea air right into the space in a delightful manner. These murals speak to a point I would like you to think about. They are fresh, incisive, original art that represents a quality and creativity so often lost in pediatric art in particular. They are not cartoon characters, butterflies, kites, pinwheels, or clowns. They have a subtlety of color range and intensity and they are enormously involving. They do not insult the discerning eye of the child or adult viewer.

It is toward this level of creativity that we need to strive. To give interest to this vertical space—which needs elements that can be viewed from many floors—amusing sculptural acrobats balance precariously high in the air. We are told that these acrobat figures can actually move back and forth on their high wire. This is a place of enchantment and delight. I think even Lorenzo de Medici would be pleased.

2. *Art in public places.* If Richard Serra's "Tilted Arc" was rejected by the common man, Zion and Breen's Paley Park at 10 East 53rd St. in Manhattan (1967) still stands today as an example of a most successful people-friendly place.

In healthcare, I have seen no better landscape architecture than the courtyard at the James Whitcomb Riley Hospital for Children in Indianapolis. The use of shadow, of strong visual elements, the human scale, sculpture, water, and healing herbs combine to create a most welcoming and restful experience.

And in sculpture, I believe that abstract expressionism has become a relic of the 1960s and that the human figure will return, as it did in the Renaissance, not in the overblown monumental grandeur of the high baroque, but in simple forms that speak to our common denominator—memory.

As far as interactive art goes, those from Boston are familiar with the installation at the Kendal Square station of the MTA—those large metal chimes hanging between the tracks that can actually be "rung" by passengers waiting for a train. In fact, I have personally let trains go by while I enjoyed moving the lever that rings the chimes, just to hear them reverberate through the tunnel. I loved it.

Sculpture, like toys, can be interactive—to touch—as for example, the revered toe of St. Peter in the great basilica in Rome, or the simple figure of a horse at Duke Medical Center's Low Vision Touchable Art Gallery. This is a new approach to art for health, and one that holds much promise for the future.

Art in healthcare should address our commonality, our need for each other, our love of life, and the physical and spiritual world we all share.

3. *The contribution of art.* I have given some examples of how an active arts and humanities program can contribute to a patient-driven healthcare facility. But its contribution goes much further than that. The arts improve staff morale, pride, and performance. The arts involve the local community, without regard to race, color, creed, or country of origin. The arts project the image of the institution as a caring place—a place for healing. The arts extend to development—to marketing and publicity. The arts speak to the whole person, and to the institution and its place in society.

In the words of Dr. James Semans, professor emeritus, department of surgery, Duke University Medical Center, "During . . . periods of anxiety, neither the physician nor anyone else can give the patient the reassurance that he would have if he could be transported by personally experiencing some art form, whether his particular preference is visual, auditory, or both. It is for this reason that the idea [of an arts and humanities program] has been so attractive to physicians and nursing staff who care about the feelings of patients in this strange environment."

4. *The new design team for the 1990s.* How can these influences we have discussed be implemented? I believe only by an integration of all creative disciplines—the architect, interior designer, landscape architect, *and* healthcare arts consultant—can optimum results be effected. When the dance is worth

the candle, I have found that many architects and designers are willing to share areas of exclusivity that used to divide them.

Then what is the objective of this team approach? Earlier, I talked about perception. To me, "art" is the building, the landscaping; the signage, sculpture, or other images as wayfinding, the art on the walls; plants, flowers, and trees; the furniture, carpeting, lighting; the music, performances, and poetry; the staff uniforms, volunteers' attitudes, handouts and graphics, pride and performance—the aggregate that makes up the way we perceive the delivery of healthcare services in America today.

The credo of a healthcare arts consultant is: "Let the healthcare environment reflect the quality of your protocol."

Years ago, I had an Uncle Gus. Every child should have an Uncle Gus. My uncle taught me to recite poetry—or at least the favorite poems he learned from his mother—and my favorite Uncle Gus poem by Arthur O'Shaughnessy says something about why we are all here today:

We are the music makers,
We are the dreamers of dreams,
Wandering by lone sea breakers.
And sitting by desolate streams;
Yet we are the movers and shakers
Of the world forever, it seems.

An art consultant and interior designer, Helen Orem is principal of Orem Associates in Chevy Chase, Maryland. Prior to establishing her own firm, Orem worked at the National Institutes of Health in Washington, D.C., for 20 years. She is a founding member of the Society of Healthcare Arts Administrators.

Chapter

SIX

PROJECT EXAMPLES/PEDIATRICS

NEW REGIONAL CHILDREN'S HOSPITAL AT STANFORD

Third Symposium on Healthcare Design, San Francisco, CA, 1990

Felicia Cleper-Borkovi, AIA
Diana Kissil, AIA
Derek Parker, FAIA, RIBA
Langston Trigg, Jr., AIA

Adult: Can hospitals be scary?

Children: Yes.

Adult: What's scary in a hospital?

Children: Getting a shot.

Adult: And what would you do to change or make a hospital a nice place?

Children: Uh, I don't know . . . Make the shots feel better.

Adult: What do you like about the new Regional Children's Hospital at Stanford?

Children: It has neat garden centers and flowers on the roof and lots of wood, curves, and walls. There are louvers on the windows and they're neat to open. There are lots of windows and light. It has lots of colors and counters in it. The building looks like blocks all stacked up.

Adult: Would any of you ever want to go to that hospital?

Children: Yes!

Adult: You would? You want to be sick?

Children: No, just to go look at it. Yeah. If I have to be sick, I want to go to a nice hospital like that.

Parker: The four of us worked together for six years designing and constructing the Lucile Salter Packard Hospital for Children at Stanford, which is its official name. Lucile Packard, who unfortunately died last year, was the wife of David Packard, the cofounder of Hewlett Packard. Lucile and David actually met as students, working in the kitchen at Children's Hospital at Stanford University, Palo Alto, California, in the 1930s. There was a time at Stanford when students who broke the rules had to do community service, and David and Lucile found themselves working in the kitchen at Children's Hospital. We never did find out which rules they broke. Nevertheless, they fell in love, got married, and David went on to bigger and better things in the electronics industry; but Lucile always maintained her love for Children's Hospital. She served on the Board and later was the chairman of the board; and I think it's fair to say that without her, this project probably would never have existed in the form that it is today.

Not only did she contribute a substantial amount of money to make it possible, she also gave significantly of herself. Unfortunately, we knew she was going to die before the project was completed, so we raced through the final stages of the design to get a model built. This was so she could get an answer to the very first question she ever asked me, which was, "Derek, tell me what this place is going to look like." And at that early time, of course, I couldn't tell her.

Order of Presentors

This presentation is divided into four areas: Langston Trigg is going to cover the unusual way the client got organized in order to do this project right; I'm going to discuss how the concept developed and how we worked with

Mrs. Packard and her committee to establish some principles for the design; Felicia Cleper-Borkovi will discuss the design and the building layout; and finally, Diana Kissil will complete our presentation by discussing the integration of the interior design, furniture, and fabrics. At this time, the building is probably two months away from being completed. The carpets and plants are going in, but the place is still buzzing with contractors.

Designing a hospital for children is really a wonderfully rewarding experience for an architect, because it gives us the opportunity to enhance the humanistic elements of architecture and to develop the therapeutic role of the environment, which is for diagnosing and treating, caring and curing, and living and dying.

The Children's Hospital at Stanford has a history of 65 years of exceptional medical treatment, delivered in an ambiance of warm, personal care. Now, spurred by the new tools of molecular medicine, the healthcare industry is on the brink of some previously un-dreamed-of breakthroughs and opportunities, and nowhere is it more important than in the care and treatment of children. Healthcare providers are dealing with prenatal screening of genetic disease, radioactive probes for sickle cell anemia, bone marrow transplants, use of monoclonal antibodies, and organ transplants—all of which were not in the mainstream of medicine a short time ago. Now these treatments improve and prolong the lives of our children.

The new hospital we designed is a replacement for an existing facility and offers care to children of all ages. We have 125 beds, which includes 31 neonatal intensive care beds and a very active and fairly large ambulatory care center that includes a day hospital.

We did a lot of research and we discovered quickly that children are not little adults. They are quite different people, physiologically and psychologically. We're dealing with a broad spectrum of clients, from newborn infants, to toddlers, to school-age children, and including adolescents. Because of the success in treating childhood diseases, some of our patients are postadolescent and even early adult. Hospitals are frightening places for children—even for adults—and this stress increases as the technology advances. We've worked hard to make this place friendly to children and to their families.

Langston will now cover the early stages of this project, and I'd like to emphasize that the preparation for the planning of this project was probably the single most important aspect of the success of the project. It reminds me of a statement made about planning by my favorite philosopher, Woody Allen, who said, "Mankind is at a fork in the road: to the left, the road leads to oblivion and disaster; to the right, it leads to turmoil and death. But only by planning ahead, will we make the right choice."

Trigg: I'd like to offer the analogy that in terms of how they view their mission, hospital administrators are somewhat similar to the soldiers that went off to World War I. There's a certain amount of idealism and naivety. They're going off to end the "War to End All Wars," and two years later they sort of struggle back, the ones that made it, and they've had their trip through hell. So, knowing that this was the situation, I did try to get the owner organized before we headed out on any road. I'd like to start off by giving an orientation of the project.

I have a drawing that represents the very essence of what design professionals deal with every day. It came from a series of self-portraits by children in hospitals. A little girl in this drawing portrays herself as a person occupying a minuscule portion of the picture. She's practically lost within a giant hospital bed and she's surrounded by wires and equipment resembling snakes and wild monstrous faces. Unfortunately, this is not atypical. Hospitals are often frightening and mysterious experiences for adults and children alike; however, for a child, it is particularly traumatic and can scar them for life. The other image of a boy returning the favor by giving a nurse a shot, is fairly self-explanatory. While it is humorous, the trauma that it symbolizes is tragic.

Create a Friendly, Humane Environment

Our primary goal on this project was to create a children's hospital that is friendly and warm, soft, and humane. We did not want the typical multistory slab that's cold, high tech, and institutional. The setting for this project is the Stanford University campus, which is approximately 35 miles south of San Francisco. The campus is over 8000 acres, which is equal to the total land area of the city and county of San Francisco. I'm not bragging, I just want you to imagine the expanse of bureaucracy that can be contained within 8000 acres!

The Medical Center buildings are approximately two million square feet. The original Children's Hospital is about a mile and a quarter away from the main center. This distance, as small as it may seem, created several problems, because both patients and physicians were constantly being shuttled back and forth. Both institutions, frankly, had outgrown their usefulness and were facing obsolesence. The project is a merger of the existing Children's Hospital and the Pediatric Program at Stanford University Hospital. The new Children's Hospital will be physically attached to the Medical Center.

The Medical Center includes the Stanford University School of Medicine, Stanford University Clinic, and the Stanford University Hospital. Currently, the hospital of 663 beds contains about 65 beds for pediatrics. Up until recently, as an independent entity, there was Children's Hospital with 60 beds. The combination of Children's Hospital and the Stanford Pediatric portion is the creation of the Packard Children's Hospital. When completed, it will become the fourth entity within the Stanford University Medical Center.

We all know how complex and political hospitals can be. Add to that the academic element, the merger aspect, and the challenges to set up a process that will function and produce legitimate results in a timely fashion.

The initial hurdle of this eight-year project, and one of the worst aspects of the job that's long term and major, is getting people to enthusiastically participate in a planning and programming process that may be anywhere from five to ten years away from being a reality. In our case, I requested that no design consultant be hired for the first year of the project so that the owner could determine, from a strategic planning standpoint, what it is that we truly needed and wanted. Often, a hospital will hire an architect, head down a certain path, and then realize they picked the wrong path. This can have costly and frustrating consequences.

Key planning processes that provided a firm foundation for the architect included structuring a Board of Directors. I was the first employee hired for the new Children's Hospital. Under the Board, there was a steering committee, an academic committee, and an administrative committee. Under those three committees were 35 task forces. They involved physicians, nurses, technicians, and administrators. Some task forces represented a department, such as administration, nursing units, or outpatient clinics. Other task forces represented ancillary support services, such as respiratory therapy and housekeeping. And still other task forces represented hospitalwide systems, such as telecommunications and material management. Task force reports were developed to describe the department or function as it existed, project where they wanted to be in 15 to 20 years, assess alternative structures to achieve their goals, and, finally, recommend one of those alternatives that the architect could later translate into a functional space program. A few of the task forces, such as the Burn Service Task Force, were short lived. It was determined that there was adequate burn service coverage in the Bay Area and, therefore, it was unnecessary to include it in this project. Other task forces, such as the Patient Bed Task Force, were essential in determining the composition and distribution of the patient bed units.

We also set up feedback sessions that involved parents and patients. In addition there was a group of physician papers that came out of the School of Medicine. The dean of the School of Medicine required that each of his service chiefs provide the same kind of assessment as the task force reports of where they were, where they wanted to be, and how they were going to get there. We also had a financial consultant who tied together all of these papers with an ongoing feasibility model and decisions back into an operating financial model.

The importance of these exercises was not only to provide the architect a foundation for the programming and design efforts, but also to set up a basis for internal decision making and for the ability to revisit, reverify, or update the decision. I'm proud to say that we continue to refer to the task force reports and that the vast majority of those conclusions remain valid.

A List of Preventive Measures

We also developed a serious list of preventive measures. I already talked a little bit about advance planning by the owner. At the risk of being self-serving, I think it's very important for the owners to have someone like myself who's familiar with the field, either with the programming or planning or with the design and construction area. It's important for the owner to plan for the planning, assemble information, and set up a format that will allow that information continually to be used and drawn upon.

We made over 35 site visits to hospitals in the United States, and some in Canada, to collect information. We visited and talked to our colleagues across the United States. We tried to learn from their successes and tried to avoid some of their failures.

It's important to set a realistic and complete budget. If it is an early or preliminary budget, it's important to include a contingency. The feasibility study has to be tied into an operational financial model, so that as decisions are made about space and staffing, it's tied into some piece of reality.

It's also important to set a realistic schedule and to allow for delays, and it's particularly important to allow for internal reviews and decisions. Often, we'll slap a schedule on an architect and expect the schedule to stay on track, even though we may take six weeks to turn around a decision on design.

It's important to streamline the process as much as possible and delegate decision making to individuals and committees, as appropriate. To this end, we had a design committee as we got further into the design and a construction committee during the construction.

It's important to understand the regulatory process. Planners have to be realistic about working with the various government agencies. Try to get them to feel like they are on the same side in solving problems. In this case, we made the decision not to go to bid until the drawings were signed and fully approved.

It's very important to assemble an effective team. Set up a good selection process, clarify the roles of team members, and establish the decision process. It's particularly important to have a key contact so that one is not getting mixed signals or allowing things to fall through. We also sought for and achieved early involvement of the landscape architect, interior designer, contractors, and engineers, so that these people weren't working at odds with each other. The contractor came in and did constructability analyses for us and value engineering. The engineers worked alongside the architects to produce a creative and artistic design.

It's also important to keep accurate records and files. Minutes should document all the attendees of the meetings and the conclusions made. Once again, I find myself in a situation that many architects and designers confront: The first three levels of management at Children's Hospital that were there at the beginning of the project have left. We have a new CEO, new administrative associates, and new assistant administrators; and something like 60 percent of the department heads have changed. Approximately 40 percent of the nursing staff has also changed. So, for protection, it's important to keep a record of how the decisions were made that allows one to return to those decisions. And it's important to have them signed-off on at every stage. I'm sure many architects and designers have experienced situations, as well, in which selective memories forget that they accepted a certain amount of square footage or a certain design scheme; and it's very important to be able to pull a signature out of the drawer that indicates otherwise.

It's also important to report to the board and keep it involved in the project on a timely basis. Derek is going to talk about this in more detail later, but we actually educated certain committees of the board so that at least we were speaking the same language and making our opinions on the same basis.

Last, it's important to maintain communications in reporting. In some of our contracts, we actually required that consultants have an exact model of a fax machine, which had an 11 by 17 capability. This allowed us to send submittals back and forth during construction and to send our design drawings back and forth during the design portion of the project.

At this point, I'm going to turn it back over to Derek who will talk about architectural programming.

Parker: My firm's first major work on this project was the piece called "architectural programming." When we were interviewed for this project, not having worked for Stanford before, I estimated this might take us 60 days. Those who knew Stanford just laughed. It actually took us about ten months to complete that first process. As Langston said, there are 35 task forces that are highly participatory organizations. It was very valuable for us to develop an understanding of those physician papers, to understand the program requirements, and to establish a realistic budget for the project. We also had the opportunity to tour existing facilities and saw many hospitals with a lot of good things. We saw Sesame Street characters on walls of many adult hospitals, but we didn't find a hospital that met our particular need and model. We saw hospitals that were terrifying for children and hospitals where families were excluded from the care of children. Those were all part of the learning process for our design committee of the board.

Developing a Common Vocabulary

A word that kept coming up as we talked over that ten-month period was "ambience." Initially, we didn't understand it except in a direct sense, but eventually we realized that the client wanted "architecture." Then we discovered that, together, we had a hard time defining architecture. The classical definition of Vitruvius that states architecture has three things: firmness, commodity, and delight was an inadequate guide. So we did something that we had never done before: We presented a short course on world architecture and throughout history so that, together, we as the architects and the board members, could develop a common vocabulary. We agreed that the building, to be architecture, should give us an emotional response; that our senses and feelings should be changed in some way; and if that didn't happen, we probably had just a building and we weren't dealing with architecture.

Together with the design committee, we analyzed our emotions and feelings and looked at things that gave us a sense of awe. We looked at places like the Piazza del Campo in Sienna that gave us a sense of belonging to something larger than ourselves. We looked at protection in a small Japanese alpine village; and we looked at buildings of power and authority, deciding that they were something we wanted to avoid if possible. We studied architecture, in both its abstract and concrete forms. In the abstract, we looked at nine characteristics, including functionalism. What is more functional than a bridge? What better example than our own Golden Gate Bridge right here in San Francisco that is not only a wonderful bridge as a function, but is also a marvelous piece of architecture and, in fact, defines San Francisco Bay.

We looked at rhythm and used the Sydney Opera House in Australia as an example. We looked at color and texture and discovered how American and English architects are a little frightened of color. We don't have quite the same verve as our Hispanic colleagues nor the inclination of architects in India to create buildings that have color and texture.

We looked at concrete elements in the work of two well-known architects, American Lou Kahn in Philadelphia and Englishman James Sterling in London. We saw how several of their buildings dealt with issues like circulation, services, and natural daylight. And we looked at one building by Lou Kahn, the Salk Institute in La Jolla, California, and saw how he defined a central space of sky, water, and travertine between two laboratory wings.

Certain things were already in place that we had to recognize. We'd already talked about children. At this point, we thought we knew quite a bit about children. Stanford is a well-established university with a very strong architectural identity. The characteristics of the Medical Center were there for us to recognize. After we had spent ten months developing the program, their influence was already on our palette. We just had to recognize it and utilize it to our benefit.

Stanford has this wonderful Mediterranean character in its architecture, which is appropriate to the dry, arid, warm climate of the San Francisco peninsula. The site adjacent to the Medical Center, plus the expansion of the Medical Center, boasted winds from the north in winter and from the southwest in summer. There was a Medi-Vac helicopter combing a wide path across the site, some beautiful oak trees, and a sharply indented site caused by building an adjacent medical office.

As we developed the program, going from the reports and papers that Langston talked about through the interview process into a draft program, we were beginning to understand the building. We realized that it was going to have more space on the first floor than on the second floor, and more on the second floor than on the third floor, which gave us an opportunity for terracing.

We looked at terraced buildings, again, from all over the world. The Law Court Building in Vancouver by Arthur Erickson is a fine example of how the terrace is a strong part of the architecture. Also, we recognized that we had the opportunity for hanging gardens so, believe it or not, we went all the way back to Babylon and looked at how hanging gardens have been treated since those times—even looking at a small residential development in London as an example.

Guidelines for Design

At the end of this three-hour course on architecture throughout history and from around the world, Mrs. Packard said, as did other members of the board, "That's very interesting; now what do we do with it?" What I suggested was that we start to design. By now we'd been working on this project for about 15 to 18 months and we still hadn't drawn a line. "And as we design," I instructed them, "don't say 'I like or I don't like.' Rather, pause for a moment and use some of the words we've learned together: What's the scale of the building? Do I like the color and texture of the building? Is it appropriate for the context of the Stanford University campus?" And out of that process, we developed some guidelines which, ultimately, as Felicia will illustrate for us, evolved into six principles that drove the development of the architectural design.

In character, we were looking for something that was noninstitutional. We had a strong reaction to the Capitol building in Washington. We wanted something with a reduced scale. We wanted something to intensify feelings and develop confidence that this was the best place to be. As an aside, I want to mention that one of the most important conversations I had for getting a sense of this building was a conversation with a pediatric oncologist at UC, San Francisco, Dr. Arthur Ablin. I said "Art, I'm doing this project at Stanford. What is the best way to approach it?" He told me, "First, try to generate a sense of *confidence* for patients; that there is no better place to be than where they are. Second, convince them that they are going to be dealt with as *human beings*; they are not a research statistic or medical record. And, third, convey to patients that the hospital is going to deal with them *honestly*. If you can communicate those three feelings in the building, then you'll be helping me as a physician to do my job," he said.

We decided that we wanted a feeling of honesty in the building for patients and families, and assurance that they would be kept well informed (see Figure C–10). We wanted to stimulate the sense of sight, with views and color. For hearing, we wanted music, as well as water—flowers and textures for smell and touch.

Scale is extremely important (and now we could use that word with the design committee)—the scale of the village, surprise, intimacy, and interest; we were looking for something that was nonmonumental and would provide distraction through displays of artwork.

Since children's stays in the hospital are often long term, we paid significant attention to the development of individuality. Although we didn't invent the art cart (it was something we found on one of our trips in a hospital), our children will be able to select decorations and artwork for their rooms from a cart and supplies provided by the hospital. We also wanted to diffuse the dividing line between the outside and the inside, and we wanted special continuity of materials, vision, views, and outside vegetation.

These guidelines, of which I've just mentioned a few, were developed into the six themes that we agreed with the design committee would be our guideposts for alternative designs for the project. These included how to approach the building, how to enter it, the distinction between the inside and the outside, how to individualize the patient's room, how to provide areas for decompression for parents and staff away from the tense treatment and clinical areas, and how to provide the appropriate level of distraction for children of all ages.

Approaching the Hospital

The approach to the Medical Center is extremely busy. We wanted children to have a different entrance; so we designed an entrance to Children's Hospital that is much quieter, much smaller in scale, but still maintains the important connection to the resources of the University Medical Center, which are available to children.

As one approaches the building on an axis, it starts with oak trees, continues to a drop-off point, a garden and terraces, an interactive piece of sculpture and water at the drop-off area, and ends with the building taking an embracing form. We extended the wings out in a welcoming way and presented a small-scale terraced entrance, a fragmented arrangement of canopies, playrooms, and gardens, intended to be like transparent toy blocks (see Figure C–11). The reduction in scale assists in diminishing the level of anxiety experienced as one approaches a large healthcare facility.

Second, we wanted a gentle entrance. The child enters the building through a highly transparent membrane into a lobby that is very small; it's low-ceilinged, almost residential in scale, and overlooks a magnificent garden. It clearly says, "Here somebody cares." Primary circulation on all floors is arranged around that garden, which is a strong reference point. The garden is asymmetrical to help people maintain that orientation. Destination and waiting areas are signaled by the use of nodes in the circulation system, with emphasis on color, change of proportions, and ceiling light.

A computer study of that main garden allowed us to look at its scale and the energy conservation of the shading required for windows. The landscape architects also used this study for the appropriate selection of vegetation for sunny and shady areas.

Felicia will now explain the remainder of the principles and the details of the design itself.

Cleper-Borkovi: The third theme is the nurturing interior. The stepped toy block arrangement of playrooms, canopies, and terraces changes as one enters the building into a curved linear space that evolved from the central garden. The garden brings in daylight, movement, change, and a sense of detail. It also brings in the energizing smell of spring, conveying a sense of freedom in a protected way. It answers the human need to be active, breathe fresh air, be comfortable, and get oriented.

Sinuous forms of the landscape penetrate the building and give shape to walls, columns, ceilings, furniture, artwork, and interior finishes (see Figure C–12). The round shape is poetic, calming, sheltering, and fun, and also connotes the protectiveness of the mother's breast and feeding spoon.

The individualized patient room is the universe of the sick child. It was designed to allow each child to have his or her parents sleeping nearby. The room reflects a balance between privacy and supervision—playful and quiet, personalized and repetitive, with both order and freedom. When in bed, the child may watch a continuously changing light show as the daylight is filtered in through window shutters and reflected on the walls and ceiling. The shutters, which are operated from the inside, also provide a constantly changing exterior appearance that further deinstitutionalizes the building.

The decompression zone allows parents to get out of the highly stressful environment. The building provides numerous indoor and outdoor decompression zones such as the lobby, lounges, libraries, sleep quarters, and terraces and alcoves of all sizes, which give parents an option for either socializing or privacy. The roof terrace, in particular, is where parent and child can take a long continuous walk.

One of the six guiding design principles was to create distraction through art and artifacts. The interior architecture was designed to be light, warm, simple, and neutral: a timeless background for changing colorful elements such as toys, art, graphics, and displays. No age-specific imagery was used, allowing interpretation of nonfigurative art at varying levels of sophistication. With abstract patterns, from finishes to artwork, the child, we believe, can create his or her own images, weaving his or her imagination with light and shadows.

Guided Tour of the Building

I'll now give a tour of the building to illustrate both the integration of the six guiding design principles and the continuity between the exterior and the interiors, since it is our belief that the building exterior and its interior should work together hand in hand to complement each other.

The first floor is the entrance floor, which is gentle, gradual, and transparent. From the lobby, one travels in two directions: to the clinics, including a day hospital, or to inpatient admitting, administrative areas, an auditorium, and an outdoor amphitheater. Ambulatory care is a dominant function of the first floor. There are five clinical modules that include primary care, oncology, hematology, orthopedic, allergy, pulmonary, miscellaneous subspecialties, and the day hospital.

The design concern on the first floor was to give the outpatient a sense of discovery and detail upon repeated visits to the hospital. The main spine that connects the entrance on a diagonal with the core of the clinic represents an excellent opportunity for a dynamic interior space; again, the garden is the central point of reference. The first floor is about indoor and outdoor continuity.

The ground floor is mostly for support functions, such as medical records and a clinical lab. It also includes the dietary department and a coffee shop.

The second floor's primary circulation, as on every other floor, occurs around the main garden, with nodes along the primary circulation to mark the occurrence of key functions. This floor is the intensive care floor, which has five distinct units, each with its own point of entry: pediatric intensive care unit, pediatric intermediate intensive care unit, compromised host, labor and delivery, and the neonatal intensive care unit. It also includes the anesthesia, pre- and postop, and support functions, such as a pharmacy and respiratory therapy. The decompression zones are particularly needed on this floor, as the stress level is very high, and they have courtyards and alcoves, as well as terraces.

The challenge on the second floor was to provide continuity of circulation between the new Children's Hospital and Stanford Medical Hospital. The surgery department is in the main hospital. It was decided later on in the process to include the labor and delivery function on the Children's Hospital floor, in close proximity to the neonatal intensive care unit, so mothers and children can be together.

The third floor contains the acute care nursing unit, and it's divided by age groups into infant, toddler, school-age, adolescent, and the psychosomatic unit. The unit has been planned for modularity and flexibility to accommodate a fluctuating patient population. This floor also has courtyards, terraces, parent support, and shared recreation areas. There is a school, as well as an occupational therapy department, which share a terrace. Unlike the second floor where there are five different units, the units on the third floor have more interaction and, consequently, there is a greater degree of consistency in their appearance.

The roof terrace provides, as I mentioned before, long continuous walks and beautiful panoramic views. It is from the roof terrace that I look down and watch the construction being completed, wishing that the new Children's Hospital at Stanford will have the likeness and joyousness of springtime that never lets anyone suspect the labor it has cost.

The interior designers were responsible for the development of all the interior architectural elements of the building, including ceiling articulation, lighting concepts, finishes, and case work design. We were very fortunate to have been involved so early in the project, even as the departmental planning was occurring, and that this early involvement allowed us to develop a fully integrated environment where all the parts and pieces work in harmony for a consistent end.

I'll now turn it over to Diana to discuss the interior design details.

Kissil: In developing the interior design, we, of course, followed the guidelines that have already been discussed. In addition, we had four particular objectives: to create a comfortable, nontrendy color palette; to develop a system of orientation throughout the hospital; to create a system to organize all the elements, such as nurse call lights, cart racks, and signage, that inevitably are an integral part of the hospital environment; and to create a "patient-friendly" environment.

Four factors drove the development and selection of the color palette. First of all, there was an early and total consensus that we wanted a nontrendy environment that wouldn't look dated in terms of color. Second, we were aware of the importance of artwork as an element to provide distraction, as well as light. We wanted to maximize the visual impact of the artwork in the space. Third, in patient rooms, we wanted the elements that the children would be bringing into the environment, such as toys, artwork, and cards from friends, to be of primary importance in the room. And, fourth, we felt that strong colors were best located in the less permanent, more easily changeable elements, such as upholstery and cubicle curtains (see Figure C–13).

So, all this led to the development of a basically warm, neutral palette of beige tones. The primary finishes throughout the hospital are light-colored painted walls, carpet, and painted tile. A very important neutral element throughout the facility was anigre or maple wood. It is used on doors, handrails, case work trim, and most importantly, on flooring in patient rooms.

Pattern an Integral Element

Within the neutral palette, pattern is also an integral element. The general carpet is a combination of very small stripes. Part of the inspiration for that carpet was some of the children's artwork. In addition to pattern in the carpet, there were many areas that received a vinyl tile floor, where we created a subtle tone-on-tone neutral pattern for visual interest. To the basic neutral palette of paint, we added four accent colors of cranberry, blue, teal, and salmon. The colors, when placed on either architectural elements or floors, are done primarily to provide signaling devices. There are really only four hues that we used; however, the intensities of the hues are varied throughout the hospital.

The general circulation carpet is five-colors: accent-colors plus yellow stripe. Adjacent to it are what we call the signal carpets in high-intensity colors, which are used in very limited areas. Adjacent to those are what we call the departmental striped carpet. The sequence is always from general carpet to signal carpet, to the departmental carpet. In the general carpet, there is a small yellow stripe, which we included to provide sparkle and vibrancy to the palette. However, we also recognized that yellow was an impractical color in very large quantities. It tends to be a very difficult color to maintain, and it can adversely affect the color rendition of the patient's complexion, which would be difficult for diagnostic purposes. So, we used yellow only in small quantities, as in the carpet stripe, hardware accents, and some light fixtures.

The palettete is completed with the addition of upholstery fabrics that are also patterned, but again retain the basis of the four general accent colors. The specific color selections that were used were influenced by children's art. We spent a lot of time early in the project looking at art and realized that children have a great knack for combining colors in very unexpected and exuberant fashions. We found that they go far beyond just using primary colors out of the bottle and, in fact, more often than not, will create some very unusual, interesting combinations using secondary and even tertiary colors.

We limited ourselves to four accent colors, for a number of reasons. First, we knew, as anybody knows who deals with a hospital, that things inevitably get moved around in the course of operation. We wanted to be fairly sure that whatever was moved around would work with the other colors that it got put with. Second, we wanted to ease the maintenance and inventory problems that the hospital would run into if we had too many variations of color.

The paint colors are warm, neutral tones because we wanted to avoid a cold, icy environment. On the other hand, we made sure that they weren't too toned or too yellow, again so as not to affect adversely the coloration of patient skin tone. We did a full room mock-up of paint color after the lighting and building glazing was in, because we knew that the interior lighting and the coloration of glazing on the building would affect color rendition.

System of Orientation

To develop a system of signaling and orientation, we looked for opportunities on all surfaces: ceilings, walls, and floors. It was important to identify major destinations and decision making points, such as elevators, departmental entries, and nurse stations. We used architectural devices, as well as color. We recessed departmental entries from the main circulation with a graceful curve that leads into the entry, created a special design for the doors, and placed a series of glass side lights adjacent to the door so that it is very clear that this is a destination point and the waiting room is visible. It's also nice for the people in the waiting room to be able to see activity in the corridor.

The second floor, mentioned before, contains the critical care unit; a high-stress area. Departmental entries on this floor are more quiet, more subtle. Again, we curved the walls into these departments, created special departmental doors, and installed a series of wood patterns on the wall to serve as an identification device for the entrance to a department.

The third floor is a more active floor, so the departmental entry itself is more playful, more active. I neglected to point out that on the second floor there are special things going on with ceilings, too. On the third floor, there are skylights; on the second floor there are a series of stepped-up ceilings that occur at the departmental entry. The carpet diagram for the third floor demonstrates how the main circulation carpet and the signal carpet of the departmental entry work with the ceiling treatment.

There is also, of course, the issue of signage. A signage designer was hired very early on in the project and worked with the entire team. We ended up with a very quiet signage design. It is for informational purposes, rather than being a design element unto itself. We did pick up some playfulness in terms of the face for the tops that are reminiscent of some of the forms occurring in the architecture of the building.

Our effort to create a system of organizing what sometimes looks like a lot of junk in a hospital corridor was successful. A typical patient corridor has door surrounds that are made with an extra layer of heat rocks. They provide a location for anchoring the nurse call light, signage, as well as a location for the children's art or messages. It forms a nice live-in consistency and a sense of identification for the room.

Creating a Patient-Friendly Environment

I have already mentioned that wood is important in terms of adding a depth enricher for the neutral palette; but we wanted a lot of wood in this space also because of its warmth and because it's a familiar, homelike material. Following that philosophy, we also avoided the use of chrome and cold metal. Furniture is primarily wood, or where we do have metal, it's typically a colored, powder coated finish.

The creation of a patient-friendly environment goes far beyond the finishes, and we took a lot of care to look at the world of the patient room (see Figure C–14). In two-bed rooms, we created zones between one patient area and the second patient area. Both of them have a sleep sofa for the parents to spend the night, which also provides a second zone in the room for the child to go to, a place beyond their bed that they can be with their parents or just occupy themselves. In addition there's a desk area on the other side of the bed to provide a place for parents or children to study, read, or write. Either patient can get to the toilet room without having to interfere with or enter the zone of the second patient. At the entry to the patient room, the sink forms another neutral zone.

We also tried to break down the barrier between the nurses' station and the patient room. Half-round, cut-out windows are placed in the nurses' station so that children can come up and see the nurses. Every nurses' station has a 30-inch high round table where children can sit, perhaps to draw, or do a puzzle. It provides them another place to interface with staff so that extensive friendliness and care develops.

We also created storage for patient rooms. There's storage underneath the parents' bed; at the side of the bed is a wardrobe area, and there is a series of shelves opposite the patient's bed.

In single-bed patient rooms, which most of the rooms are, we tried to provide lots of amenities. At the back of the room there is a very large window. It's actually a raised ceiling with indirect light. To one side of the patient's sleep/storage area, there is a whiteboard that provides a place for the child to write or draw. It can also be a place for the doctor to write or diagram something. On the other side of the bed, there are open bookshelves for storage of books, or whatever the child might bring into the room. Opposite the patient's bed, there's another storage wall done in wood with a plastic laminate top. It has a tack surface and a series of open shelves, which we really tried to maximize to provide a lot of storage for the child, just as they might have in their own rooms. I should also mention that the floor is wood, which creates quite a different atmosphere in the room.

Finally, I want to talk about the cafeteria downstairs. Again, we used a lot of wood flooring. The ceiling steps up to a skylight. There's also indirect colored lights, lots of wall space, artwork, and glass that opens up to another garden area. A typical exam treatment room utilizes a pattern within a standard neutral-on-neutral vinyl tile floor. We dropped 12 by 12 tiles, kind of helter-skelter almost, in a confettilike fashion, that are playful to view as one enters the room. A lot of color was put into cubicle curtains, furnishings, light board mirrors, and also on mobiles and other active distracting sculptures in the room.

Derek will now give closing remarks.

Parker: The total project cost was almost $100 million. I think we built, for an average cost, an extraordinary hospital. Like several projects presented at the Third Symposium, this project illustrates that good humane design does not have to be that expensive.

We've talked a great deal about concept and processes but, most important, I think we were fortunate on this project to share a common vision. In addition to her generous donation, Mrs. Packard envisioned a building that served the children, the parents, and the staff. She was thinking about a building that could simultaneously provide high touch and high tech. That vision was shared by the Board, project staff, architect, interior designer, landscape architect, and even the engineers and contractor. You could go out there during the construction and find several of the construction workers wearing hospital T-shirts. This commonly shared vision has made a real difference in achieving a healthcare breakthrough.

To summarize, we have learned that children's memories are seldom of adults, that they are most often of places and related sensations, and that is why we have designed the Children's Hospital at Stanford as a building with doves on the roof and geraniums in the window.

Children's Voices: I think the new Children's Hospital should have a window on the roof, with a place to enter. It should have a garden with trees, flowers, a butterfly, birds, a pond so a duckling can fit in it, a garden on the roof, a flat roof so the garden could fit on it, and one balcony. And when I'm in the garden, I should be able to say, "Am I in or am I out?" And then, when I'm in my room, I would like to have my mommy's hand and my teddy bear, and I would like a shelf behind me with flowers, books, toys, and a television, and when the doctor comes in, I would like him to wear a clown suit and make me laugh.

The hospital should be painted all white and it shouldn't have that emergency sign to scare someone. And it should have in big rainbow letters the name, New Children's Hospital at Stanford.

Felicia Cleper-Borkovi, AIA, is a senior associate at Anshen + Allen Architects in San Francisco, California. In charge of the Art in Architecture program at the firm, she has completed projects at St. Joseph's Medical Center, Clovis Community Hospital, and the Lucile Salter Packard Children's Hospital at Stanford.

Diana Kissil, AIA, is an architect who has specialized in interior design for 16 years, with substantial experience in healthcare. She is currently director of interior design of Anshen + Allen Architects in San Francisco.

Derek Parker, FAIA, RIBA, is chairman of Anshen + Allen Architects in San Francisco. An internationally recognized expert in the architectural design of healthcare facilities, Parker has designed and planned almost 50 major hospitals, diagnostic care centers, hospices, and medical research institutes in his 30 years with the firm.

Langston Trigg, Jr., AIA, former project director at Stanford University in Palo Alto, California, is the director of facilities planning for Kaiser Permanente in Oakland.

◆ ◆ ◆

WITH CHILDREN IN MIND: NOVEL APPROACHES TO WAITING AREA AND PLAYROOM DESIGN

Third Symposium on Healthcare Design, San Francisco, CA, 1990

Anita Rui Olds, Ph.D.

By training, I am a developmental and environmental psychologist and not a designer. However, for the past 20 years, by some strange quirk of circumstance, I have found myself designing waiting and playroom areas for pediatric facilities.

I invite you for a moment to close your eyes, appreciate the sound of birds chirping, and just relax. Perhaps you can picture a setting where you are surrounded by these beautiful creatures. Think back to a time when you were a child; your age then doesn't matter. Visualize yourself at some time when you were a child. Remember the kinds of things you liked to do, play with, or places you liked to go. Really hold that in your heart for a moment.

Now recall a time, maybe the first time, when you went to see a doctor, or when you went to a healthcare facility. Just recall what such a visit was like for you, as a little one. How did you feel? Think about your body posture and the tension you may have felt. Hold on to that thought for a moment. Then hold both the feeling of being in a wonderful place doing things that you really enjoyed, together with your feelings connected with illness, injury, and healthcare. Experience both sets of feelings simultaneously. Then, when you feel ready, open your eyes and come back into the present.

What you just visualized, the inner child, is the point at which we need to start in designing healthcare spaces for children. Unlike design approaches to other healthcare spaces, when it comes to children, we have to put aside many of the customary "designer" rules and trends and ask ourselves, "Does this feel right? Would I, as a child, have really appreciated this?" If that is hard to do, then go out and find some children to be with and ask them questions. Let the design spring from the child's perspective, because the needs of children are very different from those of adults—perhaps more so these days than ever before. I don't have to cite the cases of abuse, stress, and tension that children are experiencing today, even those who are not in healthcare centers.

What we are seeking to preserve is the spirit of the child. The spirit of the child contains a sense of wonder, a sense of openness, trust, and responsiveness—an ability simply to "be." This gets shut down very quickly if the openness and trust are violated.

The literal meaning of the word "architecture" is "to use material to make the ideal manifest." In a sense, it is the task of the architect or designer to bring heaven to earth. This means that we have to ask ourselves, "What is heaven? What are the ideals, in terms of children, that we are seeking to manifest and create for them?" And we need to strive continually for those ideals, even if they differ from current political and economic policies.

The most basic law of psychology says that action follows thought. This has two consequences in designing children's healthcare facilities. First, if action follows thought, the healing process in a child will be very dependent upon what the child thinks. If the child thinks he or she is going to get well and everything around communicates that possibility, then it is very likely that healing will result. The second consequence is that designers' actions also follow their thoughts. So as designers, we must be very clear about our thoughts and goals for children in healthcare contexts.

For children, whose sensibilities are so refined and who are responding as sensory motor beings to everything in their environment, the medium is indeed the message. The environment is their food and nourishment. Everything in it matters. It communicates something about who they are, where they are, what they can do, and what their potential may be.

To heal means to make whole. Children are naturally very whole beings and have a very intuitive sense of unity with all things. Children come to a healthcare setting because there has been a breach in the integrity of their wholeness. The designer's task is therefore to create a context of greater wholeness such that it uplifts and encourages children to return to a state of wellness once again. Since healing ultimately occurs from within, a healthcare environment can be maximally effective when it affirms the capacity of children to heal themselves.

In my experience, environments that best help children to heal are those that are very homelike, soft, and familiar. It goes without saying that few hospitals have these qualities. However, to make a healthcare setting truly appropriate for children, it is necessary that designers sometimes do things contrary to their typical design practice. These contrary approaches are essential for the spirit and healing of children. They are also essential for adults; but sometimes the needs of children will be heard, whereas those of adults are ignored.

Environments are always experienced mentally and emotionally. Keynote speaker George Leonard touched upon this the other night when he said, "For every thought there is a feeling, there is an emotion." Research being done on the immunological system suggests that it is intimately linked to the emotional system and that people who are calm and emotionally in balance are less susceptible to illness and heal faster. To the degree that an environment helps someone stay calm and centered, it is directly affecting the immunological system and the person's capacity to get well and stay well.

People's emotional needs are addressed by the aesthetic richness of a space. Particularly in the case of children, we need to conceive of all the elements in the room as artistic, interactive surfaces. This includes floors, walls, ceilings, horizontal and vertical supports, objects, forms, and architectural details. Anything can be a surface to explore with the hands or eyes. Anything can be a toy, a table, a seat, a wall, a divider, or a place to lie down. The challenge is to stop thinking in terms of standard definitions of walls, furniture, and play objects and to start thinking in terms of the movements and activities children enjoy.

For example, walls can support natural and manmade textures, mirrors, light-reflecting surfaces, play panels, vertically mounted toys, grab bars, three-dimensional murals, and things at many different heights. Play panels can function as walls and low dividers, creating spaces. Building off a wall horizontally can create seats, tables, counters, high and low platforms, and angled and varied work and sitting surfaces. All the horizontal surfaces in a room, including floors and ceilings, can be lowered or raised, hard or soft, textured or smooth, solid or slatted, flat, inclined, or wavy. They can include water mattresses, air mattresses, sacks of bean bag pellets, trampolines, nets, suspension bridges, and a wide range of resilient and varied materials. Introducing variety and detail in all these dimensions creates rich and meaningful environments for children.

Rich, meaningful, playful interiors are those that are sculpted, painted, draped, and molded much the way artists paint, sculpt, and mold wood, clay, canvas, or fibers, colors, and forms. Ultimately, the environment should provide the potential for interaction at every turn. These need not be powerful interactions but ones where something happens, where there are interesting objects to look at, unexpected surprises of light and shadow, sound, warmth, and color, nooks and crannies, things that respond, and things that smell or feel inviting.

Feeling and touch, the texture of objects and the interior materials, are especially important for young children. The skin is the largest organ of the body. It is likely that we receive more information through our skin than through our eyes or ears. The younger the child, the greater his or her need to be touched and held and to feel the texture of things—many children simply love rubbing soft materials under their noses. It is not sufficient that the textures just be visual—they must be tactile, so children can interact with them at a motor level.

Four Environmental Criteria

There are four things that children, as well as adults, need in relationship to the environment. (I was pleased to hear Dr. Roger Ulrich mention very similar needs in his presentation earlier at the Symposium.) These are: the need to move about in space, the need to feel comfortable, the need to feel competent, and the need to feel in control.

1. *Movement:* When things move, it is a sign of life; when they cease to move, they are dead. When creatures and people move in an easy and fluid way it is a sign of good health and well-being. Movement is the primary way that children learn: They are constantly climbing, crawling, and moving through space, using their bodies and their large motor abilities to interact with the world. Unfortunately, adults dislike such motion and, in general, try to stop it. In healthcare settings, children's movement is further constrained due to illness, disability, or hospital protocol that says patients must stay in chairs or beds. But, movement is essential to children's development, whether they are sick or well. So, our greatest design challenge is to maximize the capacity of children to move freely about in a healthcare setting while making this movement tolerable to all.

2. *Comfort:* When people are sick, they look for a comfortable place to be. Yet, I doubt that anyone would choose to go to a healthcare facility in order to be comfortable. Curiously, ill people need comfortable surroundings that healthcare facilities rarely provide. Comfort depends upon movement, but at the sensorial rather than the large motor level. Our senses operate by moving and responding to changing stimulation in the environment. For example, our eyes see because they scan a visual field; our ears hear because they pick up vibrating air waves that cause the ear drum to vibrate. Interestingly, we spend most of our time in a static built environment where nothing changes. Yet, to be physiologically comfortable and maintain an optimal state of alertness, the body requires moderate changes in sensory stimulation that produce a quality of "difference within sameness." Nature produces excellent examples of settings that provide such difference-within-sameness, or moderate degrees of variety. For example, a fire is a fire, but every once in a while there is a flicker or flare that causes it to change; a breeze may waft warm then cold. The combination of moving elements that are predictable yet vary because of a subtle degree of difference within the sameness is the key to creating comfortable settings in the built world.

3. *Competence:* Dr. Ulrich spoke about the need for distraction in healthcare settings. I agree with this concept, but satisfying the need for competence goes a bit further than distraction. Certainly it is good to have things to look at that will take a patient's mind off pain. But children also need a sense of mastery, a sense of their ability to try something new or do something well today that they could barely do at all yesterday. They need to have a sense of doing meaningful things during the long hours spent in a healthcare facility. Adults need this feeling of competence as well, particularly parents, who require more than a two-month old magazine to read while waiting. For children to experience a sense of competence, they must have real toys with genuine play value in an ordered and comprehensible environment. Single items and toys are insufficient. Rather, the entire context must communicate to children a sense of their own self-worth and ability to interact with and explore everything that is in the environment.

4. *Control:* In healthcare facilities, patients usually experience a loss of control and of opportunities for self-help and -care. They also experience a loss of control over levels of privacy and community. Yet, being able to control encounters and personal space are vital to one's sense of well-being. Because of the recent concern about abuse, children are now forced to have adults around them at all times and can rarely be alone or have much privacy. A study at Children's Hospital in Boston, Massachusetts, many years ago indicated that within the first 24 hours of admission, the average child was seen by 100 different people. This kind of public exposure is extremely stressful and intimidating. We need to create circumstances that allow children in healthcare settings to have some control over their lives.

Some of this control depends on the orientation of one's body in space, especially the position of one's back. It is rare to see a human being standing still in the midst of a big open space for very long. Instead, people prefer to stand with their backs against a wall, a tree, or a bench so they have protection from the rear. Since we don't have eyes in the backs of our heads and cannot see what is coming from behind, it is safest to have something very solid at our backs. This gives us the ability to look at and listen to whatever is approaching head on. Protection at our backs makes us feel secure.

In most rooms, there is usually one area (generally a corner) that is more protected than any other. If the room is a classroom or a therapist's or doctor's office, that is where the teacher's or doctor's desk will be. The person who owns the space puts themselves in the most protected place. As a consequence, students, visitors, and clients who meet with them across the desk, have to sit with their backs to the door, feeling very exposed and vulnerable.

For most clients, especially children, it is important that furniture be arranged so they can feel safe and secure by having their backs face a wall or the protected zone. This is especially true for the placement of beds in patient rooms. There is no time during this presentation to talk about the issues of layout and the placement of furniture and activities in the exposed and protected zones of a room. However, there are general principles of layout that significantly affect the success or failure of a design. Chapters 1, 16, and 24 in *Child Health Facilities: Design Guidelines, Literature Outline*, a book I wrote for the Association for the Care of Children's Health, outlines many of the principles in detail.

Six Types of Activities

Six different types of activities should be present in all waiting or play spaces for children. All ages require: (1) *quiet activities,* such as reading books, listening to stories, and playing with puzzles or small toys; (2) *large motor activities,* such as sliding, climbing, swinging, and crawling; (3) *craft activities,* and opportunities to impose their own structure on materials such as paint, clay, water, and sand; (4) opportunities for *dramatic play,* such as playing house, using miniatures or puppets, dressing up in costumes, face painting, or pretending; (5) opportunities to play *games,* from simple board games to sophisticated computer games; and, where appropriate, (6) opportunites for *therapeutic activities.* (For example, a cerebral palsied child who has a hard time sitting up should be placed in a chair or adaptive device that supports the spine and helps the child to exercise and gain greater control over his or her body. Similarly, we designed a six-foot-long easel that the chief of cardiology found very therapeutic for postoperative open heart surgery children who are fearful of moving their thoracic areas but need to do so in order to heal. As children paint and reach across the big easel, they spontaneously stretch the chest area.)

In addition to these six types of activities, certain ages require special facilities. For example, infants need spaces where they can crawl, lie down, and be up high at adult eye level, to get a better view of the whole room. Toddlers, who love to toddle, need an "open corral," a large space that has changes in level and is soft and safe. Teenagers, an increasing population in healthcare, love to cook, eat food, listen to music, play all kinds of games, and lounge.

Ideally, opportunities for each of these types of activities need to be present in every play or waiting space for children, even if the space is small. A small space requires careful planning to make every cubic inch count, like designing for a boat or an airplane. Custom designs are often required both to optimize space usage, and because appropriate products are not usually available on the market.

Project Case Studies

I am now going to discuss some of the projects I have had an opportunity to work on. However, understand that the kinds of things I am going to talk about are not standard practice in pediatric design, although they certainly should be. So often, hospitals will spend $100 million to design a beautiful building and purchase state-of-the-art technology; but when it comes to outfitting the waiting rooms, lobbies, and playrooms for children, there is no money left. I usually get called in after a project is completed, when the hospital realizes the space is not supporting children sufficiently.

This situation needs to be changed. When working with clients, designers need to make it clear from the outset that waiting and play spaces are important enough to be part of the overall budget. Healthcare providers, in turn, have to put pressure on designers to ensure that their budgets and plans include provisions for a highly differentiated space with opportunities for quiet play, gross motor play, dramatic play, crafts, and so on. This presentation carries with it a special request: I ask that, when designing children's environments, you be willing to invest more energy and go to greater extents than you might ordinarily, so that the level of detail and thoughtfulness I am about to discuss becomes standard practice and is considered customary in settings for children.

Children's Hospital, Washington, D.C.

1. *Cardiology Playroom:* When I first saw the cardiology playroom at Children's Hospital National Medical Center in Washington, D.C., the room had lots of light, and was eventually to have bright colors, plus some tables and chairs. In addition, the architect had specified a metal cabinet that he felt was sufficient for water play and storage. It was, in fact, a tall, inappropriate metal chemistry lab cabinet.

We began re-designing this space by identifying activities and breaking it into different areas (see the planning and design chapters in my book), so that there would be separate areas for messy play, quiet play, seating, dramatic play, and the like. Although the room was to be for children from infants through teenagers—too broad an age range for one space—it was all that was available for play for all ages.

A four-inch high manipulative play platform has a panel that can be installed to close it off and convert it into a giant playpen, if needed. The beauty of the platform is that the storage is built into the playing surface and it allows several children—even a few adults—to sit and play with small toys in a protected area where they will not be stepped on by people coming through the room.

Beyond the manipulative platform is a banquette. It is a place to sit and

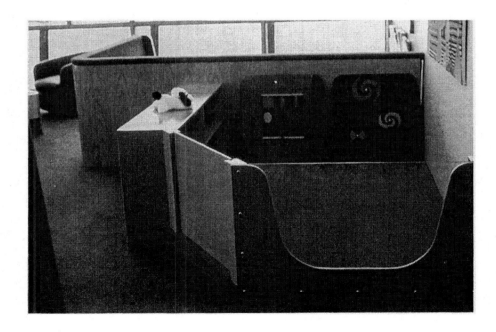

◆ **FIGURE 6–1**   The manipulative play platform has a panel that can be installed to close it off and convert it into a giant playpen, if needed. (*Project:* Cardiology playroom, Children's Hospital National Medical Center, Washington, DC. *Design:* Anita Olds and Associates. *Photo:* Anita Rui Olds.)

look out the large windows, to lie down, and to cuddle. It is also a place where teenagers can turn their backs to the room so they are not intimidated by the things for younger children. When I initially proposed upholstering this banquette with cushions, the client said, "Oh no; pillows will be stolen within a day." Knowing, however, that softness is extremely important, I said, "Okay, we'll have the pillows and we'll also carpet the banquette so if the pillows are taken, there will still be something soft to sit on." Four-and-a-half years later, I returned to the hospital and found that seven of the original nine throw pillows were still there. One had been stolen by a workman before the hospital even opened. The other one, for all I know, could have been around somewhere. The point I had made to the client was that if a place is created that shows tremendous care for people, they will, in turn, respond by caring for the place. The fact that those pillows, which easily could have been taken, had stayed there for four-and-a-half years, is testimony to this.

The little table facing the banquette was originally designed as a footstool for an orthopedic clinic at Boston Children's where there was no place for someone with a cast on his or her foot to put it up to rest. It is also an end table and a game table. The top divides into two flaps that open up. Inside, there is a little trough where a game can be placed. If a child has to stop playing to see the doctor, the flaps can be closed up and the game resumed when the child returns.

The playframe is a four- by four-foot, eight-foot tall free-standing unit that has as many as 15 to 20 different panels that can be suspended from its sides to provide a range of interactive possibilities. One panel, called a "busy board," has many interactive devices mounted on its surface. Another panel is a house front. Other panels include a bean bag toss panel and a puppet counter.

A fiberboard barrel lined with fake fur and mylar can become a private bubble for a child. It has been Rapunzel's castle and Batman's cave, as well as a place to crawl inside for some much-needed privacy and time alone.

A tall white cabinet behind the barrel is for storage of staff materials. However, I have a rule that anything at child height should be child accessible. So the doors with mirrors on the lower portion of the cabinet open up to display dress-up clothes, hats, and masks for children to put on. Children can look at themselves in the mirrors and then play within the 16-square feet of the playframe, or throughout the room.

Some items on the busy board are marble spinners, lock boxes, standard kinds of hardware equipment, noise makers, and a threading toy. These busy boards are extremely attractive. However, designers should be aware that it is hard to find commercial toys that are durable for hospital use and that can function when mounted in a vertical orientation.

Water play troughs are at stand-up height and wheelchair height for a seated child. There is also a sink for staff. The mirrors behind the troughs are lexan and distort the image. It is much better to use tempered glass rather than lexan and is equally safe. Lexan scratches and fogs after a brief amount of time, while a tempered glass mirror lasts forever.

2. *General Medical Playroom:* The next room, for general medical patients from infancy to six years of age, had about 50 linear feet of glass from floor to ceiling, with an incredible view of the reservoir. It was important to maintain some sense of relationship with the outdoors, as well as provide comforting things for infants and toddlers, especially. A feature of the room was a water mattress with surrounding platforms at 5, 10, and 15 inches. None of these levels, therefore, is as high as a chair.

A number of studies indicate that premature babies raised on water mattresses mature significantly faster than those raised on a standard crib mattress. Many of the children using this room are failure-to-thrive and abused babies who need gentle sensory-motor stimulation. This was one reason for using the waterbed, as well as the fact that it is a nice soft place to sit and cuddle. The third is that parents in healthcare environments are often very tired and very stressed. Waterbeds are one of the few places upon which it is acceptable for an adult to recline in public.

When I first proposed to the client that we put in these levels around the mattress, they were very concerned about the safety of the children. They said, "What about these toddlers; won't they fall and get hurt?" I felt it was safer for toddlers to crawl over 5- and 10-inch high levels than to crawl on the tables and chairs, which they would use if no other options were available. The hospital was willing to risk putting this in to see how it would work. It has worked very well. For instance, a blind child learned to negotiate this room without any difficulty. The room subsequently became one of the showcase rooms of the hospital.

The room also has a "pit," formed by 12-inch high risers that enclose a space, where children can sit to read books or play with toys. It is often filled with pillows. People can sit on the risers or in the enclosure. This is also a place where babies can pull-up to stand and hold on to things as they walk about. While all the risers forming the pit can move, we designed one that was smaller and easier to move so that, for example, a child on an IV could be rolled in on his or her IV pole to sit inside with the other children.

Risers are a very useful device for defining space, establishing boundaries, creating sitting surfaces (for adults as well as children) and work surfaces for playthings and materials. They are a versatile way to deal with some of the design issues that come up in rooms like this.

We designed the wall-mounted cabinets, which were to hold the types of play materials that would be used, and insisted they be built of wood rather than laminate to soften and warm the environment as much as possible.

The water play troughs below the cabinets have covers so the troughs can be used as table and play surfaces as well. The Child Life worker controls access to the water by means of keyed turn-offs under the wheelchair trough. The orientation of these troughs—placed parallel to the wall—is poor, because it forces children to turn their backs to the room, an uncomfortable position. The mirror over the troughs is essential, therefore. It allows children to see what is happening behind them so that they feel more secure, and it becomes a surface that is fun to paint on or cover with soapsuds.

3. *Burn Playroom:* This room for severely burned patients, many of whom were in isolation under a tent, was originally not a very pleasant space. It was 10-foot wide and 20-foot long, surfaced entirely in vinyl, with poor natural light. Children receiving treatment in this room have tremendous pain and only come in one at a time. The staff wanted both a water mattress and a playframe for this room. Since there wasn't space to do both, we opted for the water mattress because it had been originally designed for burn patients in England. We put foam around the frame of the waterbed, then covered it with vinyl, and added a vinyl quilt and vinyl pillows so that everything was washable. The room also has a manipulative play area and a crafts area.

When we realized there was no place for a playframe, I got the idea that panels could be suspended from the wall instead of the frame. This is a less successful solution because it forces children to turn their backs to the room and loses the space-making properties of the frame. But when there is only one child in the room, it works fairly well. There is an easel panel, a blackboard panel, a mirror-and-sketch-pad panel so a child can look in the mirror and do a self-portrait; if the child is left handed, the whole thing can be turned upside down.

4. *Convalescing Burn Playroom:* This playroom, located at the end of two corridors, could not be blocked off because it provided access to bedrooms and exits. It was to be a playroom for convalescing burn children, many of whom may have been in isolation for one or two months and needed to be in the hospital for one or two months more until they were fully healed. Since most of the children were under three years of age, the nurses were concerned about them wandering down the corridors. We decided to design the furniture to orient the children toward the windows, with the corridors at their backs. One custom-designed piece of furniture was a small couch; something similar is now commercially available. Although children come to healthcare settings because they are ill, there are few places available in waiting rooms where they can lie down. The little couches were orginally designed for that purpose. Eventually, they were moved to the emergency room where they were extremely successful.

While we were struggling with this space, Respite Care took over the area, leaving the Child Life Department without a playroom for these burn patients who had been hospitalized for so long. We searched and searched this brand new building for an alternate playroom, but the only thing we could find was a 10- by 15-foot area in the corridor opposite the nurse station. A typical architectural solution for enclosing this corridor territory would have been to make floor-to-ceiling glass walls. However, these children had been isolated long enough and they needed protected exposure to activities within the building. So we designed a low, wavy wall as a partition.

The back wall of the room holds the storage cabinets for play materials; the doors of the lower sections come off so that children can have direct access to the materials. There are two tables that come down for crafts and meals and flip up securely at other times so that the floor area is cleared for wheeled toys and movement activities.

A modified playframe enclosing a play kitchen, was a critical design element because many of these children received their burns in their kitchens at home and need to work through that experience psychologically. We intentionally introduced a wooden textured roof here to offset the flat vinyl textures and bright colors of the corridor. When the low risers in this room were spread out to create levels varying by three inches in height, children were stimulated to start to move, which is what they needed so badly because of their long confinement.

The wavy wall is very much like a giant busy board. It has a racetrack panel with two cars on it, and some areas with Plexiglas lenses that children can look through to see the outside world in different colors, or multiplied by Fresnell lenses, or magnified. Children use it extensively and even moms enjoy coming there to play. These things encourage children to see variety and change by taking advantage of the movement down the corridor that happens outside the wall.

5. *Hemotology/Oncology Playroom:* The original hematology/oncology playroom, for children ages six through 12, many of whom are in various stages of dying, contained an awkward 4 1/2- by 10-foot space, as well as a wheelchair sink and chemistry lab cabinet. We replaced these sinks with a staff sink and a water play table in an appropriate perpendicular orientation to the wall. The messy play area included the water play table—with or without a cover—a low cabinet for crafts materials, a table to do art work on, and a place to tack up paintings. Because one door needed to remain closed, we used the wall behind it for an easel and a blackboard panel.

One morning, five boys ages 18 months to 10 years of age spent one hour and 20 minutes at this water play area. These children are very weak, and water is very soothing for them—even for a 10 year old, if given appropriate toys. I wonder what they would have done had it not been there.

We introduced carpet into this room because there was none and, in some cases, ran it up the wall to make the corner softer. There was not space to put a playframe in here, but we suspended panels perpendicular to the wall to create enclosed spaces. Eventually, the 4 1/2- by 10-foot space became the cozy corner with curved risers, pillows, book display, and shelves for manipulative toys. It was the only place of retreat in the room. Both this playroom and the one for convalescing burn patients are woefully inadequate amounts of space for the children they serve. The children deserve more than this. We tried to make maximal use of the little space there was.

6. *Hemotology/Oncology Clinic Waiting Area:* For the Hematology/Oncology Clinic waiting area, which most children come to prior to becoming inpatients, the design committee had selected cold, plastic furniture. When someone sits on the edge of it, it hits them on the back of the head. It looks to me like a toilet bowl. In redesigning this room, we put in soft furniture, without arms, so people could stretch out. Many Hem/Onc patients are extremely weak and tired. Although necessary for sitting, the waiting area included couches because many diverse needs must be served in most patient areas.

We also installed a playframe, an art table, and a waterbed in this waiting room. The day I took photos of it, the waterbed was unused because it had a leak. The night custodial staff had left a Coke-can metal tab on the mattress, which had fallen through and sliced the water sack. Fortunately, this would not have happened today because waterbeds have a different construction. A tape recorder is built into the frame of the water mattress so that children can lie there and listen to stories or tapes. The room also has a manipulative play platform and an area called an "exploratorium." The exploratorium was an attempt to provide interesting things to observe and handle that would not be taken from the room. It has a Speak and Spell device; a marble maze; a microscope through which children can look at slides that tell them about their bodies; a kaleidoscope; and a magnet art game where a child can move a large magnet across the lexan top to rearrange the pieces of metal underneath and create designs.

One child spent eight hours in this waiting room receiving her chemotherapy drip. Her mother described to me what a difference the waiting room had made in the child's attitude toward coming for therapy. Prior to the completion of the waiting room, they had waited alone, in a sterile exam room, while undergoing this painful and tedious procedure. Therefore the child had never wanted to come. Now she looked forward to being in the midst of other people and participating in some of the activities while she was receiving therapy.

Nearby, we permanently mounted a device that spins and allows fluid to flow, to provide some passive visual stimulation. We also tried to do things that would give children a sense of hope, such as installing devices to measure their feet and height so they could see how much they had grown since their last visit.

Generally, three people accompany every ambulatory care pediatric patient. This presents a challenge in waiting areas, where there are many individuals in a small amount of space—adults, well siblings, and sick children—of all ages. The exploratorium and the playframe are attempts to meet this challenge.

The reception desk is kept low so children can make eye contact with this very important person.

7. *Preoperative Playroom:* The pre-op playroom, which had no natural light, is a room to which children come 15 to 30 minutes prior to sedation. The hospital performs some 7,000 operations a year. We tried to make the playroom like a big living room, a comfortable place to be. It had a playframe, a manipulative platform, and a raised banquette in the hopes that teenagers sitting on it would feel "above it all" and not be offended by the playthings for younger children. It is beautiful to see families playing together here and to see people smiling. Sometimes this is the last contact the parent and child ever have. Hopefully, that doesn't happen often, but presurgery can be a very emotional and intense time.

When I was taking photos of this room, a mother lying on the banquette sat up. She did not know who I was, but I told her she did not need to sit up on my account. She said, "I have a very bad back and when my daughter is finished with her surgery, I have to go into the hospital for mine." I smiled at her and said, "Isn't it nice that there is a place where you can lie down, too." As designers, we think about the patient using the healthcare center, but tend to forget the other people who also use it and who may be in various stages of wellness and illness themselves. They, too, need support. Having places where adults and kids can stretch out, where parents can nurse or can cuddle with one or two children together, is extremely important.

Usually parents and children waiting in this room play together; sometimes they play separately, but there is a real sense that they are all part of the same community. One mom spent the first 20 minutes of her time in the room hiding behind the newspaper, just like her husband. I think she was very scared and didn't want to show it. Eventually she calmed down and just before the physician came to get them, she was sitting in the rocking chair holding her child.

Anesthesiologists and doctors come into this room to talk about procedures. This is a much more pleasant environment than in the corridor or an examining room over a stretcher while the child is going under. It is the close, loving relationship between parents and children and staff that we are striving to create in healthcare environments.

Alberta Children's Hospital, Calgary, Canada

A speech and hearing clinic at Alberta Children's Hospital in Calgary, Canada, is part of a long avenue that extends the length of the building. The challenge was to create an interesting place to wait that would also provide some therapeutic experiences. The children can see well, but their speech and hearing are impaired. Thus one of the reasons for creating two towers with play lofts at five feet above the floor was to give them a view of the hallway so they could see things coming toward them that they could not hear. Eventually the staff added communication devices between the two towers so that children could speak to one another. The lower portion of the right-hand tower consists of a counter and storage for speech and language-related games and devices, such as language masters, that will encourage children to use whatever speech and hearing capacities they have. Behind the tower, built around an existing pillar, we put a little slide, a pit to sit in, and a puppet stage that faces the area where adults sit.

Children's Hospital, St. Paul, Minnesota

The lobby of the Children's Hospital in St. Paul, Minnesota, has a two-story structure that was installed to give children an experience of being up high and to separate and protect the lobby from the front door. On the front-door side, the underneath area of the structure holds three folded wheelchairs so that they are accessible to the entry but do not make visitors feel like they are coming into a "wheelchair park."

Another, more refined version of the exploratorium was used here, which includes a Casio music player permanently mounted on the table. Within the seating area, there is a playhouse, with a doctors' area on the front porch, and a slide hut. Seating is interspersed in and around these structures. There is also a manipulative play area in the middle and an area with vinyl flooring at the back for messy play, which includes an easel, craft tables, and a water play area. I know of no other hospital in the United States that has a water play area in its lobby. This area is both the hospital lobby and the waiting area for all the ambulatory clinics. So it gets a great deal of use and it is supervised. Knowing how important water play is for children, this hospital was willing to risk putting in the lobby a water play trough, which is used one to two hours a day.

The playhouse appears small, but it will hold three children inside; mom can sit outside and do her own thing, or if she chooses, she can interact with them. The slide hut provides gross motor play and has a busy board on one of its sides.

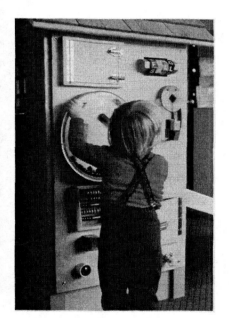

◆ **FIGURES 6–2 and 6–3** A slide hut provides gross motor play and has a busy board on one of its sides. (*Project:* Lobby, The Children's Hospital, St. Paul, MN. *Design:* Anita Olds and Associates. *Photo:* Anita Rui Olds.)

University of Maryland Hospital, Baltimore, Maryland

Our most recent playroom is at the University of Maryland Hospital in Baltimore. It was created out of three adjoining rooms, two of which are quite narrow. The middle room became a kitchen and crafts area. One end room is a quiet area for a waterbed and manipulative play; the other end room is a dramatic play area, intended to appeal to older children. The water play table has built-in faucets and a drain, but it is free standing so that it can be wheeled around the room. The kitchen allows children to make snacks and enjoy the experience of smelling food. There is some storage in this area for crafts and games that are played on the tables.

A 39-inch high infant deck, or raised playpen, where babies can be safely put, enables them to look out the window. An infant or toddler on an IV can sit there quite comfortably, see the whole room, and make eye contact with adults. Space underneath the deck is valuable for storage. Some interesting toys and sound-making devices are permanently mounted inside the platform.

Next to the infant deck, we installed a stair and slide. Just beyond that, there is a permanently mounted ceiling hook for suspending things like a baby swing, preschool swing, a rope to shimmy up, or a punching bag. These provide varied possibilities for gross motor play for different ages, at the discretion of the Child Life worker.

There is also a manipulative play area and a crawl-in hideaway underneath the slide and stairs. The hideaway has a mirror at the back and on the ceiling, and its walls are decorated with all kinds of things to touch and manipulate. Built-in closets provide storage for sound equipment, television, books, and also a staff desk.

In the dramatic play room, we built a little car, that can accommodate one or two drivers, complete with steering wheel, dials to push and move, a bell to ring, a hood that lifts up, and wheels that turn. It can be turned flush with or perpendicular to the wall. Beyond the car is a playhouse with housekeeping equipment and a puppet theater. There is even a light in the kitchen with a switch children can turn on and off at their discretion.

There is also a computer in this room, and we are working with Apple Computer to program educational games and experiences for children of all ages. Last, there is a busy board and a fish dive panel where the fish comes down the "stream."

Los Angeles Children's Museum

"Sticky City" is an exhibit I designed for the Los Angeles Children's Museum in California a number of years ago. My intention was to provide children with a large array of building materials; thus are over 300 large, but extremely light, blocks that seem to defy gravity by the way in which they stick to things. These blocks of foam are upholstered in a soft fabric and Velcro so that the blocks stick to each other, as well as to the walls and ceiling. Children initially treat them as a large mound of snow or a haystack. They love to pile the blocks together and climb up on top of them; throw their bodies in them; and generally go a bit wild. That is a very important motor response. However, eventually they begin to pay attention to the different shapes and colors of the blocks and start building things.

One 11-year-old boy spent eight hours playing with these blocks. I never thought a child of that age would be so interested. The blocks empower children in wheelchairs and on stretchers, and they encourage children with braces to move about and start using their bodies in novel ways. I have had letters from schools for the blind saying that this is the first time that blind children really felt safe enough to let their bodies go in space. Children using

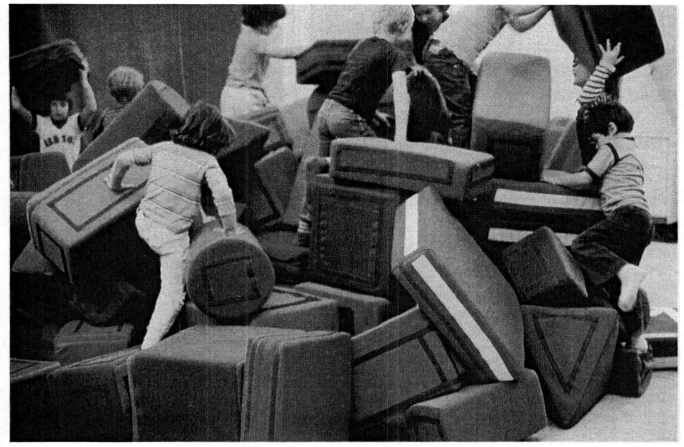

◆ **FIGURE 6–4**   Children loved to pile the large blocks of "nerf" foam and velcro together and climb up on top of them; throw their bodies in them; and generally go a bit wild. (*Project:* "Sticky City," Los Angeles Children's Museum. *Design:* Anita Olds and Associates. *Photo:* Anita Rui Olds.)

this exhibit give their creations names like "Velcro Man." Examples of a horse, cart, and chair show how extremely inventive children can be!

DuPont Institute, Wilmington, Delaware

An unusual project we did for the DuPont Institute was to design a court-yard for handicapped infants and toddlers. These children were under three years of age but none of them was developmentally above 18 months. A quarter of the children could use no extremities whatsoever, a quarter of them could toddle, and 50 percent of them could use only their arms. They were severely disabled children.

I started by asking myself, what could be done for these children? What were they missing because of their disabilities that a normal child would experience? I thought back to the experiences of my own children and about the nature of infancy, and I was reminded of the poem written by architect

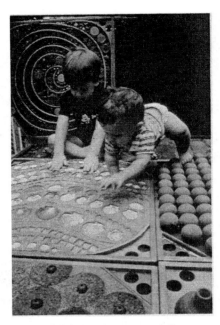

◆ **FIGURE 6–5** A courtyard for handicapped infants and toddlers features 20 different boxes that allow children to experience nature. (*Project:* Alfred I. DuPont Institute, Wilmington, DE. *Design:* Anita Olds and Associates. *Mosaic tile:* Lilli-Ann Killen Rosenberg. *Photo:* Ken Wittenberg.)

Ben Thompson in which he very beautifully captures something of the nature of childhood:

Harmony among many things was so apparent to us then.
We had frogs as friends.
Our hearts were ever open to continued discovery and surprise.

This captures some of the sense of wonder of the young child. Most children get the opportunity sometime in their first few years to wander on a beach, play in the sand and water, climb rocks, discover trees, roll in the grass, and sniff flowers. But, most of this is not available to disabled children. So we arrived at a concept of a set of 20 boxes that are from 3 to 18 inches in height; they can be rearranged to create a varied physical landscape of highs and lows.

In addition, each of the box tops is of a different texture so that both the physical and the textural landscape can be varied. I worked with Lilli-Ann Killen Rosenberg, a mosaic tile artist in Newton, Massachusetts, to produce these box tops. Some of them are intentionally very simple perceptually; all are impervious to weather and can be used indoors or out. They are soft enough so that children with no clothes can move upon them comfortably.

One top has all blue balls on it except for one pink one. On one panel, some of the standard bathroom plungers have holes underneath so that as children move across them, they deflate in unpredictable ways. Lilli-Ann's artistry was used to create textures with marbles, cork, rope, unglazed clay, wood, sea shells, seed pods, and stones.

Indeed, this equipment is very special and very beautiful. All children deserve this beauty; everything around them ought to be this way, not only one special project. It is this level of detail, aesthetics, and function that children deserve.

University of Maryland Hospital, Baltimore

The last project I'm going to present is a dream come true. For at least five years, I had been hoping to create not just a built environment for children, but also a crafted one, which involved artistry and related to nature. Last winter, the University of Maryland Hospital in Baltimore presented me with a challenge. They had a 31-foot in diameter, eight-sided rotunda with an eight-foot high ceiling, which was a massive transit zone. It had no natural light, four doors to the four major corridors of the pediatrics department, five elevator doors, and one stairwell door.

The challenge was to: (1) create something that tells children, as they get off the elevator, "This is a place for children," in a way that is not offensive to teenagers; (2) make the space useful, because there is no communal space on the four corridors, and people need a place to gather; and (3) create a "signature piece" so that pediatrics at the University of Maryland Hospital would become a recognized department of the institution.

We submitted three designs, and the hospital chose the one that I liked the best but was the most risky. We call it the "Enchanted Forest."

We started the Enchanted Forest on April 1, 1990 when Chance Anderson, a New Hampshire craftsman, contractor, and builder went out into his woods and cut down a number of real, but dead, trees, including a portion of a 150-year-old maple that stood 30 feet above the ground and was four feet in diameter. Chance laid out all these trees on his lawn and we looked them over and chose the ones we thought would be the most appropriate. Then the trees were loaded onto a truck and taken 20 miles away to a warehouse where we set up a full-scale mock-up of the 31-foot in diameter rotunda space.

The trees were heavy. They were hauled in and moved around to one spot or another. We tried to get a feeling of how they worked together, which ones had the most graceful form, which ones could stand against the walls, and which ones could stand on their own. We measured, negotiated, talked, and moved them until we began to get a sense of what would really work. At times there was a lot of frustration, but slowly the "forest" started to take shape. At one point, we realized we needed a bench, so a board was brought in that eventually became a bench over on the right-hand side. From another log, we came up with the idea to make a slide like a dug-out canoe. We used a log to make steps to the slide platform. Then we realized that the four-foot in diameter, six-foot high hollowed-out maple and the large conch from the same tree could fit in the space and balance each other out nicely.

Laurie Nichols, a New Hampshire craftswomen who carves animals, was brought in to create little animals to put into the forest. She thought we needed a mascot, so she brought in one of her pieces called "Big Mousie" that we moved around to determine where the mascot would fit and how big it should be.

One day during this process, the hospital administrator and director of mechanical engineering came to see the mock-up. At this point—no contract having yet been signed—we all took a look at what was being created and worked together to figure out how the forest would be installed in the hospital. We had fun playing with different options.

After this visit, everything was taken apart, sent to a kiln for two weeks to dry out, then brought back to be covered with fire-proofing material— which gave it a strange sheen and unfortunately changed the color tones of the wood a bit. Next, we had to figure out a way to securely mount the little creatures that Laurie had carved. An elf, for example, got bolted through his chest first and then his arms were added on to hide the bolt. Chris Ember, a New Hampshire musician, built two wooden xylophones that needed to be mounted and tested.

On May 17th, just six weeks after we had started, the trees were taken down again, put on a truck, and transported to Maryland. The grand opening for the Enchanted Forest was on June 6th.

The Enchanted Forest is a place where children sick in this hospital can come for a special experience. Proceeding down the corridor, they can look toward the center and see something very magical, soft, and mysterious.

It is a place a child can be wheeled to in a wheelchair or on a bed.

This is a place that is very regular in the sense of being eight sided; but there is nothing the same on any of the eight sides, so it is easy to see all around and notice the differences.

This is a place where children can hide inside a tree and feel its beauty, size, and shape and come to know how it grew.

It is a place where children can experience the sensuousness and curvature of the tree's form and the different textures of its bark.

This is a place where Racoon is the mascot. Racoon wears a hospital johnny with the University of Maryland insignia. He also has an IV bag be-

◆ **FIGURE 6-6** The Enchanted Forest is a place where a child, who is sick in this hospital, can come down the corridor, look toward the center, and see something very magical, soft, and mysterious. (*Project:* University of Maryland Hospital, Baltimore, MD. *Design:* Anita Olds and Associates. *Fabricator:* Chance Anderson. *Photo:* Gail Collins and Anita Rui Olds.)

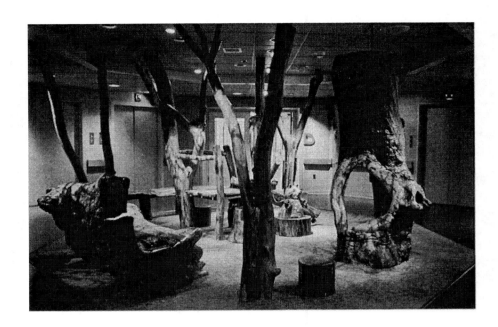

cause 95 percent of the children carry IVs; the sign on his bag says, "The medicine in this bag is to make Racoon feel better." Racoon is deeply loved—at times he is kissed and hugged by children who are about his same height.

This is a place where there is dappled light that looks like the leaves of trees, and sometimes it transforms the clothing of a friend.

This is a place where even a child 10 or 12 years old can slide down the slide, just like a much younger child.

This is a place where children can climb into a tree and where they can hug a tree.

This is a place where a chipmunk wearing blue overalls and red sneakers is reading a book of poetry, and children can look over his shoulder and read along with him.

This is a place where a 12-year-old-child, waiting for open heart surgery, and a three-year-old, waiting to go home, can meet one another, play, and explore things together.

This is a place where a mouse sleeps in the burl of a tree.

It is a place where a one-year-old has to stand on tippee toe to try and see everything.

This is a place where a great tree gave of itself to produce a beautiful bench and where a very creative artist carved squirrels underneath to support it.

This is a place where a one-year-old diagnosed with leukemia can come to sit with her grandma while her mom goes home to rest—and where grandma and child can have a few quiet moments together.

This is a place where 10-, 11-, and 12-year-olds in a day-long growth study can come and entertain themselves while they are having their blood analyzed.

This is a place where a child with hydrocephalus was totally enamored with the elf, and his nurse held him up to take a closer look at it.

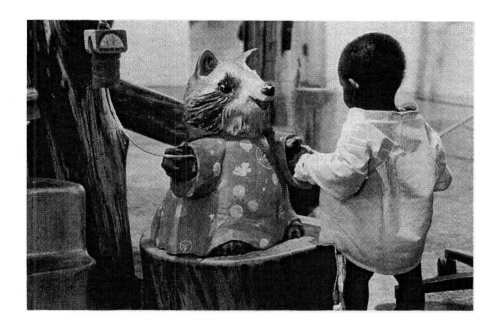

◆ **FIGURE 6–7**   Racoon, the mascot, wears a hospital johnny with the University of Maryland insignia. He also has an IV bag with a sign on it that says, "The medicine in this bag is to make Racoon feel better." (*Project:* University of Maryland Hospital, Baltimore, MD. *Design:* Anita Olds and Associates. *Fabricator:* Chance Anderson. *Photo:* Gail Collins and Anita Rui Olds.)

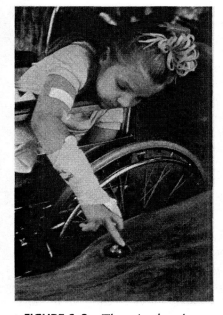

◆ **FIGURE 6–8**   There is a bench here with a magical marble that children can turn and turn to see the cosmos and the universe." (*Project:* University of Maryland Hospital, Baltimore, MD. *Design:* Anita Olds and Associates. *Fabricator:* Chance Anderson. *Photo:* Gail Collins and Anita Rui Olds.)

This is a place where there is a bench with a magical marble that children can turn and turn to see the cosmos and the universe.

This is a place where the bench also supports a very unusual kaleidoscope. It is a double kaleidoscope and it can make children goggle-eyed. It is so wonderful that even doctors are willing to drop their professionalism and sprawl on the floor in order to look through it.

This is a place where, one day, two nurses at the end of their shifts took off their shoes and stood for 1 1/2 hours just hanging out and talking with each other.

This is a place where doctors may come to hold their rounds or will bring parents to talk about things that are going on with children.

This is a place where elevator doors open and close continually and where there are beds, stretchers, and mechanical equipment going back and forth all the time. It is also a place where the birds sing 24 hours a day on a continuous loop tape. It feels quiet and comfortable even in the middle of chaos, so much so that a physician right out of surgery came here for a brief moment to review his notes.

This is a place where letters and carved animals tell children which corridor to go down.

This is a place where a child who spent several hours visiting his grandma in the hospital could come with his mom and her friends to romp and cavort together. Even grown-ups can slide down the slide!

It is a place where children can play hide-n-seek and eventually allow themselves to be caught.

This is a place where it is comfortable for a child to rest and to smile even though the child's parents are upset because another of their children is dying of cancer.

This is a place where children can come if they have no intestines and are living on an IV, who may feel faint and just want to rest in the arms of an adult. Often, there will be a friend there who really wants to talk and play.

This is a place where teenagers can hang out—and where doctors will come to find them to talk about what's going on, and maybe hang out there, too.

This is a place where doctors bring patients—IV and all—and help them get set up so they are free to climb or run.

This is a place where children can play music on one xylophone or two, by themselves or with a friend.

It is a place where children can feel very happy . . . maybe: This is a place where an eight-year-old girl whose leg had been crushed by a car was waiting for surgery. She was very unhappy; she was sad, pitiful, despondent, and even quite angry. She was interested in nothing and in going nowhere. Then something happened. At some point she noticed the chipmunk up in the tree, and then she discovered the speller down by the platform. The Child Life worker took her over to the kaleidoscope and eventually helped her out of her wheelchair so she could prop up her crushed leg and look into the kaleidoscope. Then she discovered the xylophones. Eventually she discovered the song within herself, and slowly she began to sing. She sang her song to her mom and the Child Life worker, and ever so slowly, a smile broke out on her face; and for one moment, at least, there was joy and peace and security before the uncertainty of the operation.

I would like to close by reading a statement from Goethe that has been an inspiration to me in moments of frustration and struggle in the design process, or when I could not manifest what I felt the children deserved:

> . . . Until one is committed there is hesitancy, the chance to draw back, always ineffectiveness. Concerning all acts of initiative (and creation), there is one elementary truth, the ignorance of which kills countless ideas and splendid plans: that the moment one definitely commits oneself, then Providence moves too.
>
> All sorts of things occur to help one that would never otherwise have occurred. A whole stream of events issues from the decision, raising in one's favor all manner of unforeseen incidents and meetings and material assistance, which no man could have dreamt would have come his way.
>
> Whatever you can do, or dream, you can begin it.
>
> Boldness has genius, power, and magic in it.

Please take this next step for children!

Anita Rui Olds, Ph.D., is a developmental and environmental psychologist who has pioneered the innovative design of environmental facilities for children in hospitals, day-care centers, schools, therapeutic and special-needs settings, museums, outdoor recreational areas, and medical and holistic health offices throughout the United States and Canada. She is a principal of her own design and consulting firm in Woodacre, California; a lecturer in the Eliot-Pearson Department of Child Study at Tufts University; and originator of The Child Care Design Institute, *an annual summer training seminar jointly sponsored by the Harvard Graduate School of Design and Tufts University. Olds is the author of* Child Health Care Facilities: Design Guidelines and Literature Outline, *and co-author of* The Architectural Prototype Document: Study for the Development of Day-Care Centers in State Facilities, *which details design guidelines for day-care centers in Massachusetts.*

◆ ◆ ◆

THE STARBRIGHT PAVILION

Fourth Symposium on Healthcare Design, Boston, MA, 1991

James R. Diaz, FAIA

The STARBRIGHT Pavilion encompasses all that other speakers have addressed—the values to which all of us at this Symposium aspire. I hope we can convince others to think as we do, because there are still many who ascribe little or no value to design as a means to improve healthcare.

The Starlight Foundation came together under the concept of granting wishes to sick children. It has chapters in the United States, United Kingdom, Australia, and several other countries. Its president, Peter Samuelson, is the visionary behind the STARBRIGHT Pavilion, itself a subsidiary of the Starlight Foundation. The honorary chairman of the board of the STARBRIGHT Pavilion is movie director Steven Spielberg.

Originally, the pavilion was to have been located adjacent to the Los Angeles County (LAC) and University of Southern California (USC) Medical Center, a large Gothic-style hospital east of downtown Los Angeles.

In late 1993, it was announced that the pavilion will be located in Hollywood, near the corner of Hollywood and Vine. It will be a free-standing, ambulatory care facility.

The Project

The STARBRIGHT Pavilion program has four main objectives: education, entertainment, research, and case management coordination. It will integrate every aspect discussed at this Symposium in terms of the role architecture and interior design can play in the wellness concept for children. The 115,000 square-foot pavilion will accommodate approximately 100,000 outpatient visits a year, as well as additional people who will attend performances. It is estimated that the entire project will cost approximately $58 million, of which, construction is estimated at $40 million. Construction may take place between 1995 and 1996.

The STARBRIGHT idea has been around since 1985. In August of 1989, the Starlight Foundation, with funding from the Peter Samuelson Foundation, entered into a joint venture with the Foundation for Health Services, a branch of the Los Angeles County Hospitals that manages activities not financed with county funds. It is this volunteer, fundraising foundation that engaged Medical Planning Associates (MPA) in Malibu, California, in association with my firm, Kaplan McLaughlin Diaz, to provide preliminary programming, planning, and a design image for the proposed STARBRIGHT Pavilion at the LAC and USC Medical Center.

Programming and planning criteria had been established by a report titled "A Needs Assessment and Feasibility Study of Psychosocial Needs of Chronically Ill Children and Their Families in Los Angeles County" by the USC Hamelvich Social Work Research Center. The report verified the need for expanded, complementary posthospitalization support for chronically ill children in the Los Angeles area.

Based on this study, the international board of the Starlight Foundation, along with a blue-ribbon advisory board of physicians (oncologists, hematologists, psychiatrists, and psychologists), nurses, and senior executives from relevant industries, agreed that STARBRIGHT would focus on the following four program services: education, entertainment, research, and case management. The board felt that each of these services has the potential to enhance the overall quality of life for afflicted children and families and also to influence their therapeutic outcomes.

Physical planning concepts were established by MPA through the traditional method of questionnaires and personal interviews with parties selected by the STARBRIGHT Pavilion architecture and space planning committee. Their collective vision of the program, subjective as it may have been, formed the base for quantifying the space requirements for the pavilion. From those space requirements, an interactive process (with the joint participation of the architectural and space planning committee of STARBRIGHT and the members of the planning team) determined the necessary site footprint, relationships among service components, and design concepts.

My firm's role was very exciting. We were like the "imagineers" who create physical environments for the Walt Disney Company. Our challenge was to make STARBRIGHT as exciting as an "E" ticket ride at Disneyland or Universal Studios (see Figure C–15). Naturally, we could not use exploding volcanoes, speeding carts, or things that go "bump in the dark." Instead, the entire pavilion had to be supportive of sick children, their siblings, parents, and staff.

Sparkling Jewel

Thus, the STARBRIGHT Pavilion would have become the sparkling jewel in the crown of the LAC and USC Medical Center. Set amidst a traditional hospital and physically located adjacent to the maternal/child entrance, the STARBRIGHT Pavilion would induce a smile in children who otherwise would be intimidated by their surroundings. In this prominent location, the five-level pavilion would serve not only LAC and USC Medical Center outpatients, but also those referred by hospitals and doctors throughout the Los Angeles area.

The biggest challenge for our designers was to pronounce the word "psychoneuroimmunology." Research on this topic establishes a correlation between mental health and the immune system in combating disease. Such research will be supported by the Foundation and will be an integral part of programs relating to entertainment, education, research, and case management coordination. (It is interesting to note that people from the entertainment industry who support the project want to be assured of its scientific basis.)

Within healthcare, it is instructive to see who does and who doesn't jump on the STARBRIGHT bandwagon. Medical staff who support the facility and research tend to be primary care physicians, oncologists, psychiatrists, and psychologists. Most funds today go to basic research in radiology, cardiology, surgery, and the biosciences. Very little is earmarked to study psychoneuroimmunology.

As I mentioned, entertainment is one of the four primary elements of the STARBRIGHT Pavilion. There will be a 350-seat auditorium for live and multimedia performances that will be transmitted via closed circuit telecasts to on–site pediatric patients who are unable to leave their rooms, as well as to children's hospitals worldwide. Such programs will also be taped for future use.

As for education, programs will be developed to assist patients and families in coping with the physical and emotional difficulties related to caring for severely ill children. A case management coordination service will also be available. Assistance will be provided for families to take advantage of local, state, and federal support programs. Because these programs and services may not all be funded through traditional third-party payers or government, there will be a large gap to be financed through ongoing philanthropy.

Making Children Happy

At the crux of the entire venture is STARBRIGHT's principal purpose: to make ill children happier. All aspects of STARBRIGHT's programs will support this clear and immediate goal. To interest and delight both children and adolescents, special audiovisual and live, costumed mascots will appear throughout the pavilion. The STARBRIGHT video mascot in participating hospital pediatric outpatient clinic lobbies will not only amuse the waiting children, but encourage them and their parents to investigate the services offered in the pavilion. In addition, live audiovisual mascots may be used by healthcare professionals for therapeutic and educational purposes at the pavilion.

Today, the first step has been taken with the creation of the Starlight Express Room within the LAC and USC Medical Center. Starlight Express is a room about the size of four, two-bed patient care rooms that have been remodeled into one large space. The room has a number of state-of-the-art video consoles. Children enter from the inpatient unit of the hospital. After six months, the hospital has found that there has been about a 25 percent drop in the use of pain medication for children who have been able to take part in the Starlight Express program. (That research program has now been extended indefinitely.)

Open a certain number of hours a day, Starlight Express is staffed by volunteers, including a Captain Starlight who helps children use the equipment. It is perhaps the first ongoing program that will convince decision makers that psychoneuroimmunology has intrinsic value.

While this fascination with technology can be carried to extremes, at the same time, there are a great many activities offered—such as music therapy, dance therapy, or puppets—that are usual activities for hospitalized children.

There are even more exciting possibilities for the future. The most probable is a bedside, multimedia television module that will link children to both entertainment and educational programs. These Starpods may also provide live, two-way visual and audio communication between the children and their families at home, as well as with children having similar problems in other facilities worldwide. Starpods will include a computer terminal, a television with satellite programming capability, a VCR, and a video phone. The whole idea, as Steven Spielberg describes it, is to use the fourth wall of the room to reach out to the entire world and bring something other than television soap operas to children in the hospital. The Starpod module is most exciting for its interactive possibilities.

The STARBRIGHT Pavilion will also provide child care services for young siblings whose family members are partaking of the STARBRIGHT experiences. Many other details are yet to be developed that, consistent with professional medical criteria, will enhance the overall atmosphere of participating hospitals. They will create a fantasylike environment in both the pavilion and the pediatrics areas of those medical centers.

The pavilion's basic goal is to create an expanded group of psycho-social services for children suffering from chronic and life-threatening diseases and their families. It is most important that the pavilion and STARBRIGHT enhancements are designed to complement, rather than replace, services already offered in hospitals.

Illness not only disrupts the normal development of the child, but also affects the overall quality of family life. The future will bring greater survival rates for seriously ill children. At the same time, the number of children living below the poverty line is also likely to increase, thereby increasing the association of those diseases and complications to poor living conditions.

The feasibility study cites several examples of gaps that exist in the present system of healthcare delivery. The need to provide education and resources for sick children, their families, and allied health professionals is clear. Factors that cause stress and methods of coping with them will be explored by researchers. Great emphasis will be placed on providing services to adolescents and to those suffering from mental disorders. Through these innovative programs, the STARBRIGHT Pavilion will unite the forces of entertainment and healthcare to improve the spirit and ability to cope with prolonged sickness for children and their families in Los Angeles and the whole world beyond. The STARBRIGHT Pavilion will serve as the "mother ship" for an eventual network of STARBRIGHT facilities.

Primary Concepts

I'd like to describe the primary concepts of entertainment, education, research, and case management coordination in detail.

1. *Entertainment.* There will be three types of entertainment: diversionary, educational, and therapeutic. Some of the entertainment planned is purely diversionary in nature, but its benefit to sick children should not be underestimated. Both chronically ill children and those facing life-threatening diseases need regular relief from daily routines that often involve painful and unpleasant treatments. Existing medical research, in fact, suggests that positive mental health may on occasion boost the immune system and thereby, in certain circumstances, promote healing. This entertainment aspect will also be educational, affording children an opportunity to learn more about their health challenges in creative and enjoyable ways.

Live performances will take place in the auditorium. Located in Hollywood, the pavilion will be able to take advantage of talent living in the area as volunteers. The auditorium will accommodate viewing films, children's live productions, educational seminars, concerts, theater, ballet, puppetry, and magic shows. When not in use as a theater, the auditorium will be available to the medical staff and the community for other programs.

In addition to the television production capacity, there will be an extensive audio/visual library. Education, entertainment, and therapy will be networked into this audio/visual library. We envision an extensive variety of audio and video tapes, as well as passive and interactive laser disks carrying film and television programming. All of these will be used by STARBRIGHT children and their families, as well as by researchers and health providers. Inpatients from any hospital bedroom will also be able to view these materials. Children in other facilities around the country, and around the world, will avail themselves of this resource via the STARBRIGHT Network. Viewing booths of varying sizes will permit individuals, families, and peer groups to view tapes in appropriately scaled settings. The library will include patient-friendly materials on issues like surgery, diseases, and preventive measures. Those materials exist today, but certainly the pavilion will be a depository and a place to create new ones. Facilities will also exist for children to make their own tapes, either to send to children suffering from similar diseases in other locations or to send home to family members.

2. *Education.* The deficiency in relevant education for seriously ill children and their families, is documented by medical practitioners and by associated clinical research. Families who have a sick child need supportive and instructional therapy. There is a strong tendency for families who have a chronically ill member to become dysfunctional. In particular, well siblings feel neglected and may seek attention through inappropriate and sometimes dangerous ways. STARBRIGHT therapies will deal with family groups by addressing issues that combine sickness therapy and family unity. The feasibility study notes the infrequency with which these problems are handled today. Activities in the STARBRIGHT Pavilion will be differentiated from the medical care normally received in the hospital and clinic facilities. The STARBRIGHT Pavilion enhancements are intended to be associated in children's minds with pleasant, nonpainful experiences; and STARBRIGHT will present them with a place in which they feel safe and can regain a sense of empowerment.

The pavilion will offer a wide range of therapeutic activities. Play, of course, has long been recognized for its ability to discharge negative feelings, as well as being an arena in which to practice the mastery of difficult situations. The following is only a sampling of the types of play with therapeutic potential that will be offered at the pavilion: music therapy, which all of us realize is beneficial to all age groups; art therapy, which is a useful relaxation tool; and puppet therapy. To me, puppet therapy is the most creative, because both verbal and physical activities are combined. Puppets may be operated by either the therapist or the child. The story line and dialogue are part of the therapy.

Beyond, there is the exciting area of computer play and interactive video. Today, computer play is limited to games, but interactive video offers promising directions for educating seriously ill children, parents, siblings, and healthcare professionals. Touch-screen television and multimedia systems offer unlimited opportunities, especially with the capacity for dual languages and learner controlled pacing so that progress can be tailored to the individual.

3. *Research.* The research mission is founded upon the link between mental health and the welfare of seriously ill children. A specific goal will be tracking STARBRIGHT services that lessen overall medical expenditures for seriously ill children, thereby encouraging third-party payers in the future to consider insurance coverage under certain circumstances. This must be done to extend the STARBRIGHT concept to other places. Clinical research is necessary not only to secure the backing of the American Academy of Pediatrics, but also to substantiate, it is believed, the need for additional funding and the establishment of other centers in the future. Existing studies on the impact of families on childhood illness require extensive, continuing research on psycho-social factors. Healthcare practitioners bemoan the dearth of research on coping resources that may mediate family response. Such knowledge would aid in the development of appropriate intervention strategies.

Varied research opportunities will also examine such psychoneuroimmunological issues as whether and to what extent entertainment can help pain management; specifically, which STARBRIGHT offerings motivate children to keep their appointments.

Like other centers of this type, the pavilion would have observation rooms and office space for researchers who will be attracted by the forms of education and therapies offered. The integration with the University of Southern California will also allow students to participate in the research studies of the pavilion.

4. *Case Management.* In the feasibility study, case management was highlighted as one of the most frequently requested services by parents of sick children. The study's professional resources also stress the need for someone to provide ongoing follow-up and assistance in coordinating fragmented services after diagnosis and the original disease intervention. The STARBRIGHT case management coordinator would work closely with other hospital case management providers, physicians, and the family to assist in securing the best and most appropriate referrals for the child. Basic information would be provided about free and low-fee services available in Los Angeles County, as well as on a federal and state level. The coordinator would also facilitate coordination among the various departments of the medical center, thereby justifying the importance of being located near to a medical center.

Design Concept

The design for the STARBRIGHT Pavilion originated from two goals voiced by Peter Samuelson, who said, "We want the building to bring a smile. It should look as if a parent had built the hospital and a child had designed the pavilion." Unlike the parent's serious construction, the child would build an environment for children using toy blocks, Tinkertoys, Lego, and so on. Consequently, the exterior design of the STARBRIGHT Pavilion is intended to attract the attention of children but, equally, the respect of adolescents by providing an artistic combination of generic Lego and Tinkertoy-like forms as both structural and decorative features (see Figure C–16). In contrast to heavier metal, concrete, and plastic components, there will be major sections of glass, allowing the curious to preview the activities inside. Such exterior glazing and a giant skylight will shower interior spaces with natural light. Rising above the building entrance there will be a sculptural communication tower containing both transmission and reception capability for the pavilion. The design and height of this tower will create a recognizable silhouette for the STARBRIGHT Pavilion.

A specific philosophy was developed for each of the areas of the building and its surrounding plazas. There is an entry plaza, a main entrance, and an open public court area. It is also important to note that at the rear there is a place for large trucks with technical equipment for television and deliveries made to the theater stage.

The entry plaza will be treated as a play area with large toys: perhaps a train, cognitive climbing equipment, a large doll house, and the announcement tower. It will act as a natural attraction to the pavilion.

The announcement tower is important because it will serve to herald live and audiovisual events. There will be banners, or a large screen for the display of announcements, cartoons, photographs, movies, live performances in the theater, and the like.

The plaza to the east of the pavilion will be more private and contain large, out-of-scale toy blocks that are part of a big wading fountain. The fountain is shallow, allowing children to wade safely on hot days. The water will emanate from the toys themselves through Rube Goldberg devices. This is envisioned as an activity area for the children in the program.

Visitors will enter the pavilion through a fanciful vestibule. To provide the transition from the everyday world into STARBRIGHT, the vestibule might contain a yellow brick road walkway that lights up and plays musical notes as children walk upon it. Immediately inside the pavilion, children step into a large, four-story atrium. It is here that the trolley is first seen. Traveling the height and length of the pavilion, the trolley carries perhaps 10 to 12 people at a time, stopping at the third level, roof garden, and finally a rooftop oasis. Also seen in this area are the balconies of the upper levels. Whether seen from the atrium or the trolley, the interior corridors appear to be storefront facades, or stage sets to create a flexible environment.

Functional areas lie behind these fanciful facades. As detailed design is completed, a major challenge exists to extend the child's world into each functional area. The pavilion may be likened to a Medieval cathedral in which architects, artists, artisans, and laborers will be able to add individual touches. There will be the opportunity to design everything from architectonic elements to murals, mobiles, toys, educational devices, graphics, and even signage for adults and children from all parts of the world.

James R. Diaz, FAIA, senior principal at Kaplan/McLaughlin/Diaz (KMD) in San Francisco, California, is nationally known for his ongoing work in healthcare architecture and planning. As principal-in-charge, Diaz is responsible for KMD's healthcare projects, participating in a hands-on manner in preliminary planning and design. He is a Fellow of the American Insitute of Architects (AIA) and has served as national chair of the AIA Committee on Architecture for Health. He was one of two private sector architects selected to serve on the Governor's Task Force on State Design and Construction Policy in California, with the primary task of reviewing the interface between state agencies and consumers.

SAN DIEGO CHILDREN'S HOSPITAL AND HEALTH CENTER ADDITION

Fifth Symposium on Healthcare Design, San Diego, CA, 1992

Edward Carter
David L. Noferi
Annette Ridenour
Blair L. Sadler
David H. Swain, AIA

Swain: The purpose of this presentation is to illustrate a totally integrated healing facility for children. We like to call it "A Place of Miracles." Our team goal was to interpret the owner's vision and provide a special place. Through the design team's research, experience, imagination, skills, and talent, that vision was born. This presentation will explore the journey we took and the results we achieved.

Blair Sadler, president and CEO, Children's Hospital and Health Center will begin by explaining the hospital's goals and vision. Next, David Noferi, project architect, NBBJ, will define the architectural interpretation of that vision. Then I will discuss the interior design elements. Annette Ridenour, principal of the Aesthetics Collection, will present the art program; and Edward Carter, vice president, facilities development for Children's will review the process and describe the team effort it took over a five-year period to realize this project.

Sadler: It is the 1950s: Ike is in the White House, San Diego is a Navy town, and Mission Valley is little more than a cow pasture. In 1953, Children's Hospital breaks ground for San Diego's first pediatric hospital. We open our doors in August 1954.

In the 1960s, a new consciousness begins to affect every walk of life. Children's broadens its role in the community, adding more beds, operating rooms, and X-ray facilities. Our name changes to reflect the concept of total child healthcare. Now we are Children's Hospital and Health Center.

The 1970s begin as an era of change. At Children's, new achievements mark every year. We add the pediatric intensive care unit, genetic research lab, motion analysis lab, and satellite clinics.

As San Diego enters the 1980s, the population increases and business expands. Children's becomes the regional pediatric trauma center for San Diego and Imperial counties. New structures and facilities appear: the pathology lab, the center for child protection, and the Han Surgical Pavilion.

The problem facing Children's Hospital in the early 1980s was that we were turning away many children solely because we did not have enough beds and outpatient clinic space. San Diego was, after all, the fourth fastest growing county in the country and the nation's sixth largest city. In the late 1970s and early 1980s, other hospitals turned to Children's for the care of sick infants and kids. This centralization of pediatric care was good for the community, but we were always scrambling to keep up.

From 1980 to 1985, we were able to make a series of small, incremental bed additions, bringing our total from 107 to 154. However, we had reached the limit in the existing facility. So the trustees met with the management and medical staff and decided to embark upon the most significant expansion in Children's history. We put a project team together and selected architects and contractors with one goal: to build a children's hospital that looks like a children's hospital, not like a traditional hospital. We wanted to focus not only on function, but also on feelings.

We asked ourselves, "What do we care about? What do we want this environment to feel like? What impact do we want to have on children and their families?" We realized we wanted to build a children's hospital in San Diego on a scale that would not intimidate children.

We also wanted to build a place that would provide many areas that would be inviting to children: their own rooms, the playroom, the courtyard, and the nurse station. We wanted to build a children's hospital that would be bold, unique, innovative, and creative. We wanted the place to feel like a house—a place of fun. We wanted rooms to be light, lively, and engaging to help children feel special.

In the playroom, we wanted to have individualized activity spaces. In the courtyards, we wanted to have multiple levels to provide opportunities for kids to interact with nature and fantasy. We wanted to build a children's hospital that would express a sense of caring, feeling, and stability—a place in which healing occurs. We wanted to build a hospital with a distinctive symbol that expresses the mission and becomes a true landmark. Our clock tower became that symbol of stability, healing, and peace.

We wanted to build a children's hospital whose message would be read by people entering the campus, in the parking garage, and throughout the building. We wanted to build a hospital in San Diego in which parents would have comfortable facilities so they could stay with their children. We wanted to build a hospital that would make recruiting top physicians and nurses easier. We wanted it to say, "This is a place that is committed to excellence, innovation, and caring for kids." We wanted a place where people would want to come to work. We wanted to build a hospital campus, a true campus, that would integrate the new hospital with other major buildings, such as a new doctors' office building and a 1000-car parking structure.

We wanted to have a sense of unity and continuity. We wanted to express the special characteristics of San Diego and the Pacific Rim—past, present, and future. We wanted to create a new landmark that would be easily recognizable, to take advantage of the heritage and the flora and fauna of San Diego (see Figure C–17). We wanted to take advantage of multiple views to and from the hospital; to have a hospital that felt more like home than high tech, that was not overwhelming or intimidating. We wanted to have the components of a home, a front porch, and real windows; this had to be a place of caring, because our children have very special needs.

The new hospital will be the home of the Pediatric Trauma Center. Here the sickest children in San Diego County will be cared for. A child who has been in an automobile accident or a youngster who has fallen into the family swimming pool will be treated by our multidisciplinary teams of medical and surgical subspecialists, nurses, and other healthcare professionals skilled in emergency and intensive care.

Our pediatric intensive care unit will provide state-of-the-art care for children who are critically ill or injured and usually need life support: for those who have received open-heart surgery or other lifesaving surgical procedures. This new hospital will provide the latest in technology and extensive diagnostic capabilities—all tailored specifically for children, because our children have very special needs.

Our surgeons in the orthopedic institute will take care of children with problems such as scoliosis; sports injuries; hip, knee, and foot problems; arthritis; neuromuscular diseases; and traumatic injuries. Our children have very serious diseases. They are kids with cancer and leukemia who need special care before and after surgery. We needed to design a building that was truly a place for miracles.

Interpreting the Vision

Noferi: The project included a new 114-bed hospital with a new lobby, gift shop, cafe, emergency department, and clinic spaces. Also included is a central power plant, pharmacy expansion, and shell space for an imaging department. Its total size is approximately 190,000 sq. ft. Also included is a 1000 car parking garage, connecting bridges to the main hospital, a new roadway, utilities, and finally the remodel work for all the vacated departments. The design was conceived in 1986, six years ago. The building is about 95 percent complete.

The hospital's goal statements provided a very challenging mission for the design team. In order to capture the spirit of the descriptive terms Blair mentioned, it was necessary to apply a process of discovery through documentation to allow the design team to grasp quickly the concepts. Our process began with a great deal of research about San Diego, the region, and the community. We toured some area facilities in order to find key architectural influences to draw upon. We also looked at other institutions and non-institutional building types to stimulate discussion in our search for appropriate architectural characteristics for the project.

Our criteria were essentially organized under three headings: children, hospital, and San Diego. As a point of reference, the existing facility, founded in the early 1950s, was a sprawling complex of primarily single-story brick buildings with low-pitched roofs. Most of the patient rooms were oriented toward intimate courtyards and were very residential in scale.

San Diego's roots are in a hilltop site in the San Diego Mission built in 1769, with its whitewashed adobe walls, bell tower, and lush vegetation. This was followed by the Victorian era represented by the Hotel Del Coronado, with its grand residential image gesturing toward the sea—a dominant white structure capped with distinctive red-roof forms. That era is also captured in the Point Loma lighthouse. A regional adaptation of neoclassicism is represented in the Balboa Exhibition buildings; and a regional adaptation of the Art Deco style is in San Diego's train station and County Administration Building, with their stark walls and use of tile.

Modernism in San Diego is represented by Irving Gill in the Bishop School. And then there is what we call "'40s funk," represented in the beach community of San Diego and the Crystal Pier Hotel. A cottage from this community became a model for the patient rooms, as well as the nurse stations. Finally, there are the buildings of Horton Plaza with a collision of forms and of colors, adding a great deal of visual interest.

The primary theme that developed out of our research was the notion of a home: a special place of caring, nurturing, and protection; a place of normalization that captures the essence of San Diego, children, and the hospital. The entire project became an exercise in scale—breaking down the large facility into a recognizable kit of parts: familiar residential forms; abstract forms and geometric shapes; hand-size parts and adult-size parts; and the use of regional colors.

The image of Children's to the community is that of "the house on the hill." With its variety of roofs and forms, it could be viewed as a hilltop village. The tower is quite a story—a major image for the facility and most importantly a symbol of time and healing.

Upon a closer look at the building, one can see major abstract forms.

These are, it is hoped, pleasant distractions to a child's imagination, allowing multiple interpretations—a face, an animal, or another familiar object.

Residential windows and a selection of modular materials in masonry express more house than machine. We built a mock-up to determine shade and shadow, articulating it in terms of color. We also applied the selection of materials to a parking structure, which preceded the actual hospital itself. We used tile, glass, and glass block to fit into that masonry module. Essentially, we created the kit of parts from materials and forms, addressing the scale and reinforcing a geometric motif by using squares and cubes, circles and globes, triangles and cones.

Next, we addressed the climate by planning for smaller windows on the west and south facades, where the sun is the strongest. Courtyards provide shelter from the hot sun, but they were also developed with a sensory theme in mind: sight, smell, and touch. Finally, a soft, curved cornice detail became a major decorative element, terminating at a precast cube articulated with a tic-tac-toe game.

The Interiors

Swain: To illustrate the focus of the interiors, I will use a series of short statements, followed by images that reinforce the statements. The premise is that A Place of Miracles is a healing place that is influenced by many aspects: culture, people, nature, seasons, time, and climate, which all come together with technology to heal. The interiors enhance and interpret the vision, lower anxiety, promote healing, and express the character of San Diego.

Images such as nautical forms, the sun, and the air—the feeling of freedom and life—the cityscape and waterfront of San Diego, lightness, and color reinforce regional feelings. As an example, the cultural heritage of the region is represented by the Hotel Del Coronado in its architecture and other design elements. The idea of seasonal change influences the interiors and the outer architecture through the use of color, lighting, and the "openness" of nature. The people of the region have their own unique cultural heritage; and elements of that culture were brought into the building through color, form, art work, spatial arrangement, and symbols.

So too, in this new facility, seasonal elements and the passage of seasons are represented by art work, colors, and a close connection to the outdoors (see Figure C–18). The healing aspects of nature are brought to patients through the "mini" courtyards, which allow patients and families to experience nature directly outside their rooms. Clocks and their symbols of the passage of time as a healer are used as a strong symbolic element.

This is a facility that expresses a sense of caring. Staff members offer that caring. Functional spaces, the availability of "retreat" areas, and having control over their surroundings allows staff to provide that caring.

Much has been said about the family and its important role in the healing process. The family is a very large part of healing; so the provision of comfortable waiting areas, in-room sleep-over facilities, and entertainment for siblings allows family members and friends to feel at home. Access to meals and information are important elements in supporting the family.

A visually stimulating, yet organized, lobby delights the family, patient, and friends as they arrive, which helps to lower their anxiety. Having multiple places, retreats, or areas of refuge to which children and parents want to go is important. Children and adults need these areas to provide positive distractions, as well as a comforting environment.

One of the goals of the building interiors is to be more house than machine. This house should be whimsical for patients, family, and staff. The patient rooms open up onto the neighborhood, or pod, allowing patients the choice of interacting with their neighborhood or of retreating to their house (i.e., room).

Again, the environment should provide elements of surprise and positive distraction. Imagine the surprise and wonder when a child looks out the window of his room at night and sees the stars shining over the nurses' "home" (i.e., the fiber-optic "stars" in the barrel vault over the nurse station—see Figure C–19).

Patterns and shapes as well as color are important. Floor patterns and colors relieve the anxiety of patients and their families through the unexpected. Multicolored door frames and corridors provide the element of surprise. Room identification through color association (i.e., "my room has the blue door frame,") gives a sense of control and personalization.

Providing for privacy and personal space is also important. Children should be able to retreat into their "house" with their TV, toys, and artwork; it should be a place in which children can be with themselves and their things.

Control is provided through the choice of art, lighting, temperature, noise, privacy, and meals. Choice is essential to healing. If the patient and/or the family have choices, they feel in control; anxiety is reduced and healing occurs more easily (see Figure C–20).

The clock tower is a distinctive symbol that expresses the hospital's mission and is a landmark. Symbols are elements of healing. This symbol is of time and of San Diego and its people, expressed in familiar color and shapes. It is whimsical, yet stable; soaring and uplifting. All of these characteristics are embodied in what we call A Place of Miracles.

Formulating the Art Program

Ridenour: My firm was hired just before the ground-breaking. We had been talking to the Facilities department and administration for almost two years about the project. Like many hospitals, Children's was afraid to begin an art program until the general contract bids came in and administrators knew how much money there would be for it. Art was always planned to be an integral part of the facility; it was budgeted as part of the overall building budget. This represented a progressive approach and a commitment to the value of art from the very beginning.

We started by interviewing the architects, interior designers, facility managers, and administrators. We needed to understand the planning path they had been on for almost five years. An art core committee was formed; and together we looked at a dozen facilities, such as the James Whitcomb Riley Hospital for Children in Indianapolis, the University of Virginia Children's Medical Center, Children's Seashore House in Philadelphia, Children's Hospital in Boston, and St. Joseph's Hospital Center in Mt. Clements, Michigan.

After reviewing these projects, the art core committee was able to establish some priorities for the entire art program. One priority was that this hospital should be a children's place and provide a supportive environment for the whole family. For this reason, the art needed to be engaging and reassuring, providing positive interaction and connection.

Where did we want art? We wanted it to lead patients and visitors through the building and into the building. We wanted art to establish the location of the main entrance and be part of the waiting experience, both indoors and out. We wanted to use art and sculpture to create landmarks and memorable locations that would lead people through the facility. We wanted to place art that would make patients smile in exam and treatment rooms.

We looked at artwork from throughout the country. We used art galleries and representatives as resources. We looked not just for art work to hang on the walls, but for art work that would support our goals.

The commitment of the team to the process had a lot to do with how it worked. Long blocks of time were carved out of very busy schedules. Artist selection and concepts were reviewed, rehashed, and reselected until everyone on the committee was satisfied.

After the preliminary selections were made, an art review group made up of the department managers was encouraged to give input. This process helped refine the selections. After looking at the many possibilities, we finally decided to use multimedia, multidimensional, and multicultural art.

In order to get the owners to understand the possibilities, we did many renderings of sculpture, banners, and ways of finding one's way to the building from the outside. Finally, 12- to 15-foot topiary animals were selected to border the landscaping of the campus. They were friendly, sculptured, inviting, and alive.

The sculpture fountain in front of the building was originally envisioned as the "mission piece," the one piece that would symbolize the miracle work that happens at Children's. Here again, we reviewed the work of many artists from around the country. Dennis Smith from Salt Lake City was selected because of his ability to portray children in dynamic movement working together.

Major waiting areas received an enormous amount of thought. Foremost in our minds was the appropriateness of the imagery. How will this make patients and families feel? Austine Wood-Comarow was commissioned to create 14 Polages™ that mimicked childhood experiences. Using polarized light and technology borrowed from science, Austine has been working for 25 years to produce an art form that changes imagery and color. The art allows the viewer to meditate upon an image ever changing in time and space.

George Rhodes was commissioned to create an engaging audiokinetic sculpture—a network of colorful interactive objects that bounce, chime, loop, and spiral to attract and involve the viewer—especially children.

Southern California presents the opportunity to build outdoor waiting spaces that become meeting spaces and extended living rooms. A mural was designed as an interactive mosaic, including cast bronze sculptural elements. It brought to the space visual excitement with a hands-on opportunity to reinforce the message that this is a special place.

A wayfinding graphic program was developed by the signage consultants, David Robinson and Associates, to assist in orientation in the friendliest of fashions. Rabbits, bears, and kangaroos were carefully located on the directional signs. Petting sculptures were purchased to be placed strategically on the path of window seats throughout the corridors.

Long connecting corridors linked the new hospital to the surgical tower,

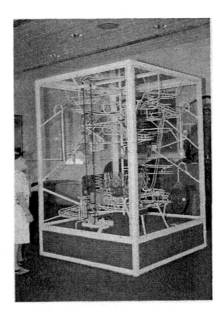

◆ **FIGURE 6–9** George Rhodes was commissioned to create an engaging audio-kinetic sculpture. (*Project:* San Diego Children's Hospital and Health Center Addition. *Architecture/interior design:* NBBJ Architects. *Art consultant:* The Aesthetics Collection. *Photo:* Courtesy of The Aesthetics Collection.)

medical office building, and parking structure. What could we do to make these corridors feel like linking elements? Hands-on, interactive art was designed by artist Bob Mason. This art amplified the themes of time, growth, and discovery.

We wanted the patient rooms to be personal spaces for each child. In order to facilitate this, each room has been provided with changeable art frames to display the child's personal art or picture, or to hold a picture selected from a catalog of changeable art.

Exam rooms and treatment rooms are some of the most difficult spaces for children and their families. Working with the staff, we commissioned playful and engaging mobiles, birdhouses, and fanciful mirrors to be placed in these spaces.

We even wanted the donor recognition system to be a work of art. We challenged many artists for solutions and selected a Tiffany-style window that shows the geographic boundaries of San Diego County from the ocean to the desert. Custom French doors were designed to be placed in front of the window with the names of the donors printed on them.

In conclusion, the art program at Children's serves several functions. The Dennis Smith sculpture serves as a reminder of the miracle work performed at Children's; it inspires, reassures, and lets people know that they are entering a special place. The interactive art of George Rhodes, Bob Mason, and others strategically placed around the building is playful, creative, and happy. The Polages™ designed by Austine Wood-Comarow placed in key waiting areas are restful, soothing, and relaxing. All elements tie together, reinforcing the goals of creating a special environment for children.

The Process

Carter: What the previous individuals have described indicated the challenge in translating this vision into a process with contractors, designers, and hospital staff and in keeping the momentum of what was going to be a very special project.

Those involved included the following: (1) the board of trustees, who were the visionaries and key leadership; (2) the traditional board leadership that oversees the entire project and makes sure that it continues its course; (3) the planning groups within the residential community surrounding the hospital; (4) the medical staff; and (5) the hospital staff.

To involve all these people, we established six core focus groups that included staff, auxiliary, physicians, parents, and, of course, children. One of the groups was an outpatient group that included physicians, nursing staff, and families who had used the hospital's services in the past. We wanted to build a user-friendly environment—to make the "in and out" convenience of visiting our outpatient clinic something that would avoid the unfriendliness or the complexities of a major hospital campus. Again, we focused on scale, making sure that patients and visitors feel, upon entering our outpatient areas, that they are entering a physician's office or a smaller clinic built just for their needs.

We formed a second group for the emergency room. This was composed of hospital staff physicians, as well as community physicians. Children's was building the first and only dedicated pediatric emergency room in San Diego. Many of our community physicians wanted to know what was going to be done, how they might make use of it, and how it was going to help them improve the care that they have been providing to San Diego children for many years. We involved them every step of the way, and continue to involve them with monthly reports, updates, and tours.

Another group, the inpatient focus group, concentrated on staff and parents' concerns about a child's stay in a hospital. The hospital is a child's temporary home, and the scale and design should aim toward making that environment as friendly and comforting as possible. We spent a lot of time communicating with the nursing staff and families through feedback surveys and other vehicles.

We also had a public areas group. This committee was concerned with the design of the graphic system and helped us to understand how a parent reads hospital signage. The group also helped us to design special parent and child features, even to the point of testing our new waiting room furniture.

A support services group included the necessary hotel services, as well as information systems and other hospital services. This group was instrumental especially in the working drawing stage, when many projects die and go into the "black hole" of state review and contract documents. We spent many hours reviewing the contract documents and listening to this group's input regarding outline specifications. We wanted the new environment to be energy efficient and as user friendly for our staff as it is for the families.

Another factor in the process was the regulatory agency and agency staff. The project needed city permits, so we had to work with the city and the community planning groups. We had to go through the state review process, which can be very lengthy in California. We conducted several presubmittal conferences with the design team and the state plan check staff to help the state understand how we were going to go about the submittal process and to get their feedback to help the process go more smoothly.

The second area of process development is the work plan, which the design team developed early on. To do this, we first conducted design review meetings with as many people as possible. There are several schools of thought as to how many people need to be involved in design, but the level of enthusiasm and commitment of our staff encouraged us to invite as much involvement as possible. We had several conferences, and on a few occasions we conducted "charettes," in which we had open houses to review plans and designs. There was outstanding staff turnout. Involvement of this nature will not guarantee success, but failure to involve many of these people could have guaranteed failure.

We had to develop a strategy on how to submit the plans to the state. We decided on a strategy of submitting in phases, which allowed us to construct the project in a logical fashion. Since there were four construction increments, we submitted in four phases. The early increments allowed us to relocate the entire infrastructure to the present hospital, which meant that interruptions to vital services needed to be carefully coordinated.

By submitting our project in phases and receiving multiple permits, we were able to stay on-track and keep every sequence on schedule. Submitting in phases also allowed us to take advantage of a very competitive bid climate: We were able to bid the project in increments and realize significant savings by hitting "windows of opportunities" in the marketplace.

A project that is developed with a multiyear, multiphase approach still works with a lump sum budget. And in the case of Children's Hospital, that was certainly true. We did have one budget figure that our board had authorized and, as we proceeded through the process, we had to keep it in mind. One of the strategies we used was to defer decisions on various components of the project. We would keep our options open as long as possible and then revisit those decisions when there was a critical opportunity to reinstate those components.

Again, by achieving a savings via the multibid approach, Children's Hospital was able to add several components, such as a helipad, pneumatic tube systems, energy management systems, connecting bridgeways between parking structures and office buildings, and bridgeways between office buildings and the existing hospital surgery area.

Of course, there are many decisions about components that cannot be revisited. Those need to be rejected or accepted at the key time. But those decisions that can be deferred should be left on the table for discussion. By doing this, we were able to add approximately $1.5 million back into our project during the construction phase.

In summary, bringing the themes and the concepts from the design phase to reality—a reality in which the men who buckle on the belts and carry the tools do not always understand flowery words or good intentions—needs to be handled carefully and done in a way that keeps enthusiasm high.

My advice is to get the entire design team on board as early as possible. Get a commitment from the design team at the principal level to maintain stability. Set up operational committees early and keep them involved. *Celebrate every milestone.* If there are multiple phases and multiple deadlines, when one of these is achieved, celebrate it.

Staying flexible is important. By being flexible and maintaining momentum, we were able to add features back into our project that we formerly thought were lost. We were able to incorporate new ideas because we had established critical dates when those features could be reinstated. We were able to incorporate new research and designs at the last moment. By involving the people, as I have described, and developing the groups, I think we were able to keep the project fresh.

The End Result

Sadler: So what have we accomplished? We have achieved our twin goals of function and feeling. We have added 114 new beds, bringing our total to 220. We have doubled the number of outpatients to 36 and opened the region's first emergency room designed exclusively for kids. No longer will a child ever be turned away in San Diego because our hospital lacks the space.

But we were also true to our feelings in designing a building that is not intimidating. It is bold, innovative, and creative. It expresses a sense of caring. It is a place to which parents want to come and in which people want to work. We believe all this was achieved by keeping these qualities at the forefront throughout the entire project.

We think our team has been very successful in turning these dreams into reality—into The New Children's Hospital: A Place of Miracles.

Edward Carter, now vice-president of facility planning and construction for The Medical Center in Winston Salem, N.C., was vice-president of facilities development for Children's Hospital–San Diego from 1982–1993. During that time, he was respon-

sible for construction improvement projects totaling more than $40 million and a new $58.4 million Patient Care Pavilion expansion, which opened in early 1993.

David L. Noferi joined Seattle-based NBBJ in 1979 and has since distinguished himself by his hands-on management style, as well as his ability to plan, organize, execute, and control large complex projects. He has been a key participant in two of the firm's largest healthcare projects, and since 1991 has served as principal-in-charge of operations for NBBJ's Los Angeles Studio.

Annette Ridenour is principal-in-charge of The Aesthetics Collection, a professional art services company she founded in 1980 in San Diego, California. An entrepreneur in the art world since 1972, she is nationally recognized for her creative work in developing cohesive artistic environments and visual statements for healthcare facilities and corporations.

Blair L. Sadler is the president and CEO of Children's Hospital and Health Center of San Diego and its affiliate corporations. Prior to his appointment at Children's Hospital in 1980, he served as vice president and director of the hospital and clinics at Scripps Clinical and Research Foundation for three years. Sadler holds a law degree from the University of Pennsylvania and has served as a medical-legal specialist for the National Institutes of Health; co-director of the trauma program at Yale Medical School; and assistant vice president for the Robert Wood Johnson Foundation.

David H. Swain, AIA, joined NBBJ in Seattle in 1969, and began his career in commercial architecture and interiors. He has led the NBBJ interiors practice since 1984 and began to focus his energies solely on healthcare in 1987. Since that time, Swain has spearheaded the interior design for a number of NBBJ's national healthcare projects.

Chapter

SEVEN

PROJECT EXAMPLES/HOSPITALS AND MEDICAL OFFICES

THE AGA KHAN UNIVERSITY HOSPITAL AND MEDICAL CENTER

Third Symposium on Healthcare Design, San Francisco, CA, 1990

Mozhan Khadem
Iqbal F. Paroo
Thomas M. Payette, FAIA, RIBA

Payette: It's quite an honor for me to be at the Symposium to talk about the Aga Khan University Hospital and Medical School project in Karachi, Pakistan. I have put many years of my life into this exciting project and feel very attached to this medical center.

The focus of this presentation will be on design. For me, there is a dilemma regarding the way we think about interior and exterior design. Today, we intend to describe how this particular project forces the focus on that dilemma.

Let me just say a little bit about the two key members that are here. Iqbal Paroo is President and CEO of Hahnemann University in Philadelphia, Pennsylvania, which is a university just for the health and medical sciences. Iqbal was born, and spent his early years, in Kenya; he came to the United States to get his undergraduate and graduate degrees in healthcare management at Georgia State University. Iqbal was the project CEO responsible for setting up the management structure in Pakistan to oversee this project. He was the owner's representative, involved in that crucial period of time when we were designing the totally new facility and thinking about the people who were going to work in it and use it. Mozhan Khadem, now a partner in Payette Associates, was at the time this project was initiated, the partner in charge of the design work at Perkins and Will in Chicago.

Background

Let me just provide a little bit of background relevant to the project. First of all, the project was actually one man's vision: the vision of His Highness, the Aga Khan. He brought about the creation of this new medical center and school in Pakistan. For those unfamiliar with him, the Aga Khan is the religious leader of 15 million Shia Ismaili Moslems worldwide. He was educated at Harvard. From his own business ventures, he has put millions of dollars back into the Moslem community. This particular Aga Khan has a major interest in healthcare and architecture. He has set up all kinds of healthcare outreach programs. He has given $22 million to Harvard and MIT for the Third World Islamic Architectural Study Program. He has also given millions of dollars to a once-every-three-year award program for architectural development in the Islamic communities. He is truly a great benefactor to healthcare and architecture. We were very fortunate to be able to work for him, and it has been very rewarding.

The Aga Khan University Hospital and Medical School includes a 250-student nursing school, a 500-student medical school, and a 750-bed teaching hospital. At the time we were introduced to it, which was the end of 1971, the owner had a team in place that was mostly comprised of Europeans located in London. There was a management team in place for budget control, scheduling, and costing, and there was also a construction management firm.

My architecture firm, Payette Associates, which is located in Boston, was selected in January 1972 in a joint venture with an engineering firm based in London to design all the new facilities.

The Aga Khan's major goal for the project was to attain the highest possible level of standards for education, medicine, and patient care treatment, comparable to standards found in a Western institution. He also wanted to create an environment that was compatible with and respectful of Pakistani culture, both in a historical sense and in the way in which a society in Moslem countries lives today.

Let's talk a minute about contracts. The contract we signed with them included services for architecture and interior design, as well as for all the engineering disciplines. We worked very hard to get interiors incorporated into that initial contract. What we ended up with was a statement that said, "Interiors will, at some later date, be discussed."

We started the design work in 1972 and the university and hospital were operational by November 1985. By December 1974, the entire design construction document package was completed, and some site construction began in 1975. In 1976, reevaluation of how far medical technology had evolved brought about program changes and a process of redesign.

In 1976, a construction manager was hired, Turner International; and in 1977, construction began on the nursing school. Nurses were needed before the hospital could be opened, so the nursing school was under way early and completed before the opening of the hospital in 1985.

Iqbal arrived in 1977. In 1978, Kaiser Foundation International was engaged to do the equipment planning. It wasn't until 1978 that interior design discussions started. Of course, the construction documents had been fully completed and the nursing school was well under construction. At the time, the Aga Khan Foundation decided to have a design competition for the interiors and three firms were engaged: Hellmuth Obata and Kassabaum in St. Louis; Payette Associates in Boston; and a small international firm that has a U. S. office in Cambridge, Massachusetts. Believe me, it took a real effort for us to win that competition. Construction on the major project, with a large British contractor, started in 1980 and wasn't finished until 1985.

Issue of Culture

I'd like to address the issue of culture once more. I explained earlier that the client was very concerned about this project fitting their culture. At the direction of the client, Mozhan Khadem joined the team at the onset of the project, in 1971, as a design consultant. In fact, he led a tour of the design team through Islamic countries, where we studied historical and cultural issues relative to design. That expedition took about one month: we started in Spain, visiting Cordoba and Granada; then went through North Africa and Persia and ended in Pakistan. Although it was a rather forceful way of getting indoctrinated, it was extremely effective.

In addition to gaining a greater appreciation of the architecture and culture of the region, we saw firsthand how the urgent need for hospitals with Western standards had brought forth glass skyscrapers in the Saudi desert. The inappropriateness of these buildings reinforced our goal to design the Aga Khan University Hospital and Medical School in a way that was culturally responsive, while providing all the required technology of a state-of-the-art medical center (see Figure C–21).

Delving into our historical study, we uncovered patterns of lifestyles and related environments repeated throughout time. For example, in this region the courtyard becomes central to the active living space. The design of the

Aga Khan University Hospital and Medical School obviously is a courtyard design. We deliberately avoided a formal tower building, which one often associates with the Western world.

The Indus River comes through Pakistan from the Himalayas and empties into the Indian Ocean at Karachi, which is located in the desert. Throughout Karachi, there is very little air-conditioning; natural ventilation has brought much comfort. The buildings also have a second skin to act as a roof protector for heat reflection; and they allow breezes through to create a cooling effect, with the possibility of water evaporation from pools in the courtyards. There are a few months during the year where there is only high humidity, and several other very hot months. The use of water as a cooling element, both physically and visually, is needed to meet those kinds of climate demands. Intense sunlight is also an issue. Screens and other blockers have to be provided to reduce the amount of light, allow shade, and still let the breeze come through.

The plaster used for construction is called "weeping plaster." Its roughness covers up the deformation of the imperfections in construction, but it also allows for a darker tint because the "drips" create tiny shadows over the surface of the wall. Other construction technology that we had to work with was very basic. There are normal concrete forms, but workers carry buckets up in their bare feet. This culture is truly different; it has an imagery all its own; and it's deeply based in many centuries of a rich heritage.

I now welcome Iqbal to present the owner's position; and then Mozhan will address our design approach to this project.

Paroo: My comments this afternoon will not only represent the thinking of the owner, that is, the client, but also my own thinking. Over the past two decades, the experiences I have had with architects and designers, in North America and abroad, has changed the way I practice from a client's perspective.

The Aga Khan University Hospital and Medical School was probably one of the most ambitious and successful projects ever undertaken by the Aga Khan and his foundation. This wonderful complex is a tribute to the professionals who designed it, the people who built it, and the people who are there running it today. Most of all, it is a tribute to the philanthropist, the Aga Khan himself, whose ideals it truly represents. It started with a dream, as a $15 million project and a 120-bed hospital in 1964. And in the two decades that elapsed, between the announcement of the project and its actual inauguration, the scope of the project was widened and adapted to reflect the changing needs and circumstances of a very different world that Pakistan faced.

This project also represents an extraordinary synthesis of tradition and modernism geared specifically to respond to the Moslem world and the Third World environment. The university also serves as a beacon of excellence for the Aga Khan health services worldwide and, in fact, today, as a not-for-profit institution, serves over one and one-half million patients a year.

If there is one message that I would like to leave, it would be to say that, as a client, I see architecture encompassing the interior, exterior, and the landscape. It is all a single package to me. I have found too many cases of fragmentation, resulting in a nonintegrated final product that results in many change orders, which always cost money.

From an architectural point of view, the Aga Khan University not only is an extraordinary achievement, but it's a prototype of facilities in that part of the world. For patients and visitors, it is a spacious, comfortable, and attractive complex that reflects an outward appearance of professionalism and devotion to quality and standards.

When the Aga Khan first started thinking about this project, he wanted it to reflect Pakistani and Islamic culture and heritage. At the same time, he insisted that the institution be more than functional; it should be consistent with 21st century medicine. To put it simply, he was marrying Islamic tradition to 21st century standards, and I believe that's why many of us from the West were recruited.

His Highness was also impressed with the concept that was presented to him, since that concept was very similar to his own thinking about what architecture should be about. His Highness considers architecture as one of the most important elements of culture. He used to tell us that, "man lives in his home by architecture." Over time, I, too, have come to consider architecture as a "space" for man's physical and spiritual needs. And, clearly, Payette's design concept for the Aga Khan University Hospital and Medical School captures the spirit of the people who were and are expected to use it (see Figure C–22). Over the years, I've also recognized that space must respond to the changing needs of people, the changing culture, and the environment that surrounds us.

When I arrived on site in the fall of 1977, it became very clear to me that the one piece of the design that was not integrated, as Tom mentioned before, was the interior. Because it had been postponed, it affected a major portion of the project that had already begun—the nursing school. Because construction had started, we ran into problems when we started to deal with the interior. We had to go back and rethink some of the design pieces, and that's when the message came through loud and clear. Fortunately, because the rest of the project had not started construction, we had the opportunity to integrate interiors and make the necessary corrections in the design, rather than having to do it postconstruction.

The Aga Khan's vision required enormous collaboration. There were people from 20 different cultures working on this project, and to get all those people thinking together required enormous cooperation. One of the key elements of our success was that there was an excellent relationship between the client and the design team. This special relationship also resulted in very refined communication between the Aga Khan and the design team. Throughout the whole process, whenever the design team advised His Highness, he always listened because he was interested in improving the quality of the project. I always felt we were on the "cutting edge" of what we were doing.

Let me close by saying that there are few men who can conceive an idea as grand and noble and as revolutionary as the Aga Khan University Hospital and Medical School and turn it into a reality. The creation of the design, meticulous construction, and the soothing landscape show a commitment to academic excellence and a resolve to revolutionize higher education in the Islamic world to meet the challenges of the 21st century. His Highness is a great believer in the enrichment of the environment, and the Aga Khan Hospital and Medical School is truly a flowering of that conviction. I was proud to be a part of that team, and it taught me a lot.

In conclusion, the single test of a successful project for a design team is to ensure that the owner's vision and intent is achieved in the final product. So if a design team is dealing with an owner who does not have a clear vision or clear intent, they should insist on going through that process first. In the final analysis, without that clarity, the end result will be a product that they'll never be satisfied with; and the reason they won't be satisfied is that they didn't know what they were asking for to start with.

I am grateful for the opportunity to be at the Symposium. Mozhan will now go through the part of the project that brings it into a reality.

Kadem: This project was truly an exciting experience for those who participated in carrying it out. It developed in us a certain attitude toward architecture, environment, interior design, and landscaping. As Tom said, we cannot separate these aspects of design; they are all parts of the same exercise. Architecture is the organization of spaces, which deals with the way people live; and the treatment of surfaces, which deals with the cultural memory and heritage of the people. Sometimes these surfaces are vertical, such as the walls inside of a room, exterior facades of the streets, or of the courtyards; and sometimes they are horizontal, such as the floors, ceilings, or the landscaped areas. We learned on this project that when we pick up pencil and paper to start the design concept, at the very same moment we should also be thinking about the rosebush in the garden and the aspects of the interior surface finishes as well as the environmental implications of our basic conceptual thinking.

Guiding Principles

Before I go into the main discussion of this project, I would like to convey two principles that the design team of the Aga Khan project, have come to believe in. I have such a profound commitment to them that I believe they should be the guiding principles for design professionals in the closing decade of this century. I would like to share them. We certainly are going to carry with us the good lessons we have learned from the modern movement and postmodern movement, but those are now relics and cannot lead us into the future. The fad of deconstructivism simply does not have any positive philosophical energy proven to be of any significance.

The first principle really deals with something that we hear about often from politicians. They talk about the "new world order." They really do not understand its full significance. The new world order has to do with the fact that we are at the threshold of a global consciousness with regard to the universality of man and the oneness of mankind, and that all nations and races have to live in harmony and peace in the coming century. That is the agenda for the 21st century.

World peace will be the by-product of the unity of mankind. Such a vision means that all cultures of the world, with all of their diversified aspects, participate as equal members in a global forum. It means that every one of us has to learn to appreciate each other's beauty and individuality. America, itself the setting of so many diverse cultures, should not be considered a melting pot. I like America because of its diversity. It's like a garden with many flowers and plants; they are all different, but by proper design, they can be unified. It is the unity in diversity that we seek. As design professionals, we should respond to the diversity of human cultures. Therefore, the first principle that is going to guide us into the next century is *culturally responsive architecture.*

The second principle which is perhaps even more important is *environmentally responsive architecture*. In order to clarify that, I would like to go back to the scientific revolutions of the 18th and 19th centuries. Scientists somehow convinced us at that time that qualities of nature can be quantified, and they presented this science as final and definitive with one object in mind—to use it as power. In fact, Francis Bacon said science is power. Power over whom? Power over nature and over people. Now, our 20th century knowledge tells us that our science is neither final nor definitive. At best, it is a way of knowing an infinitesimal aspect of "quantifiable" nature. But, there is much to nature that is mystical and beyond our comprehension. Thus far, in order to maximize our power over nature, we have compartmentalized it into different disciplines and specializations. We were able to develop massive instruments of power over nature that have resulted in the destruction of the environment—the pollution of the air and water, deforestation of the Amazon, and so on.

Architecture has followed a similar path. I would submit that we, as architects, have not done any better than the scientists. We have used scientific methods and attitudes and have shown very little respect for nature. We are responsible for another level of pollution that has happened on our landscape, the "visual pollution."

To illustrate my point, I will tell a story about visiting the Sea of Galilee last year. Although I'm not from a Christian background, it was a very profound experience for me. We visited the beautiful scenic area in Israel where Jesus delivered the Sermon on the Mount. I was overwhelmed by the fact that I was in the same beautiful spot 2000 years later, looking at the same sea, and seeing the same mountain. There are some parts of the Sea of Galilee that are so virginal that you can actually imagine the scene where Peter would be casting his net and Jesus passing by telling him to stop fishing and become the fisherman of men. When you resonate against such a memory field of history, it becomes very powerful and it shows you an aspect of life that is really what living is all about.

When I turned around to the other side of the Sea of Galilee, I saw a Coney-Island-like chaos of commercial development. I felt completely violated. There are many other examples. There are certain sites that by virtue of history—whether religious or secular—become sacred and we have to respect them. Unfortunately, we don't.

There are two levels of response with regard to environmentally responsible architecture. If the building is on a virgin site, I believe we have to respond to the natural requirements of the site. We should never assert ourselves over nature; we should deal with natural elements like water, light, and air with the respect that they require. When we deal with the built environment, we are usually adding something to an existing urban site. In a good number of urban sites, we are dealing with a lot of existing visual pollution. Therefore, our first obligation is to do "corrective surgery." I have examples that demonstrate how we have tried to do corrective surgery in some of our projects in the States, but this is beyond the scope of this presentation. Since our subject is the Aga Khan university and hospital, I limit our discussion to environmentally responsive architecture on a virgin site.

This idea of culturally and environmentally responsive architecture means that we have to find out what are the environmental and cultural forces that affect the project. Unlike what we have been taught in our universities, we have to put aside our egocentric attitude, which is our obsession with producing a sensational piece of work, and concern ourselves with the discovery of these forces and their proper architectural representations. Let us start to become discoverers; the path of discovery is much more arduous and will lead to greater creativity than we have ever dreamed of. This shift of attitude is necessary, because with it we can produce architecture that has a sense of place, that responds to culture and nature.

Project Description

In the Aga Khan university project, we have tried to produce a work of architecture that is culturally and environmentally responsive. I would like to read to you a letter that I wrote to the Aga Khan in 1971, at the time when the modern movement was dominant. The vision of His Highness, the Aga Khan, was to produce a work of culturally responsive architecture which would reflect the latest functional and technological thinking. The following are quotes from what I wrote to him:

> What is currently happening in the Middle East, from an architectural and artistic point of view, is quite upsetting. A region that once produced truly original and significant examples of architecture is currently witnessing the desecration of its landscape by either a multitude of foreign imports or a vulgar display of superficial design motifs, decorations, and arches that have been copied from Eastern historic examples.
>
> The philosophical basis of modern architecture in the Middle East should be found in the architecture and the cultural heritage of its people. A great number of Islamic historic monuments that contain living functions, especially those in the Indo-Persian world, do not have a comprehensive exterior geometry and, therefore, are not objects in space. They literally merge with the fabric of the city and are integrated with their surroundings. Their architectonic value is that of the continuous interior spaces and courtyards that surround the observer; not an isolated building that stands apart from him.
>
> In this kind of planning, the diverse physical requirements of human society are incorporated into one organic whole and the significant architectural episodes, such as the mosque, the university, the hospital, etc., are represented through the identification of appropriate entrance portals, fountains, changes of levels, vistas, etc. The beholder, therefore, is not aware of the exterior of any particular edifice. His architectural experience consists of his entry through a magnificent portal and the interlocking procession of the interior courtyards and spaces. The sequence of spaces is not simply a series of mechanically laid-out courtyards connected with links, the policy that has led to many abortive architectural attempts in the East and in the West. It is rather a procession of a variety of enclosures with differing scale, proportion, and function. This variety of treatment evokes moods of meditation, interaction, privacy, repose, and motion.
>
> The manner of transition between courtyards is most significant. These spaces of transition have been handled with supreme artistry. Each provides for a different function, which psychologically prepares the observer for the succeeding architectural event. Each has its appropriate entrance portal that partially or completely conceals the full impact of the magnificent court behind it. As these delightful courtyards unfold in a rhythmic and hierarchal

sequence before the bedazzled eye of the beholder, he gains a profound artistic experience that cannot be attributed to any singular architectural episode or any specific point in time. The experience is derived from the whole of the complex while observed in a state of motion. This is truly kinetic architecture. It would be marvelous indeed to bring modern technology to the service of such an idea. We are convinced that such an attempt would produce a unique architectural and artistic statement worthy of the noble intentions of His Highness, the Aga Khan.

In the architecture of continuous enclosed spaces that surround the observer, we are not talking about the exterior of an edifice. We are talking of the roofscape. Sometimes these roofscapes have organic curvilinear forms, similar to the one in the Indo-Persian subcontinent. In North African examples they have geometric forms. The courtyards usually have highly embellished surfaces.

Traditional windscoops that catch the wind and take it inside for cooling reasons were a source of study for us. In Pakistan, the windscoops in the city of Tata are very famous. In Indo-Persian examples of Islamic architecture (i.e., the mosque) the buildings literally emerge from the fabric of the city and disappear into it. A mosque in the Indo-Persian subcontinent, unlike a cathedral, had multiple functions: It functioned as a library, a university, a community center, a place for eating and drinking, a hostel, and so on. It is interesting that the exterior geometry of a traditional mosque is not easily comprehensible and corresponds to the multiplicity of its function. One notion that I want to correct right now is that the Taj Mahal is not a typical example of Islamic architecture. It is an example of an Islamic tomb.

In this kind of architecture, the elements that take the place of "exterior facades," for identification purposes, are entrance portals. These entrance portals are not just openings to walk through, they are architectural experiences. After the entrance portal, there's a transition space that is handled with great artistry. It prepares the visitor psychologically for the succeeding architectural event. It leads to other spaces.

The spaces themselves all have a function, whether they are large formal courtyards or intimate rooms, or passageways. Courtyards are part of the building program. In the Aga Khan facility we incorporated many open courtyard spaces that function as lobbies and living rooms.

Another aspect I want to talk about is light. If our goal is to be environmentally responsible, when we design for light we have to realize that light is not just a quantity of foot-candles. Light is a mystery. When you really think about it, light is a profound mystery. There is more to light than a certain amount of foot-candles. This means that we have to explore light and show it in architecture in the multiplicity of its manifestations—the way it appears to us and the way it evokes a sense of awe and wonder about life itself. It's very interesting because many philosophical or mystical schools devoted to the idea of light have originated in that part of the world. Sohrevardi, who was known as the "master of illumination," was a great mystic. He was executed, as mystics usually are. He developed a whole school related to the philosophy of light. It's interesting, also, that he was influenced substantially by the Manicheans and the Neoplatonists. Abbot Suger was influenced by similar ideas about light, as demonstrated in the writings of Dionysus the Areopagite, and built the Church of St. Denis to exhibit his philosophy of light. Thus, the Gothic movement was born. As we all know, light is treated with a sense of mystery and wonder in Gothic architecture.

Landscaping in that part of the world is quite different from the great French axial landscape or the informal landscaping of the English gardens. In Islamic countries, many examples of landscaping are based on the Sasanian courtyard. These courtyards were called "pardis," which is the word that was brought to the Western world by European travelers and is the root word of "paradise" (see Figure C–23).

In these gardens, water is used in a most delightful way, manifesting in qualities of intimacy and charm as well as awe and wonderment. Again, when we use water in architecture, we have to convey its enigmatic nature, rather than flaunt our technological ability to manipulate a certain quantity of "H_2O." Who says water is not sacred or mysterious? Try going without it for four days—the first sip would convince anyone who doubts its mystery.

Surfaces in environmentally and culturally responsive architecture are very important. This is true of surfaces in architecture in America and Europe as well. Before we fell into the trap of compartmentalizing life, when all of the arts were together, buildings had a soul; they had memory. The surfaces evoked memories of the past; they communicated with people. That is when architecture was art and when buildings spoke to people.

Unlike what many of us were told in school, surface decoration is not skin deep; it is culture thick. It evokes a past. Each of us resonates against a vast field of memory. This memory gives sense and meaning to a piece of architecture. Let us look at surface treatment of entrance portals at the Aga Khan University.

The entrance portals are always adorned with calligraphic or some other symbolic surface treatment. The calligraphic design around the portal is based on the literary and artistic heritage of the region. Sometimes it is legible and sometimes it is coded. It produces a memorable effect.

We could have designed the Aga Khan facility as a box. Putting the program in the form of a box was a very popular thing to do in 1970. The architectonic quality of a box design is that it is space exploitive. It demands attention, it needs to be seen and appreciated; and if there are too many of these buildings in too small a space, we will have the mess that is urban America.

On the other hand, the same program can be organized around man in the form of a series of courtyards, as is the Aga Khan university and hospital. Just imagine being in the center of one of these courtyards. When we open them up to relate them to each other and to outside space, we develop entry portals. And when two entry portals are connected, transition spaces develop; thus a hierarchal system of spaces is produced, evoking different functions and different moods. The exterior geometry of the Aga Khan facility is not comprehensible. It requires its meaning when one walks through it. It is kinetic architecture.

The courtyards have various scales and proportion for different functional requirements. The lobby of the hospital or its "living room" is partially under cover, and partially open to sky. Classrooms open up to spaces for interaction.

There are many gates and fences that separate different areas of the facility from each other. Every one of them has a design that has symbolic calligraphic significance. Calligraphy, as it is known in that part of the world, is as important as painting was to 17th century Europe. Schools of philosophy and poetry have developed around calligraphy. Each letter of the alphabet is endowed with certain attributes; again, this represents a level of mystical insight that also exists in Western tradition, but it is not acknowledged. For example, the letter "alpha" (alef) is the symbol of the beloved. There are numerous poems in which the writer refers to his beloved's stature as an alpha. Being a vertical line, an alpha is aloof; it never attaches to another letter.

Lambda (lam) has at times been considered the symbol for the lover. And since I am a romantic person at heart and am very fond of the mystical and earthly references to lover and beloved, we developed a calligraphic design of interlocking "alef" and "lam" (in Kufic tradition). So the lover and the beloved became united. We chose a specific saying from the classics that had the alpha and lambda repeating. We believe that when a sick person comes from a remote village with an extended family to get cured and sees the lover and beloved embracing, he gets well and goes home faster. In the cultural tradition of that part of the world, this union has a great deal of philosophical and symbolic meaning.

The saying I chose for the intermediate panel of the gates says, "Enter Therein and Peace Will Be Upon You." This saying, is flanked by the lover and the beloved symbol at the top and on the sides. The saying at the top of the entrance portals and the gates is from the Koran, saying "La Elaha Ella Allah," (There is no god but God.) The mystical symbols of the lover and the beloved come from the great Sufi tradition of the area. This symbolism is stated eloquently in the work of the great poet Rumi.

We developed a series of tile designs that are unique to this project; each one of them has a different story. The client was amused when I told them we wanted a great quantity of Halla tiles. I went to Halla and found tile-producing shops consisting of two old men who made beautiful tiles, producing only a maximum of 20 a day. When I told them how many thousands we wanted, they escorted me out of their hut. Nevertheless, we still wanted those tiles. Another problem was that they were not very durable. So we took the tile makers to the factory in the city where they produced mechanical looking tiles, and the old men agreed to work for us there. They sat on the floor—they didn't want to sit on benches—and started drawing our designs on these tiles. They had some problems with color running in the high temperature kilns of the factory. But this problem was resolved. Now, a legacy has been left in Pakistan: These tiles that look handmade are being produced in factories and are of world class standard.

Corridor walls and other surfaces are tied together with these tiles. We felt it was very important to have symbolic designs on them so that the users can recollect the beauty of their cultural heritage.

The story behind one of the tile designs is interesting. Even to this day in Pakistan, when one looks at decorated surfaces of buses and houses, one often sees a depiction of the story of "Miraj" along with a rose. The story of "Miraj" is Mohammed's heavenly journey. Legend has it that when Mohammed went to Seventh Heaven, a drop of his perspiration fell on the ground and a rose grew; this is the origin of the rose. We felt it was a beautiful story to put into a coded calligraphic design.

Ismaili Moslems invoke the name of Ali, who is supposed to be the lion of God. So we used calligraphy to depict the face of a lion around the edge of the ceiling in the medical school auditorium.

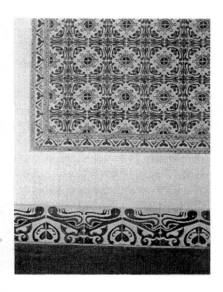

◆ **FIGURE 7–1** Each one of the tile designs, which were developed especially for this project, has a different story. (*Project:* Aga Khan University Hospital and Medical School, Karachi, Pakistan. *Architecture:* Payette Associates. *Photo:* Paul Warchol.)

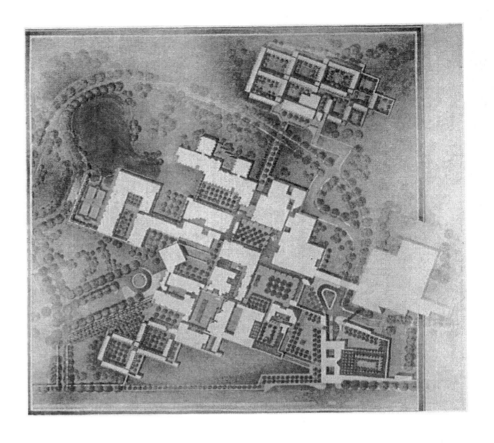

I could go on forever, but I think it is time to turn the platform back to Tom.

Payette: The Aga Khan University Hospital and Medical School is exceedingly interesting because it has affected the way we now think about the approach we take to all of our work. The Miami project Mozhan mentioned demonstrates what we learned about culture and history from that month-long tour of Islamic countries. It brought back the fact that when we design a project in our own community, we assume that we already know everything about it. In reality, we must step back and look at the cultural roots of each individual community, so that what develops is a true reflection of the people it serves. Each institution, community, or country has its own special image, the richness of which must be brought forward. Cultural identity should not be stamped out.

In closing, I want to emphasize the remarkable effect the Aga Khan University Hospital and Medical School has had on our firm and express my gratitude to the Aga Khan for the opportunity to design it, and to the Symposium for the opportunities to share our experience with a larger group of people.

Mozhan Khadem is a principal with Payette Associates, a Boston, Massachusetts, architecture and design firm internationally known for its healthcare expertise. With over

30 years of architectural experience, he has been with Payette for 13 years, providing high-quality, culturally responsive design direction for projects in the United States and abroad.

Thomas M. Payette, FAIA, RIBA, is president and CEO of Payette Associates. With more than 25 years of experience in the design of medical institutions, research laboratories, and academic facilities, he has provided design direction for numerous projects in the United States and abroad.

Iqbal F. Paroo is the president and CEO of Hahnemann University in Philadelphia, Pennsylvania. The university has a 621-bed hospital, medical school of 800 students, graduate and allied health professionals schools of 1600, a staff of 4600, and an annual operating budget of more than $400 million. His 20 years in the healthcare field have included positions with the Aga Khan Hospital and Medical College Foundation, Charter Medical Corporation, Hospital Corporation of America, and Healthcare International.

◆　◆　◆

LAMBETH COMMUNITY CARE CENTER

Third Symposium on Healthcare Design, San Francisco, CA, 1990

Robin Nicholson, MA, MSc, RIBA

In November 1980, two doctors, a community leader, and a physiotherapist came to our office in Camden Town in North London to look at slides of our work and to offer their vision of a new kind of health facility. The chemistry was immediate—we were thrilled at the prospect of designing a new, socially useful, "missionary" project, although our enthusiasm was tempered by previous experiences of other visionaries' great ideas and subsequent lost dreams.

Two weeks later the junior Minister of Health, in his short, but radical reign, unlocked the funding of the construction and 18 months' running costs of the Lambeth Community Care Center. Nearly five years of hard work had already passed, and it was to be another five years before Prince Charles and Princess Diana formally opened the center. Every month in the life of the project was a struggle, and today both the center's very success and the present economic regime continue to threaten its existence.

Located in a quiet 19th century back street of terraced houses, the center provides patient centered and preventive care for those living nearby within the National Health Service, which provides over 90 percent of all healthcare in the United Kingdom. In a small but modern and accessible building, there is a dentist, chiropodist/speech therapist, social worker, occupational and physiotherapists, but no resident physician. At ground level is a day center that is also available for community use; and upstairs are 20 beds. Both floors relate strongly to a large garden. Critical to its success are its small size and design focus on the patient, and democratic structure. It aims to provide good health service for local people; its modest but revolutionary attitude toward people and their health makes it an "in-between" place, more an extension of the home than a hospital.

The Beginning

I want to connect you to that place, the London Borough of Lambeth, 1980–1990, to illustrate the center's ambitions and very real achievements. People in the United States and United Kingdom speak the same language, but sometimes with different tongues; we both have our separate myths and dreams. What is certain is that we are all changing and the greater certainties are often the most vulnerable.

The project was developed in the turmoil of Margaret Thatcher's revolution—an economic and social upheaval that, like General Pinochet's in Chile, has clearly shown to most of us the poverty of monetarism and the Chicago school of economics; like him, she was reluctant to let go. Today we have an enterprise culture of unrestrained greed and a pitiful lack of investment in production, education, and health. Against this acclaimed "economic miracle," it is ever more difficult to remember the selfless service that traditionally allowed the public health system to work in the United Kingdom and be one of the most economically efficient in the world.

Lambeth, like many of the one-time villages that make up London, has developed with a complex physical and social structure. It would be perfectly reasonable for a visitor to Bedlam, the original mental asylum and now the Imperial War Museum, to drive down between the plane trees of Kennington Park Road, lined with its 18th century brick terraced houses and feel sure that London was the most civilized of places. Yet only a few blocks away that same visitor would walk over the vast Aylesbury estate, a 1960s state-of-the-art public housing development, and wonder how the human race could survive the self-abuse.

In such a typical inner city area, the effects of ten years of radical conservatism shows more clearly the social state: homelessness and poverty right alongside gleaming Porsches and Volvo station wagons. Meanwhile, the population is aging, the family unit is dissolving, and the traditional sense of community responsibility is overstretched. Optimism and idealism are rare, but essential, commodities at such times.

The Lambeth Hospital

In the early 1960s, the authorities decided to demolish part of Florence Nightingale's own hospital, St. Thomas's, and build a new, modern, air-conditioned hospital block with small wards around a deep plan on the most spectacular site on the River Thames opposite the Gothic delights of the House of Commons. It is easy, with hindsight, to mock other's follies, but the effects of North Wing were to be controversial; and one of the first was to make "The Lambeth," as the old hospital was called, redundant.

The Lambeth had developed out of a 19th century workhouse, where Charlie Chaplin's mother spent some of her less fortunate days, and had grown into the kind of hospital that we all know, depend on, and yet sometimes love to hate. But without a doubt, the community felt the hospital was theirs.

In 1974, the previous Conservative government had invented Community Health Councils (CHC) to act as "watchdogs" to the National Health Service (NHS). Within their remit was the power to challenge the disposal of surplus land and buildings, and the old Lambeth hospital provided just such an opportunity. The Health Authority wished to build a 1000-bed hostel for their nurses, but the CHC doubted the wisdom of that. They proceeded, through public meetings and a one-in-five household survey, to establish the local community's requirements for sheltered housing for the elderly and disabled and a new community hospital.

Over the next four years, a model for a new facility emerged that would offer a local service complementary to that offered by St. Thomas's one mile away, a service that was seen as a necessary consequence of the concentration of high-tech treatment of illness in such a district general hospital. Recalling the dominance of hospital-based consultants over the local general physician (GP), this project will be seen as a testament to the determination of the principal players and the support of the local community.

The desire for attention when one is ill often demands total submission, because people are naturally fearful of the outcome. The concepts of "care" and "good health" may at best be considered to be dangerous distractions from the serious intentions of the surgeon Hippocrates; and is it 20 years since Ivan Illich started illuminating the self-contradictory nature of all institutions, which he claims progressively deteriorate into self-justifying elements of the Establishment?

The Caring Ambitions

Increasingly, as one GP wrote in an introduction to Lambeth Community Care Center, "many people working in fields of primary healthcare were thinking about new methods of caring for isolated members of the inner city population—people who frequently needed general practitioner care, supported by acute nursing and rehabilitation services, but who, for want of such a facility, were usually inappropriately admitted to the local district general hospital. It was also envisaged that the facility would act as a center where frequently isolated individuals (especially GPs) working in primary healthcare would be able to get together with the aim of improving coordination of activities and collectively raising standards of practice."

The Target Client

The center has two principal parts—a day unit and 20 beds for inpatients. In addition, there is a strong commitment to the local community, which has use of the center for meetings.

The operational policy of the center sets out the criteria for admissions to the inpatient beds, as follows:

- Any person aged 16 and above who is on the list of a contracted GP and who requires short-term (less than 28 days) inpatient care
- Patients who need basic observation and assessment in order that decisions about their future treatment and care can be made
- Patients who need inpatient admission because they cannot be cared for at home, but who do not need the facilities of a district general hospital or other specialist care
- Patients discharged from district general hospital wards who need rehabilitative care before returning to the community

- People living on their own or with carer(s), who require either planned or crisis relief respite care
- People requiring terminal or continuing care, but who do not require specialist acute hospital care

The center does not accept patients suffering from acute psychiatric conditions, with notifiable infectious diseases, or those requiring specialist care.

The Project Team

All NHS building projects have multidisciplinary project teams to pull together the brief and operational policies and to monitor the design development. Inevitably, the pressures of work encourage many such teams to turn into "rubber stamps" and often their changing membership prevents the nurturing of true visions.

The Community Care Center had built up an ad hoc team over a period of time; but once the money was allocated and my firm was appointed as architects, the team acquired health authority officers and began to meet on a much more regular basis—approximately every six weeks.

The project team principals were not interested in monitoring our design of the project or rubber stamping anything; they wanted to design it with us.

The core team consisted of four general physicians, two community nurses, one sister, one occupational therapist, one physio-therapist, CHC secretary, one administrator, one hosptial building officer, and a project team secretary.

My senior partner, Ted Cullinan had been in practice for over 15 years and the practice was known for designing careful and composed buildings that drew support from the Arts & Crafts tradition while enjoying the freedoms of later "modern architecture." These are buildings for living and working in; buildings that enjoy the way they are made; beautiful buildings.

Although we had been selected on the basis of our past work, our experience as a cooperative practice in sharing the design process was important. The original brief requested "a domestic building" that might have summoned up images of little houses with thatched roofs and coach lamps outside the front door, but the team readily accepted our proposal that the center could better be seen as a large country house set in the city. Such concepts had to be argued through with a group of up to 17 people who exhibited the classic dynamics of any group. In retrospect, we were embarking on a nearly impossible and rather dangerous path: four years of assertion and argument, often tense, but eased by laughter, and in the end transformed with love.

Participatory Design

At this time, there was an idea developing in the United Kingdom called "community architecture," which grew out of the increasingly popular dissatisfaction with the state housing program. It claimed that by involving the user or occupier in the design of buildings, they would be more appropriate and people would therefore look after them better; indeed, the world would become a better place. This claim is as vulnerable as all such deterministic claims.

While we had long argued that architects should be more willing to seek and accept criticism during the design process, the results of the practice of community architecture are hardly encouraging. And to that extent, the Lambeth Community Care Center does offer a more modest, but effective model of "participatory design."

The community had invented the concept and was supportive, if somewhat incredulous, throughout. "This isn't bloody Monkton Street, because it's so bloody beautiful" was a typical local response to the completed project.

The project team represented the principal disciplines and the community was represented by the secretary of the CHC, who was well known and in regular contact with an impressive number of local people.

At each meeting, we would present ideas in the form of drawings, which were not initially for approval, but to enable discussion to take place. Discussion was needed not only between ourselves and the team, but also among members of the team, who frequently misunderstood one another. This process meant that every aspect of the building and its use was discussed, although we could never predict which aspects would be most closely scrutinized.

We feel that this is a critical part of the architect's role that is frequently ignored for the benefit of entropy, or at least the status quo. A kind of Parkinson's logic operates as follows, "Any organization tends to decline at the point at which it builds a building for itself." This argument asserts that many briefs for buildings are drawn up by asking every member of the existing organization what they require in terms of accommodation. And most of us, when asked such a question, always at an inconvenient moment, look at the space we are in, add 10 percent; look at the size of the window, change its direction; look at the furniture and ask for a more adjustable chair, a deeper carpet, and double the filing capacity. The result fixes a situation in which they have had to adjust to circumstances as they have developed; they are frozen into the concrete frame and steel filing cabinets at one point in time.

One of the reasons we were chosen as architects was that we had no previous experience in hospital building or procedures. We finally persuaded the Regional Health Authority to give us permission to proceed on condition that we did not ask to join their list of approved architects; but we were well ignorant of the many NHS procedures, many of them long outdated and still strangling the procurement of good health facilities.

Of course we had all had our own encounters with the health service; and we had guidebooks to tell us what not to do by proposing lowest common denominator solutions, the general being promoted at the expense of the particular. But we believe that all buildings are part of a five-thousand-year-old tradition of making spaces for people as life-enhancing and as beautiful as we collectively know how and that the particular often provides the clue to the general.

Our ignorance had a further direct consequence: We had no option but to question everybody on the team and many others who were not about their present accommodation and its shortcomings, in order to learn the functions. By asking each person to be as critical as possible, we learned not only about bed making techniques, but also what a sphygmomanometer was.

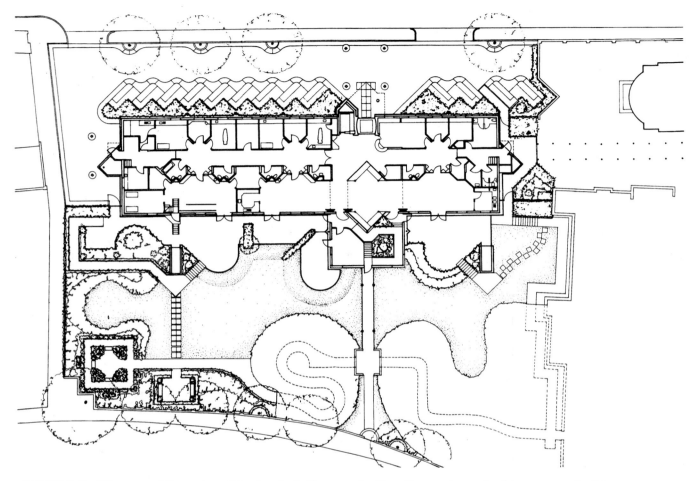

◆ **FIGURE 7–3** The ground floor plan of the Lambeth Community Care Center shows the "compactness" of the space. (*Architecture:* Edward Cullinan Architects.)

This period allowed us to get to know the team members as professionals in their own right. The nurses would always defer to the doctors in team meetings, but on their own they were clear headed, independent, and often critical of the doctors' habits.

Having chosen a new site with the team and having introduced the idea that it was not only more domestic to go upstairs to bed, but also more appropriate to build a two-story building on Monkton Street, we were able to begin to design the building form, plan a layout, and decide on the materials all at the same time.

Arriving at the basic form of a wide house on the street facing south over the garden with a large terrace in front of the wards was fairly straightforward; but to find the key pattern was extremely difficult and was distilled over a number of stages.

Not only does this building break many conventions in line with the philosophy of the center, but it also is on the absolute limit of smallness. Our financial advisors insisted that there was only enough money to provide 80 percent of the area recommended in the various government guidelines. I am sure that this situation is familiar; but to save 20 percent on a four-bed ward and make it "homelike" at the same time is impossible.

The approach was through discussion and bargaining:

- Eliminate certain spaces, such as the waiting room.
- Reduce the sizes of others to a real minimum: One room that would have suffered most from its small size, the physiotherapy room, is one of the few at the size requested.
- Overlap some activities: It was clearly unnecessary for 35 people to sit in one room, move into another adjacent to eat lunch, and then go back again.
- Time-share some spaces: The occupational therapist (OT) and physiotherapist immediately understood the game and allowed the OT's practice bedroom, which in our observations was often used for staff bicycle storage, to double with a physio cubicle for postural drainage.

The GPs had asked for two consulting rooms because, in Parkinson's logic, doctors work in consulting rooms. Only very late and only when no one else would share the part-time chiropodist's space did they realize that they could. In practice they have never used that space, but rather have consulted their patients as though they were in their own homes—that is, wherever they are in the building.

Not all the moves were to squeeze, as an examination of the plans will show. In particular, passages and corridors are not sized for the largest object ever likely to pass down them, rather they are places for sitting and talking or watching that allow the building to be enjoyed by those using it. The most extreme example is the placing of the main staircase within a conservatory.

The Site and Building

Not far from Bedlam, down the Kennington Road, the old Lambeth hospital lies like a banana across this part of Kennington, effectively dividing the neighborhood once the old hospital and its grounds were closed. In 1979, Monkton Street appeared to be a run-down cul-de-sac; but it was also an important, if dangerous, pedestrian link. One side was lined with empty factories and the other by an eight-foot-high brick wall behind which lay seldom-used hospital tennis courts.

When the wall came down, and fortunately the factories had been occupied, this rather squalid dead end was transformed into a "place" and the 24-hour occupation of the Community Care Center ensured a safer passage for everyone.

Some patients find the street side less friendly than the garden; but this is a correct response, because it is north facing and deliberately reserved onto the public realm. The glazed porch is formed by extending the roof of the building over to the back of the pavement, giving generous protection to ambulances and the sister's office that hangs from it surveying the street. On entering, people are welcomed by the receptionist and invited into the sitting room, the heart of the building.

This internal space is made with two glazed bay windows for sitting in. It was devised partly to satisfy the team sister, who insisted that her patients must be able to see the ambulance draw up to take them home. From here, the dining room opens up with sliding screens.

The key to the pattern, which took so long to find, lies in the typical nine-meter-wide slice through the ground floor plan that is repeated three times. Each day room, such as OT, faces south onto the garden and has French windows opening onto its own terrace (see Figure C–24). Its door is in a glazed screen flanked by two seats in a space formed by them and three doors set back opposite—two to larger consulting rooms and one to a smaller office all on the north side. Thus, daylight is brought into the center of the building where people are moving, and where, without it, it would be so easy to get lost. At each end there is, as in a traditional country house, a (metaphorical) green baise door to allow the staff through to service spaces and to go upstairs.

The processional public route upstairs passes the seminar room, ramps up around a tiny lushly planted jungle, up a flight of stairs into a transparent world of steel and glass. The upper conservatory is, strictly speaking, outside the building and is particularly enjoyed for the protected exposure to the garden that lets the patient be in nature (life) but also inside (shelter).

Upon reentering the building, people used to be welcomed by the nurse station, controling the elevator, stair, the drugs cupboard, and the sister's office. It offered both total vision down the corridor and an important closeness to the patients in single rooms, as well as the prospect of being able to enjoy a full moon through the skylight above it! So successful was this focus, that staff were drawn to it at all times. Therefore the nurse station has now been removed. Since the sitting room at one end is not especially popular, I have recently begun to imagine a combined nurse station and sitting room as a focus in the main social space. The staff room is at the other end to provide privacy, coffee, and a view of the garden.

Gathered around the nurse station are the four single rooms for the most dependent patients. Beyond lie the four-bedded wards, which all open up through large French windows onto the terrace overlooking the garden. Clerestory lighting not only allows for cross-ventilation of these rooms, but more importantly, allows the evening sun to wash down the cross walls.

Opposite the ward doors, two bathrooms form an alcove with two seats opposite one another and a large window. These seats allow the most intimate conversations and consultations to take place in public as well as allowing the patients, therapeutically, to spy on the activities in the street below.

The Interior

Our brief was inevitably full of conflicts—to design a "homelike" building as unlike St. Thomas's hospital as possible and to be maintenance free. The first instructions of the district building's officer were to cover all doors, frames, and walls up to three feet six inches with indestructible plastic. This provided us with the clue to the interior: the raising of the skirting to take the points of wheelchairs, the installation of a dado rail to take trolleys and chair backs, and a picture rail in those rooms with an apparently endless supply of pin boards, white boards, key racks, and dressing racks, all as a means of containing that chaos. These rails were then turned into chunky architraves around doors and access panels, and the result is a net of limpid green stained wood laid onto the plastered walls.

The lighting was an area of structured conflict—determination to have tungsten lights by the users against the insistence on the economics of the fluorescent by the building officer.

While suffering from normal use and lack of maintenance, the building is slowly being enriched with artwork. We started by painting plaques of medicinal herbs as part of the external composition. We added a Steiner-based fountain in the conservatory, a series of eight paintings by Tom Philips painted for their particular positions, and most recently a stained glass window by Jonathan Butler in memory of a young patient who died in the center.

Patients

One of the key concepts in the center is the belief in the need for relative patient autonomy. This and other aspects of life in the center are discussed anecdotally in Gillian Wilce's book, *A Place Like Home,* but it may be helpful to describe some of these aspects here.

Since the center is in part seen as an extension of people's homes and is aimed at enabling people to live in those homes, it is crucial for them to grow independent of the center. This is the exact opposite of most hospital regimes that sometimes have no option but to move the patient from one of total dependence to total aloneness at home. Furthermore, most patients are frightened of their illness and of doctors.

These two strands are brought together in the program at Lambeth. Each patient has a key worker who carries prime responsibility for that patient at all times and who can advocate on behalf of the patient. The special relationship of staff and patient is seen to be important, as is the multidisciplinary team who works out the care plan with each patient. The key worker is usually a nurse, but not always; and like all staff, they wear no special uniform. It is, after all, meant to be like home.

Understanding one's condition is seen as essential for healing, as well as a democratic right; and so patients' medical notes are left at the end of the bed. These notes, far from being sanitized placebos, are serious and seen as an important form of communication. Wilce quotes from one, "S: 'I feel old and useless.' P: Suggests lots of cuddles." Not only do the notes record what is wrong, but the patients, their families, and friends are encouraged to contribute to them.

The patient's timetable is determined by the patient, except that meals are provided at conventional times. Getting up, bathing, and going to bed are completely according to habit and only sometimes cause problems, for example when a patient announces that he or she always showers at 5 A.M.!

At the center, it was realized that the self-administration of drugs would be essential in the preparation for going back home, living independently, and being able to take the correct number of the right pills. This is a typical example of the center's challenge to the dependency inherent in ill-health practice.

It is difficult not to mention the experience of the center as a place to die in. The concept was often discussed in project team meetings, but the mechanics of body handling was better understood than the concept of the permission to die. Each case is different and strikingly challenges our present "Waspish" ignorance and fear of death—perhaps a consequence of the commoditization of death.

By now, a significant number of people have felt sufficiently calmed by the attentions of the staff and by being in the place in which they have decided quite deliberately to die—sometimes at terrifying speed.

There is in death, a rare sense of belonging and responsibility. Wilce quotes, "When a patient died before her relatives could get there, it was her fellow patients who picked a flower to put on her, said prayers 'round her, and then asked that she stay with them in the room, in her own bed, for a while."

The Garden

Although England may have been a nation of shopkeepers, it is now a nation of gardeners. So, when the project team inquired as to when the garden was to be designed, the fiercest battles were only just beginning.

Five years after completion, there is now a wonderful chaos of plants, many propagated and planted by the staff and neighbors, but all faithfully planned with the project team. The original schemes incorporated a bridge from the conservatory to the back gate and a pair of planted ramps made with the excavated material from the foundations. This would enable patients to wheel from upstairs across the bridge down and around through the garden into the ground floor and back up in the elevator. Although these features still dominate, they are just the framework for a valley, a seat, a homage to Lombard Street, San Francisco; another to the laburnum tunnel at Bodnant, North Wales, a green room to hide in, a rose garden, and a lawn, all in less than an acre.

Does It Work?

From the first admission, there has been an extraordinary atmosphere in the center. A real optimism pervaded, but was this a function of its genesis or just because it was new? Its inventors' ambitions were critically insistent and included a program of research, which was completed in 1990.

In practice, the center serves a population of 80,000 in a 1.5-mile radius with 39 contracted GPs. The resident staff presently consists of 19 nurses, three physiotherapists, two occupational therapists, one social worker, one dentist, one chiropodist/speech therapist, one part-time dietician, four administrators, and two porters.

To date, bed occupancy averages a staggering 92 percent; 63 percent being women, 82 percent over 65. The average length of stay is 16 days.

These statistics, a detailed description of the center at work, and its unfashionably, but crucially democratic structures are contained in an assessment study published in 1990 by Gregor Henderson and Maryrose Tarpey.

They carried out two sets of interviews with patients, caregivers, and representatives from the community and Health Authority to establish the aims of the center and test its success in achieving these aims. The three main aims were indentified as: (1) good quality of care, (2) effective multidisciplinary organizational structures, and (3) community participation.

Although the second two aims are integral to the center's philosophy, the most revealing to me, as an architect, are the conditions perceived necessary for the achievement of good quality care: (1) that the service should be provided in an atmosphere and environment that is friendly and informal, and (2) that the patient care should be individualized—using a key worker approach, giving appropriate treatment, and promoting patient autonomy.

While identifying certain problems, the researchers reported:

> Generally, the building itself, including the garden and the canteen, were seen as a condition for achieving good quality care in the center. People praised aspects of the building, such as the use that has been made of natural light. Users in particular, praised the accessible and homelike physical structure of the building. Community representatives and service providers suggested that the design of the building and its influence on the work of the center was so significant that it should be taken into account if the center was to serve as a blueprint for the establishment of other community care centers (see Figure C–25).

The Future

In 1990 we celebrated the center's fifth birthday in an atmosphere of great enthusiasm. Although the economic knives are still flailing and the catering arrangements prejudiced, the recent threats to close the center for the ease of saving a half a million pounds a year seems to have been lifted.

The center has had its teething troubles, but probably they are a necessary feature in any such public program for change: change of attitude for patients, change of attitude for the staff, and in this age of scepticism a rare example of architecture popularly seen as contributing to the caring process.

In a special issue of the *Architect's Journal* in October 1985, historian Jules Lubbock summed up his research on the project:

> I base my evaluation largely on the views of the present users, staff, and patients, none of whom were on the project team. Above all, the building not only assists therapy, but is therapeutic in its own right. Ward patients ask for the curtains to be opened, look out at trees, and want to get out of bed. Its beauty and intricacy teases one to explore and encourages patients to walk and become independent.

And, as one of the center's own leaflets asserts on its front cover, "The Lambeth Community Care Center facilitates a community environment for giving, sharing, receiving . . . enabling people to maximize their capabilities to live a full life."

Footnote

In October 1992 the Government published Professor Bernard Tomlinson's Report on London's Health Care Service, in which he uniquely singled out the Lambeth Community Care Center as follows:

We have been impressed by the concept of the "Community Hospital," which has been implemented in West Lambeth, and which provides, on a planned basis, access to low-intensity care for the patients of a group of GPs. We recommend that this model should also be more widely adopted.

References

Henderson, G., and Tarpey, M. 1990. Assessing the Lambeth Community Care Center. Research report published by the Lambeth Community Care Center.

Lubbock, Jules. 1985. A Patient Revolution. Special issue of *The Architect's Journal*. 42 (183).

Wilce, Gillian. 1988. *A Place Like Home, a Radical Experiment in Health Care*. London: Bedford Square Press.

Robin Nicholson, MA, MSc, RIBA, has been a director of Edward Cullinan Architects in London, England, since 1980, where he has worked on a wide range of projects in health, education, and urban design. He is a vice president for Public Affairs at the Royal Institute of British Architects and is a member of the NHS "Environments for Quality Care" working group that is developing guidelines for improving the healthcare environment for patients and staff.

◆ ◆ ◆

MEDICAL OFFICE DESIGN: THEORY AND TYPES

Fourth Symposium on Healthcare Design, Boston, MA, 1991

Jain Malkin

The topic "theory and types" allows us to recognize the vast network of services under the heading of healthcare. Facilities designed to deliver these services are specifically adapted for the equipment that needs to be housed and the type of care or treatment provided. Design professionals who do not specialize in healthcare facilities tend to view the field generically. In the 1980s, those of us who specialize in the field became very good generic healthcare designers. We learned how to create hospitable healthcare environments that are soothing for patients and families and easy for environmental services staff to maintain. The 1990s, however, provide a great opportunity to truly refine these skills and recognize the subtle differences among specific patient populations.

Under the general heading "ambulatory care," for example, there are several types and subtypes. At one end of the spectrum are physicians' and dentists' offices. Also under that heading are neurologists, pediatricians, allergists, and a variety of other subtypes. Medical conditions of their patients dictate functional design features that should be accommodated. All too often, medical offices have the same generic look—it doesn't matter whether it's for a neurologist, an allergist, or a family practitioner.

People who suffer from allergies, for example, are sensitive to dust, mold, pollen, and many airborne irritants. They may also be sensitive to wool and bonding agents used in carpet backings, as well as to solvents in paints and to any number of other environmental pollutants. Heavily textured surfaces, such as shag carpeting or nubby upholstery fabric, make these people itch just looking at them.

Neurology patients may be confused, dizzy, and unsteady and have trouble with balance or coordination. How does this affect design? Highly contrasting surfaces, busy patterns, or highly saturated colors can exacerbate these conditions; therefore, a neurologist's office should be soothing and comfortable, offering no architectural surprises. This doesn't mean that the design cannot be visually interesting. Too often, medical offices have a sameness about them that reminds me of a formula fast-food restaurant. The basic elements of a medical office are there, but the fine tuning for patients with special medical problems is lacking.

If ambulatory care is the "theory," there are at least five specific "types" of healthcare facilities, such as physician and dentist offices; diagnostic medicine, surgery, and recovery care centers; and large clinics. Under each of these type classifications are various subtypes, such as clinical lab and radiology. MRI and mammography, which require highly specialized design treatments to meet the equipment requirements and patient comfort needs, are subtypes under radiology and diagnostic medicine. Under surgery is dental surgery, pediatric surgery, and women's surgery. Recovery care centers is a new category in which a postsurgical patient can remain up to 72 hours for extended care. These numerous headings and subcategories should remind design professionals of the special needs that cannot be met by a generic healthcare design formula.

Productivity Studies

I had the pleasure of attending a presentation by Michael Brill from the Buffalo Organization for Social and Technical Innovation (BOSTI) at the symposium's Executive Forum meeting last June in California. Brill is also one of the speakers at the fourth symposium. Well known for the BOSTI studies on office productivity, Brill is a professor of architecture at State University of New York at Buffalo. His research has been published in a two-volume book that answers these three questions:

- Does office design affect productivity and the quality of work life?
- Which facets of the office have these effects?
- What are these effects worth in terms of economics?

After the Executive Forum, Wayne Ruga, the founder of the Symposium, challenged me to study Brill's research and try to find an application for medical office design. This body of research is very well respected, although none of it is related specifically to medical office design. I read those two volumes and tried to extract some principles that would provide a different perspective on medical and dental offices.

For many years, medical offices have been viewed as a collection of rooms precisely sized to accommodate various pieces of equipment and types of procedures. In addition, the flow of patients through the suite and the shortest possible route for physicians and nurses are equally important. As I studied Michael Brill's research, I realized that the biggest difference between a corporate office and a medical office is that in the corporate office, most of the interaction and communication is between teams of people from within the office; whereas in the medical office or clinic, the principal interaction is in the coming and going of outsiders, the patients.

In terms of office layout and space planning, it's difficult to apply Brill's principles to the design of a medical suite. However, with respect to the individual's work space, there are a number of interesting parallels. I have often marveled at the amount of work that somehow seems to get processed in the typical medical business office. In many physicians' suites, it's not uncommon to find workstation sizes so small that they resemble pigeon holes—perhaps 20 square feet per person with almost no horizontal surface area to lay out work, and no privacy. There may be four people working elbow to elbow, all on the phone simultaneously, in a 12 by 12 foot space that also accommodates a copy machine, office supplies, and medical charts.

In contrast a nonmedical office, or business with similar annual revenues, would generally provide staff with more privacy, larger workstations, and more sophisticated equipment for accomplishing tasks. Yet physicians have rarely expressed a concern about front office staff productivity or job satisfaction. This may soon change. The past few years have seen the gradual erosion of physicians' incomes, which means that now there may be the impetus to design offices that place a premium on efficiency and productivity if this results in higher profit margins and greater job satisfaction. In spite of what are often very poor working conditions, physicians' front office staff tend to be loyal and dedicated. It is not uncommon to find people who have worked for the same physician for ten years. Many staff members are motivated by a sincere desire to help people who are sick, and they often feel tremendous loyalty to an individual physician.

So why fix something that isn't broken? If the staff shows up for work and

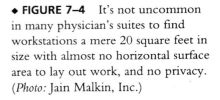

◆ **FIGURE 7–4** It's not uncommon in many physician's suites to find workstations a mere 20 square feet in size with almost no horizontal surface area to lay out work, and no privacy. (*Photo:* Jain Malkin, Inc.)

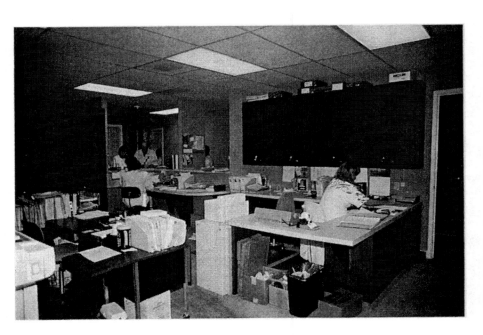

seems reasonably happy, is it worthwhile to consider any alternatives? This leads to something I've been thinking a lot about lately. For the past two years in preparation for writing my book, *Hospital Interior Architecture*, I read a lot of research about the environment and its influence on healing. And I learned that it is possible to create a physical setting that is actually therapeutic. This has the greatest relevance, of course, in an inpatient setting because people are not in an outpatient facility long enough to be healed. But what these studies made me aware of is that human beings respond chemically to everything they see, feel, and hear. The body responds to energy and vibrations that people are not conscious of. Things like noise, vibration, poor lighting, or lack of privacy have a cumulative, negative effect—a logarithmic multiplication that over time causes workers merely to survive, rather than thrive. It's sometimes hard to convince clients of the benefits to staff (as well as patients) of natural light, access to nature, or furniture that adjusts to an individual's body because, from outward appearances, the staff seems just fine. Human beings are amazingly adaptable and they are able to survive under the most adverse conditions; but I'm talking about productivity, not mere survival.

I propose that design professionals look at ways of creating harmony in the medical office environment. If a negative work environment is created for people, they will interact negatively with co-workers, patients, and even their families when they get home at night. A work environment that meets their needs and makes them feel well cared for positively affects energy levels, as well as physical and psychological health. If we begin with the assumption that most people are in some way striving for happiness and productivity in their work environment, then we need to look at the physical environment as a tool to accomplish these objectives. Apart from functional considerations such as privacy, size of work space, and quality of lighting, there are symbolic meanings: what the environment says about its attitude toward the staff and toward work.

There are costs and benefits of both poorly and well-designed environments. Poorly designed environments do have costs in terms of loss of productivity and morale. Well-designed environments offer many benefits that one must weigh financially. According to Brill, over ten years the capital cost of an office represents seven percent of the total mission. People and operational costs, on the other hand, represent 93 percent. It is this type of information that needs to be brought to the attention of decision makers so that they can put capital costs into perspective and realize that spending an additional $10,000 to enhance the quality of the environment is really negligible over a ten-year period.

According to Brill, the four principal facets of the environment are the work space, ambient conditions, psycho-physical constructs, and facilities design and management. The *work space* includes the amount of physical enclosure and floor area, layout, furniture, and access to windows or natural light. *Ambient conditions* are what can be sensed in an environment and are controlled by specific building systems such as temperature, air quality, lighting, and noise. *Psycho-physical constructs* covers issues such as privacy, communication, wayfinding, comfort, communication of status, and opportunities for display or personalization. *Facilities design and management* deals with policy issues about the design and use of the environment, such as participation, flexibility, and occupancy.

Brill uses four measures of productivity:

- Job performance: the amount of work processed, the number of errors, seeing opportunities for improvement.
- Job satisfaction: feeling rewarded, a sense of dignity, and fulfilling a mission, which results in less absenteeism and turnover.
- Communication: visual observation of co-workers, face-to-face communication, electronic and telephone access, co-examination of medical charts, X-rays, and reports.
- Environmental satisfaction: dealing with issues of privacy.

Privacy is not just four walls. It's defined as being able to control interactions with others. Other facets include the amount of enclosure of the work space, physical comfort, adaptability of furniture, human factors parameters, noise level, adequate storage for paperwork and personal effects, a view of the outdoors, and opportunities to socialize with co-workers.

To summarize, according to Brill, the most important facets of the environment are:

- Amount of enclosure—the capacity to concentrate requires four walls high enough to provide visual screening.
- Layout or arrangement of work space—so that it works as a tool.
- Ability to adjust furniture—no person has a body that is the same as anybody else's: the armrest, seat height, slope of chair back, and mounting bracket for the VDT and the keyboard pad all need to be adjustable.
- How well noise is suppressed—noise is defined as unwanted sound.
- Capacity to display things.

Brill emphasizes that staff must be trained to use furniture and workstations properly, that this is not an intuitive process and it is something that designers often overlook. People are trained to use a computer and other equipment and they also need to be taught how to be wise users of their workspaces. Don't assume they know how to adjust chairs and manipulate other tools of their environment to help them become more productive.

Brill advocates a periodic evaluation to keep the environment fit. He says this is not a one-time exercise after the project is completed; it requires continual tweaking and reevaluation. In a depressed economy, this might be a new service for designers to offer: assessing offices in terms of new measures of productivity, and suggesting ways to make it easier for people to do their jobs well.

In summary, the design of medical offices has been a relatively stable commodity in spite of much change in the healthcare industry at large. Many think of the office as a cost center only, not an investment with a return—a place to house tools, but not a tool itself. Thus workstations often reflect decisions based solely on cost, rather than cost versus benefit. If the medical office is viewed as a manipulative tool rather than a static setting, it becomes possible to imagine a number of environmental amenities that can, and do, affect performance.

Medical Office Buildings

Let's shift gears and focus on the fundamental principles of medical space planning. As I discuss completed projects, think about the symbolic meaning, what attitude toward the staff and toward patients the environment reflects. Efficient medical offices begin with an intelligently designed medical office building. Too often, buildings are planned by designers or architects unfamiliar with special requirements of medical suites. Things such as the locations of structural columns, the placement of stairs, elevators, mechanical shafts, public restrooms, and the window module can either impede or facilitate the layout of suites.

Other factors influencing the design are the size and the shape of the lot, the view, specific requirements of a particular anchor tenant, the architect's desire to impose a unique design, the budget, and zoning restrictions. The key point I would like to make is that a medical office should be thought about in terms of a planning module. Four feet or four feet six inches are the two typical planning modules. This means that window mullions then need to be placed at four feet on center or four feet six inches so that partitions do not end in the middle of a panel of glass. Experienced medical space planners know that medical and dental offices are comprised of many small rooms. There is a high density of partitions; therefore, the placement of window mullions is critical, as is the height of window sills so that cabinets can be placed under them.

The building should have a minimum of 12,000 square feet per floor for a certain level of efficiency. If a building has less than this, the owner may not be able to get a good mix of tenants and it will limit flexibility. The locations of stairs and columns, obviously, is very critical: Stairs make a difference because sometimes they impede suite layout.

Within the suite there cannot be more than a 20-foot dead-end corridor. Columns should be laid out on the grid to fall within the walls. Columns on the exterior should be flush with the face of the interior wall if possible so that they do not extend into the exam rooms running along the exterior wall. A two- by two-foot column at the foot end of the exam table is undesirable because a physician cannot stand there and perform an examination. On the exterior, the columns can be worked into the architecture as a design feature.

Keep the core factor (the public area space that is nonleasable) to no more than 14 percent. A beautiful, spacious atrium lobby eats up a lot of space. Separation of fire exits is something most designers are aware of: If there are two stairs on either end, a third stair in the middle of the space allows one-half of the building to be leased to a single tenant, while still maintaining two required exits for the other tenants.

Knowledge of feasibility or marketing studies is critical for medical office building developers. A building with numerous 3000- to 6000-square-foot suites is very different from one that has many 1500-square-foot spaces.

A suite planning guide shows that a 28-foot depth is recommended for small suites. And unless the building is very small, I wouldn't recommend doing that bay depth. "Depth of bay" is the space between the exterior wall and the public corridor. Twenty-eight feet would work for suites less than 1000 square feet. It allows for two rows of 12-foot deep rooms and a four-foot corridor. A 32-foot bay depth is the most common. It works for suites ranging in size from 800 to 2500 square feet. A double-loaded corridor is established with one row of 16-foot deep rooms that may include the business office, special procedure rooms, or waiting room. Along the window wall there are exam and consultation rooms (private offices), which are typically 12 feet deep with a four-foot corridor.

For flexibility, consider having a 32-foot bay depth on one side of the public corridor of the building and a 44-foot bay depth on the other side. Larger suites can then be accommodated on the 44-foot side and small-to-medium size suites on the 32-foot side. A 44-foot bay depth works well for a suite from about 1800 to 4500 square feet and provides space for a center core or island, as well as another corridor.

For large suites ranging in size from 6000 to 10,000 square feet, a 60-foot bay depth is best. There are problems putting a 6000-square-foot suite in a 32- or 44-foot deep bay, because the layout won't be efficient for the amount of walking that will be required. For large clinics of 10,000 to 20,000 square feet, a 72- or an 80-foot bay depth is necessary. Typically, these may take up an entire floor of a medical building.

Common Characteristics of GPs

I'd like to discuss the things that are common to all medical offices by evaluating a general practice (GP) suite. This is the foundation for more specialized suites. A fairly typical size is 1500 square feet. The business office and waiting room have to be close to each other. Sometimes it works well to have the nurse right up front so that the nurse can pick up patients in the waiting room and usher them to an exam room. Minor surgery, more often than not, is at the rear of the suite in a more private area. There is a blood drawing lab that may also do urinalysis.

To simplify, there are three functional units of a medical suite:

- Administrative
- Patient care
- Support services

Now, think about image or symbolic meaning. First impressions are very important to patients: The way an office looks and feels has a significant effect on the way they view the physician and the quality of the care provided. In one example (see Figure C–26), patients are connected to nature, which research has shown to have many stress-reducing benefits. Few people can actually evaluate the clinical care they receive but, nevertheless, they make a judgment based on the "body language" of the office environment. There are certain nonverbal clues. Dusty plants with dead leaves, burned-out light bulbs, torn drapes, old magazines, and faded or dirty carpet can give a strong message about the physician and the kind of medicine that is practiced.

The next example (Figure 7–5) shows a neatly designed space, very well organized, with some detailing on the ceiling. It gives patients a very good impression. This was done by a physician in La Jolla, California, where I work and live. He's a general surgeon—a sweet, wonderful guy who loves Mexico. When I sit in this room, I feel the physician's concern for my well-being and comfort. His personality comes through in the wonderful photos he has taken of people in Mexico. Traditional Mexican carved wooden seat-

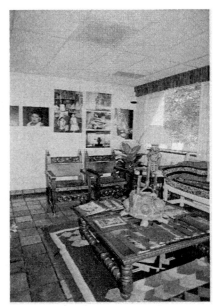

◆ **FIGURE 7–5** In this neatly designed room, the physician's personality comes through in the wonderful photos he has taken of people in Mexico and other thoughtful details. (*Project:* Surgeon's office. *Design:* Alan Berkenfield, M.D. *Photo:* Jain Malkin, Inc.)

ing with colorful handwoven fabrics and a superb selection of magazines make waiting more pleasurable.

I would challenge designers to avoid standard furnishings and try to create an environment that expresses orginality. This same physician actually does a lot of surgery in his office. And instead of a very clinical, sterile room, he has a surgery room with wonderful Mexican folk art on the counter along with syringes and scalpels. And he tells stories about Mexico and visiting the Indians. It's such a nice experience that I bet this man never has any malpractice suits—people love him.

Too many medical suites have narrow corridors and the perfunctory three-by four-foot reception window with a plastic laminate transaction shelf at a 42-inch height. Compare that with another suite in the same building that was remodeled to allow light to pass through from the exterior wall into the corridor. It presents a much nicer appearance.

A large 30,000-square-foot clinic was designed with a corporate look, with a consistent appearance among different departments. Although it was built within a modest budget, there's a lot of interesting detailing in the ceiling. Nurse stations in corridors are where nurses and physicians spend a good deal of time. Most large clinics have miles and miles of corridors that are very boring. To address this problem, sections of walls were recessed, to create niches and establish a rhythm in corridors enhanced by concealed lighting. Indirect cove lighting throughout corridors creates a nice ambiance. When clients say they can't spend money on good lighting, I say, "Okay, I'll use inexpensive furniture and forget wallcoverings, we'll just use paint. But I want to put the major portion of the budget into lighting." That usually wakes them up to the fact that lighting is really important.

Typically, business offices in medical suites have a two-foot deep counter and little cubby holes that work very well for storage of forms. This arrangement allows staff to organize things nicely. It's not uncommon for these practices to generate millions of dollars in annual revenues. But in most nonmedical offices with that annual dollar volume, employees would be working in far better, more organized, well-designed work spaces. In the medical business office I just described, there's absolutely no space to lay things out. The people working here are billers. A biller sits at a desk and bills for a two-million dollar surgical practice in a very small space, with boxes all over the floor and obviously little concern for productivity. There is only about a two-foot space for the biller even to push her chair back.

The design of the exam room is very important. If the exam table is turned so that the foot end or the stirrups are facing the door, every time someone walks by or opens the door the patient is totally exposed. There are some large clinics that have this exam room layout as their standard. There must be a reason but it's never made sense to me. What seems to be the best layout, in terms of privacy and function, is to have the foot facing the window. The physician comes in, greets the patient, washes his or her hands, and sits down. The patient occupies the other half of the room, longitudinally. Most physicians examine to the right of the patient even if they are left handed. The sink cabinet would be straight ahead on the right, as the physician enters the room.

Designers always need to ask physicians if they are right or left handed. A right-handed exam room allows the physician to sit between the cabinet and the patient's right side, reach for instruments from the cabinet with the left hand, and examine the patient with the right. It's critical that this relation-

◆ **FIGURE 7–6** The best layout for exam rooms, in terms of privacy and function, is to have the foot of the exam table facing away from the door. (*Project:* Exam room. *Interior design:* Jain Malkin, Inc. *Photo:* Robinson Ward Photography.)

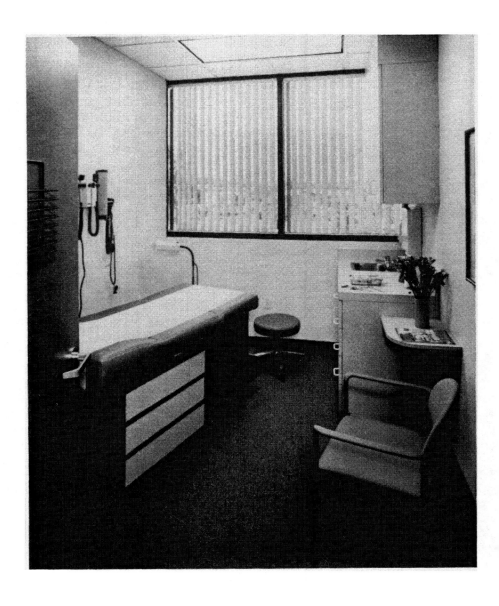

ship is understood: that the physician, nurse, or technologist is typically on the right of the patient.

For many years in California, we've had to preserve an 18-inch handicap set back on the pull side of the door. This will now become standard with the federal Americans with Disabilities Act. When the door is offset 18-inches from the wall in a small room, the door is almost in the center of the room. This disrupts the layout of the space by preventing the exam table from being moved back far enough. So, maybe exam rooms should be 8-feet clear in width rather than 7- by 6-feet. Generally, an 8- by 12-foot room (7-feet, 6-inches by 11-feet, 6-inches clear dimensions) is fairly standard and works well.

For larger family practice suites, one of the things designers need to think about is the basic organization of space and whether rooms will be arranged in pods or clusters, or have centralized support services. If the decentralized pod concept is used, a physician consultation room, two or three exam rooms, and a nurse station would be clustered together.

Another way of organizing space that also works well for some suites is to cluster all the consultation rooms together with the staff lounge at the rear of the suite, in a quiet area, out of the patients' path of travel. The exam rooms—there may be 12 or 15 of them—may be placed together in a cluster around one or two large nurse stations. Support services (nurse station, X-ray, and lab) will all be centrally located.

A decentralized plan uses the pod or cluster concept in which three or four exam rooms, a nurse station, and a consultation room form a unit. In large clinics, I prefer the cluster concept because the patient has the feeling of greater intimacy. All over the country, smaller practices are merging into large groups to take advantage of the economies of scale and to be able to offer patients access to specialists for consultation. Nevertheless, patients do not want to feel they are entering a big clinic, because it's intimidating. Anything that can be done to create a feeling of intimacy is worthwhile.

Primary Care Specialties

Some physicians put a great emphasis on the consultation room and want a beautiful design. Others don't care about it; they use it simply to read mail and take phone calls. Since they don't consult with patients there, they don't care too much about it. In the exam room, it is desirable to have casework that hides the medical equipment so that the patient, while waiting for the physician, does not get anxious.

A "weights and measures" area of pediatrics suites may have a baby scale and a full-size adult scale, perhaps recessed into the floor. Sometimes pediatric exam rooms will have a baby scale on a lowered portion of the built-in exam table.

Staff areas are very important, and increasingly so, with the kinds of stress that the staff is working under. It's very important to provide a comfortable, attractive place for the staff to have lunch and take breaks.

One pediatrics suite is designed in a pod concept. I have talked about things that were common in general practices, common to all suites and although pediatrics is a primary care specialty, there are many obvious differences. For example, it's an extremely high-volume specialty. A pediatrician can see six to eight patients an hour. Sometimes a pediatrician will examine two siblings together in a larger examining room designed for this purpose.

There needs to be in such a high-volume specialty a separation between incoming and outgoing patients. People should be coming in one way and going out another to avoid cross traffic. In a pediatric suite it is not uncommon to have one nurse who primarily answers the phone, responds to prescription refills, and decides whether a patient needs to be seen or not. There may even be a separate switchboard operator because there is such a high volume of calls. There should be a separate cashier and appointment counter that is at least six-feet wide so that there is plenty of room for people to check out.

Many pediatrics suites have separate waiting rooms for sick children and well ones. This is somewhat controversial. Some pediatricians argue that it doesn't matter because the children mix together in school anyway. But most prefer that separation. Each waiting area needs a play area, reception window,

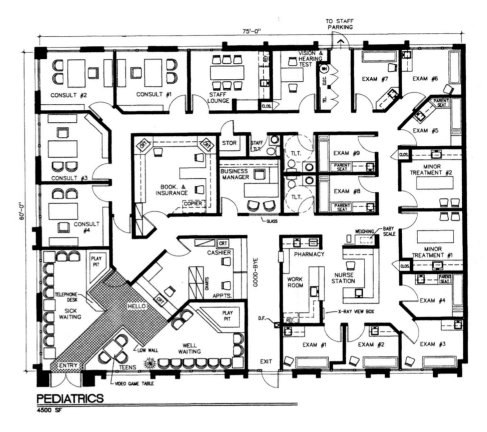

PEDIATRICS
4500 SF

and check out area around the corner. In one suite plan, the rooms are arranged in clusters or pods with a consultation room and a row of exam rooms dedicated to a specific physician. Each one has a nurse station. Nurse stations require excellent visibility of exam rooms because the nurse controls traffic and needs to know where the physician is at all times.

The building shell of one 60,000-square-foot multispecialty clinic works very well with two 44-foot bay depths on either side of the public corridor. The clinic is organized into separate departments; so even though it is a very large clinic, it functions like separate medical suites except in the main lobby where there is a large, central registration area for checkin and checkout.

In another example, a nicely designed gastroenterology suite has many symbolic meanings and messages. It's neat and orderly, contemporary, highly original, with considerable attention to detail. It shows that the physician cares about his staff and patients. A soffit has been created with postformed plastic laminate and there is a lot of attention given to bringing light into the suite. Very interesting things were done with artificial light focused on art objects. It's obviously not an inexpensive suite design, but its beauty seems worth the expense.

OB-GYN Suites

OB-GYN is another high-volume practice, in which a nurse practitioner often does the more routine examinations. In this specialty, the ratio of staff to physicians is quite high. Every woman knows that there's probably no specialty where she has to wait longer than in an obstetrician's or gynecologist's office. Therefore, seating should be comfortable and easy to get out of for pregnant women (see Figure C–27). The nurse station needs to be quite large because there is a lot of lab work: Practically every woman who visits the suite is asked to leave a urine specimen. Several toilets are needed, with specimen pass-throughs to the nurse station or lab. Because many women are sensitive about being weighed, the scale should be located in a private area. Four exam rooms per physician are often provided because of the high volume in this speciality. A minimum of three exam rooms per physician is essential.

There are a number of options in OB-GYN with respect to the placement of casework in the exam room: Either locate it at the foot of the table, along the short-end wall, or along the long wall, on the right side as one enters the room.

Dressing areas are also very important in this specialty. In one example, although it has only a 32-foot bay depth, the layout is interesting because the examining rooms are quite large. The casework runs along the foot, which is not uncommon in an OB-GYN suite. The stirrups face away so that the patient is visually screened. In one suite, large dressing rooms create spacious niches in corridors, which are not typical of most medical suites. There are numerous toilets scattered throughout. Ultrasound, fetal monitoring, and minor surgery are other special rooms in OB-GYN suites.

Women's health centers have come about in recent years. They differ from OB-GYN suites because they're not just OB-GYN—they may offer internal medicine, primary care, mammography, bone densitometry, and a variety of educational programs. Usually, they have an all-female staff and feature an emphasis on prevention and education. Women's health centers grew out of the women's movement and respond to the fact that women make most of the healthcare choices for their families; if hospitals can capture this market, it assures them of many other referrals. Women's health centers offer designers opportunities to break away from conventional ideas about what medical offices should look like. It's really hard to predict whether gender-specific healthcare for women will continue to be provided in high-profile specialized facilities or if these programs will ultimately become integrated into primary care networks.

The attempt in one mammography suite in a community hospital was to create a kind of sophisticated, yet playful, design. Education is important in these facilities, so there is often a book niche, reading room, or lending library.

Other Specialties

Plastic surgery suites are very different. It's important to understand how the suite functions: There is an examination/presurgical consultation area and, on the other side, a surgical suite. It works well if these can be separated into two distinct suites by the reception area. In one layout, the nurse station is placed so that it relates to both suites.

After surgery, patients have bruises and bandages, which sometimes makes them self-conscious; in addition, one wouldn't want to expose presurgical patients to this. Therefore, there should be a separate postsurgical waiting room.

It is always important to think about staffing. A reception area should be located so that one receptionist can communicate with people in both waiting rooms. The concept here is that patients are seen in one area for presurgical consultation, often in a high-profile physician's private office with a built-in slide projector and screen. When patients arrive for surgery, they check in at the reception desk and are escorted to the surgical suite, where there may be one or two operating rooms, a scrub area, clean and dirty work rooms, a recovery room, and a bathroom. The nurse station divides the surgical suite from the examination suite. On the surgical side, the nurse station abuts the recovery room, providing excellent visual access to recovering patients.

For obvious reasons, plastic surgery suites should be the ultimate in high-profile design. This is an example of an impressive office that gives patients confidence in the surgeon's skills. No one wants to go to a plastic surgeon who is not successful. It is important to have the trappings of success: unusual furniture, unique art objects, and so forth. Prospective patients want to know that the surgeon has good taste, as aesthetics are very much related to the plastic surgeon's skills. The suite design of a plastic surgeon should not be trendy: There are many interesting things to look at. And there is an emphasis on detail. Nothing is more essential to a plastic surgeon's work than detail, and this suite says attention to detail is important.

A typical plastic surgery exam room in another suite does not have a standard exam table; a chair that reclines is used instead. Things like diplomas can be handled in a more interesting way, such as using a variety of frames, rather than all matching. Some have glass "mats," allowing the wallcovering to show through.

Refraction rooms are typical in ophthalmology practices. Many designers understand the concepts of refraction rooms and refracting lanes. A data collection room may contain a visual field area and various diagnostic equipment. There may be a laser procedure room. An optical dispensing area contains frame bars and fitting tables and will, of course, have a small lab.

In one very beautiful orthopedic suite, the designers have incorporated well-balanced seating that people can get out of easily. People should be able to rest their entire weight on one arm of a chair without it tipping. Sofa-type seating, which forces strangers to touch one another, is undesirable; individual chairs, with arms, are much more desirable. The focus in the waiting room is a 420-gallon saltwater aquarium (with a room for servicing it outside the suite so that the service people never have to enter the waiting room).

A typical orthopedic exam room may have a table that is perpendicular to the wall rather than parallel. Some orthopedists specialize in hand surgery and need "hand rooms" where they can examine hands at a special table. Of course, X-ray view boxes are critically important in this type of suite.

I take issue with seating that doesn't have arms, but in one large orthopedic suite in California various types of seating were tried, and the surgeons felt that this was appropriate for their patients. There is nice attention to detail and many interesting angled walls.

The nice design features aren't just concentrated in the waiting room, either. The designer carried them through all the staff areas and the business office as well. Some of the things Michael Brill spoke of concerning privacy have been implemented here. This is different from most medical suites: There are plants, privacy, good lighting, and really nice work spaces. A great deal of thought has been put into the design of this suite, and it makes a very nice impression on patients. The design might be more contemporary than some people would feel comfortable with, but that's a stylistic issue.

Good physical therapy suites are rare. Designers attend to other parts of the office, but they rarely extend their efforts to the therapy areas. They usually look so clinical. In this same orthopedic suite, the designer has carried the design theme through the gym, locker rooms, and a beautiful sunken spa area.

In this presentation, I've examined some key planning issues in the design of medical offices. I hope that the information will be useful in marketing design services to physicians, or that physicians will be inspired to return to their offices and evaluate them from a new perspective.

Jain Malkin is president and founder of Jain Malkin Inc., a design firm based in La Jolla, California, and specializing in interior architecture for healthcare environments. A pioneer in the healthcare design field, she has taught medical space planning at Harvard University and lectures widely on creating healing environments. Malkin is the author of Hospital Interior Architecture, Medical and Dental Space Planning for the 1990s, *and* The Design of Medical and Dental Facilities.

Chapter

EIGHT

PROJECT EXAMPLES/LONG-TERM CARE

THEORY AND TYPES

*Fourth Symposium on
Healthcare Design,
Boston, MA, 1991*

Martin H. Cohen, FAIA

Healthcare environments for the elderly is and promises to remain a robust growth area for knowledgeable and experienced design professionals. In this presentation, I will review state-of-the-art facilities designed for the aging; discuss the fundamental goals, principal design issues, and emerging problems in design for the aging; and imagine future possibilities of healthcare venues for the aging.

I'd like to begin by sharing the 1991/1992 Design for Aging Facilities Review presented by the American Institute of Architects (AIA) and the American Association of Homes for the Aging (AAHA) at AAHA's annual meeting in San Francisco just ten days before this Symposium. AAHA is the professional organization of not-for-profit providers of healthcare and residential services for the aging, including nursing homes and continuing care retirement communities in the United States and Canada.

In what is expected to be a biannual program, the jury for the 1991/1992 Design for Aging Facilities Review and its related exhibit was charged with evaluating the programming and design of 56 entries in the categories of continuing care retirement communities (CCRCs) and nursing homes (including Alzheimer's units), assisted living facilities, and independent apartments.

The program statement and data submitted with each project were used to review plans and photos of completed works and works nearing completion, or about to begin construction. The jury attempted to screen the projects so that an up-to-date picture of the aging industry's best responses to design and programming issues would be presented. Five of the 43 projects selected for the exhibit were judged to be outstanding and worthy of citation.

Design for Aging Facilities Review was the first exhibition of environmental design ever presented at an AAHA annual meeting, and it was very warmly received. The exhibition included panels describing all 43 projects selected by the jury. A publication titled "Design for Aging Review" is available from both AIA and AAHA. The exhibit was prominently featured in the main registration area of the convention center and 150 people attended a two-hour presentation by the jury, which included: Ron Blitch, AIA, president, Blitch Architects, New Orleans, LA (chair); David Green, CEO, Evergreen CCRC, Oshkosh, WI; Tim Johnson, COO, Presbyterian Homes, Evanston, IL; and myself. I've collected all our notes and will attempt to give a reasonable, but somewhat briefer, facsimile of that presentation.

The projects range from modest additions and renovations to complete $60 million complexes. Only 32 are represented, not because the remaining 11 didn't deserve to be shown, but because the jury felt the quality of their slides didn't measure up to the standards of the rest. The entire exhibition will travel in 1992.

The Projects

The Design for Aging Facilities Review projects vary in scale and site planning concepts. Several CCRCs successfully used grand classical campus plans to differentiate the project components, such as Arbor Glen in Bridgewater,

NJ, designed by Cannon Architects of St. Louis, and Terrace Gardens in Milpitas, CA, designed by the Steinberg Group of San Jose, CA.

Other projects responded to regional differences and historical cues to shape the site development concept, such as Kirkland Village in Bethlehem, PA, designed by Reese, Lower, Patrick, and Scott of Lancaster, PA.

High-rise solutions illustrated a careful layering and vertical integration of functions such as assisted living, independent living, and common areas, as at the Seasons of Pompano, FL, designed by William Dorsky Associates. Urban sites generated high density, high-rise solutions with shared common spaces on lower levels, such as the Jefferson in Arlington, VA, designed by Cochran, Stephenson & Donkervoet (CS&D) of Baltimore.

Some projects successfully adapted and reused existing structures to create familiar buildings that comfortably fit into the neighborhood context. This included saving the facade of an existing building at the Argyle, which is an assisted living nursing facility in Denver, CO, designed by Oz Architecture of Denver. A national historic landmark was renovated to create the public areas of a CCRC at the Stoddard Baptist Home in Washington, DC, designed by Oudens + Knoop Architects of Washington, DC.

Adaptive reuse can also be applied to affordable housing solutions, as in the conversion of a school into an assisted living and adult day-care facility at the Lincolnia Senior Center in Fairfax, VA. The architect was Herbert Cohen & Associates of Washington, DC. Renovation can be used to breathe new life into existing long-term care facilities. In the Hebrew Rehabilitation Center for Aged in Roslindale, MA, architects Huygens, DiMella, Shaffer & Associates of Boston designed the entrance to be visible and exciting and updated the main public corridor to add informal seating for patient socialization and to bring the outdoors in.

New residentially scaled noninstitutional environments can be created to blend into their neighborhood context. An indoor/outdoor porch adds to the feeling of home in the Sunrise Retirement Home of Arlington in Arlington, VA, and provides traditional lounge space. The architect was Heffner Architects of Alexandria, VA. For Canterbury Place in Pittsburgh, PA, designed by the Design Alliance of Pittsburgh, a residential ambience is created in an urban environment via a garden terrace and an upper level dining room with a panoramic view. In larger CCRCs, such as the Argyle in Denver, a residential feeling is created with seating nooks and prominent stairs. These public spaces are used as an available alternative to elevators and to create a sense of place. (The architect was Oz Architecture of Denver.)

Diffused daylight is used to warm visually a large public space, bring the outdoors in, and add a sense of time and season, as in Brookridge in Winston-Salem, NC, designed by Calloway, Johnson & Moore of Winston-Salem. A clerestory can also be used as a source of daylight and to create a dramatic space, as at the Cedar Nursing Care Center in Portland, ME, designed by Tsomides Associates of Newton Upper Falls, MA. Properly designed, indirect lighting can effectively overcome glare and provide a lighting level appropriate for the aging, as in the Masonic Home Independent Living Community in Elizabethtown, PA, designed by Sherertz, Franklin, Crawford & Shaffner (SFCS) of Roanoke, VA.

Interior pedestrian malls were used as a recurring theme, to organize circulation, focus resident and staff socialization, and provide orientation cues to residents and visitors at the United States Air Force Association (USAA)

Towers and Nursing Center in San Antonio, TX, designed by HKS, Inc., of Dallas. An atrium can also be used to achieve similar results as in the Franciscan Village in Lemont, IL, designed by O'Donnell, Wicklund, Pigozzi and Peterson Architects of Deerfield, IL.

Designs for the aging that engender warmth, richness of space, and fulfill resident needs can be achieved in a variety of styles. Consider the Argyle in Denver (by Oz Architecture); and the Dyrness Building, apartments for the elderly in Quarryville, PA, designed by SFCS. Scale is an important factor in outdoor spaces to differentiate between public and private space for residents, such as in Erlandson Square, apartments for the elderly in Holdredge, NB, designed by Richard D. Nelson & Co. of Omaha; and the Argyle in Denver (by Oz Architecture).

Developments that offer small-scale cottages can provide the advantages of congregational living within the context of a single family home, such as Erlandson Square in Holdredge, NB (by Richard D. Nelson Co.) or Brookridge CCRC in Winston-Salem, NC (by Calloway, Johnson & Moore). In many projects, the commons building is the focus of the design and the program of activities for the CCRC, including health clubs, convenience shops, banks, craft studios, dining and club areas, barber and beauty shops, etc.

In Arbor Glen CCRC in Bridgewater, NJ, designed by Cannon Architects, travel distances for residents have been minimized by using relatively short corridors in a pinwheel-shape plan. At the Menorah Campus in Amherst, NY, adult day-care and child day-care add to the variety of activities in the commons building. The commons is the element that binds together the nursing, assisted living, and independent living apartments. The architect was NBBJ/Rosenfield of New York City.

A variety of options in environment, circulation, and activities is important to residents, as exemplified in the diversity of dining in Orchard Cove CCRC in Canton, MA, which features a formal dining pavilion, an informal garden dining room, and alternate dining options, such as a deli and a breakfast room. Independent apartment design for the aging demands careful attention to issues of furnishability, accessibility, and resident choices. Subtle details mark the difference between successful and unsuccessful environments for the elderly. In the typical kitchens at Orchard Cove, details such as the low, shallow pantry shelf above the counter and a desk-height work counter respond to the special needs of the elderly. This facility, designed by Huygens DiMella Shaffer & Associates of Boston in association with Korsunsky Krank Erickson of Minneapolis, was completed and occupied in 1993.

Other elements of good apartment unit design include well-proportioned, flexible rooms and efficient circulation. Long-term care environments need to recognize issues of territory and privacy of residents, as at Kirkland Village CCRC in Bethlehem, PA, designed by Reese, Lower, Patrick, and Scott. Issues of territory and privacy can be dealt with in a variety of configurations and include spaces scaled for small groups of residents. Resident control and accessibility can be achieved by elements such as individual lavatories in a shared bath and a private linen closet, as in the Rockynol Retirement Community in Akron, OH, designed by William Dorsky Associates of Cleveland.

Territoriality, privacy, and access to exterior views for each resident can be accomplished in traditionally shaped rooms with minor modifications (such as increased width), as in the Cedar Nursing Care Center in Portland, ME, designed by Tsomides Associates. Furnishings and finishes can make the difference between an institutional setting and a homelike environment, as in Barnes Extended Care at Clayton in St. Louis, MO, designed by Hellmuth, Obata & Kassabaum (HOK); and the USSA Towers and Nursing Center in San Antonio, TX, designed by HKS.

Social interaction, privacy, patient control of the environment, and a humanistic residential image are achieved in the Musquodoboit Valley Home for Special Care in Middle Musquodoboit, Halifax, Nova Scotia, Canada, through the use of a bay window in the corridor. The code limitations differ somewhat from those in the United States. The architect was William Nycum Architects Limited of Halifax.

A good approach to long-term care facility design is the creation of clusters with private and common spaces interspersed throughout, as in the Menorah Campus in Amherst, NY, by NBBJ/Rosenfield. A family room, sun room, therapy room, nurse station, and other small-scale spaces enable staff to provide more personal care.

Even large-scale providers, such as the Veterans Administration, are developing facilities using cluster concepts and providing residential-style amenities, as in the Huerfano County Medical Center and Colorado State Home in Walsenburg, CO, designed by the Davis Partnership of Denver.

Special populations, such as dementia and Alzheimer's patients, can be provided enriched environments with plans that include walking paths and secure transitional areas between private and active spaces, as in the Washington Home in Washington, DC, designed by Oudens + Knoop Architects. Wayfinding is an important issue in facilities for the elderly. Subtle cues such as artful arrangements of familiar objects throughout Barnes Extended Care at Clayton in St. Louis, MO, are an imaginative and effective solution. The architect was HOK.

Returning to issues of overall design and scale, theme-oriented developments, such as the Fleet Landing Retirement Community in Atlantic Beach, FL, create an environment for a specialized market (retired Navy personnel). Since people retire from the Navy as early as age 45, a variety of active spaces are provided to accommodate the unique needs of the residents. The architect was the Haskell Company of Jacksonville, FL.

Gabled roofs and articulation of facades are design techniques used to provide a more residential scale and appearance, such as in the Villa Rancho Bernardo Convalescence Center in San Diego, CA, designed by the Stichler Design Group of San Diego. Familiar forms can help soften residents' transitions into a CCRC, as in Collington in Mitchellville, MD, designed by CS&D.

Landmarks, such as towers or arcades, provide a sense of place. Materials and architectural detail help to express the vernacular of the region, as in the Masonic Home Independent Living Community in Elizabethtown, PA, designed by SFCS and in Terrace Gardens, Milpitas, CA, designed by the Steinberg Group.

Worthy of Citation

Five of the 1991/1992 Design for Aging Facilities Review projects were judged to be of outstanding quality and worthy of citation. First and foremost, they display an understanding of the needs of residents and utilize current knowledge about the aging process. The scale and design are residential. They provide accessibility, privacy, familiarity, functionality, and community.

The projects respond to staff needs for an efficient, effective working environment. They also relate appropriately to their sites and adjacent buildings and give a pleasant overall feeling. In summary, these projects successfully combine the design elements I've just reviewed.

1. *Rosewood Estate*, Roseville, MN, designed by Arvid Elness Architects of Minneapolis, is a free-standing, assisted living facility that combines home-like apartments with support in an unmistakably residential style and scale. It has 68 one-bedroom and efficiency units with kitchenettes. Apartment sizes

◆ **FIGURE 8–1**   This assisted living facility recalls a traditional colonial house. Sensitive to its neighborhood, the three-story wood frame building is broken into components to diminish its mass. (*Project:* Rosewood Estate, Roseville, MN. *Architect:* Arvid Elness Architects. *Photography:* Franz Hall.)

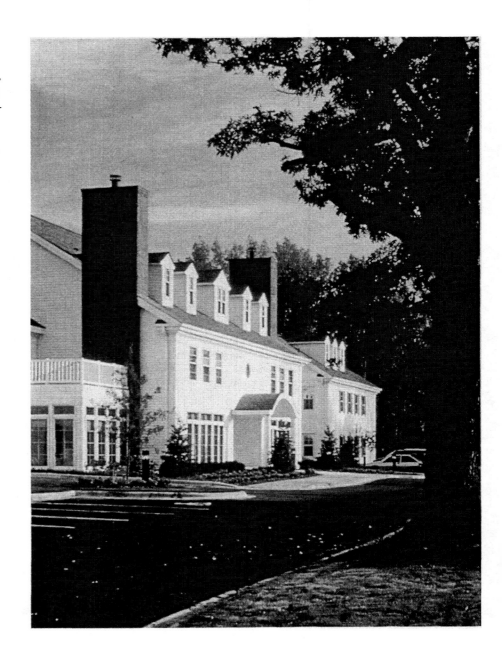

range from 362 to 629 square feet. The average cost was $50,000 per unit, which the jury considered reasonable because of the high quality achieved. It's a classic, colonial residence configured as a large home and out buildings, to conceal its size. It has two stories in the front and three stories in the rear, overlooking a lake.

Completed in 1989, it was considered appropriate for any upscale residential neighborhood. The residential feeling carries from the outside through the interior, with fireplaces in the drawing and dining rooms, which open on either side of the central entrance hall. Each room also opens up to a three-season porch. The facility has good residential detailing throughout and there's also the protection of full sprinklers and smoke detectors.

The plan makes good use of the site. Because of the slope down to the lake, there are grade level entrances on two floors. All three floors provide areas for a wide array of social and special-use spaces, in addition to the living and dining rooms. A greenhouse, beauty/barber shop, aerobics exercise area, television lounge, laundry, card room, patio, storage, and, most significantly, a single office for a home healthcare agency are located on the lower level. The home healthcare agency is a contracted service that occupies a space equivalent to an office in the home. It was considered a key to the success of this development because, thanks to its use in lieu of dedicated medical space, code officials viewed the facility as a multiple residence, not as a health facility.

Apartments are clustered in groups of four or eight around a lounge. French doors open between the living and bedroom areas in one-bedroom apartments. There are also unique bed alcoves in the one-room apartments. The lounges encourage social interaction and minimize corridor length. It was considered a well-planned project, totally focused on providing a pleasant, residential environment for occupants. Its success is indicated by the fact that it's 100 percent occupied.

2. *Bruening Health Care Center*, designed by Herman Galvin Gibans of Cleveland, is an addition to the Judson Retirement Community in the Chestnut Hills area of Cleveland, OH. The Judson Retirement Community began with the original mansion on the site, and later added a ten-story residential, independent living facility with 150 units; an adjacent parking garage; a community building with a kitchen and dining facilities, as well as an auditorium and administrative services; and a skilled nursing unit (SNF) that is being renovated into a 22-bed assisted living unit and a 24-bed Alzheimer's care unit.

The existing CCRC was accessed only from Chestnut Hills at the top of the hill, even though the property was bordered by a street named Ambleside that falls 70 feet down the hillside on its way to the city below. As a result, before the Bruening Health Care Center was built, the entire area of the site on the hillside was inaccessible to the residents of the CCRC. A new bridge connects the existing community and healthcare facilities to the top of the new Bruening building. The Bruening building houses a healthcare pavilion and commons facility on the top floor. There's an exercise gym, OT and PT rooms, a hydrotherapy pool, and community facilities, including conference rooms, classrooms, lounges, and a rooftop terrace—all with spectacular views of the city below.

The facility is located on top of three SNF levels, each with 42 beds per floor, for a total of 126 new SNF beds. The SNF levels in turn are on top of two levels of parking (with a total capacity of 150 cars) and new on-grade receiving storage and materials handling facilities. Stacking the health pavilion above the nursing units with parking and service below makes excellent use of this steep urban hillside while maximizing the views of the city from both the nursing levels and the healthcare pavilion. It also expands the commons facilities for the existing residential community at a very strategic location; integrates shared use of existing kitchens for all facilities of the CCRC; provides new centrally located healthcare parking and general support facilities; and expands the total capacity of the CCRC without intruding on the views from the residential units on the top of the hill.

Nursing, parking, receiving, and stores are all conveniently, but unobtrusively, located below the main campus level and with direct on-grade access from Ambleside to each of the parking levels and receiving levels. Thus, a formerly inaccessible part of the site has been turned into a superb asset. The jury considered this to be a brilliant planning solution, providing a unique response to a complex program on a very challenging site.

The configuration of the nursing levels is driven by an innovative and sensible staffing model. There are seven-bed clusters grouped around nurse aide stations. Each cluster and nurse aide station has its own decentralized linen and supplies back-up. Patients can be nursed on a 1:7 ratio for morning care on the day shift, a 1:14 ratio on the evening shift, and a 1:21 ratio on the night shift. Each 21-bed group incorporates decentralized tub rooms and support facilities, such as clean and soiled utility rooms, supervisory offices, and a team leader/reception station. There are also opportunities for socialization, decentralized group dining, and activities on each floor.

To stimulate long-term memory retained by many dementia patients, the decor of these facilities recalls the ambience they may have enjoyed for years in the independent residential units they previously occupied in the CCRC. Single-bed patient rooms afford privacy and opportunity for personalization, such as using one's own furnishings and memorabilia. Public spaces (for example, the hydrotherapy pool) and the design of the building exteriors reflect the urbane context of the existing retirement community, whether seen from below on Ambleside or looking down the hill from the existing CCRC.

3. *Woodside Place* in Oakmont, PA, designed by Perkins, Eastman Partners of New York in association with L.D. Asterino & Associates of Pittsburgh, is a free-standing, assisted living facility for people with Alzheimer's disease and similar forms of dementia. There are 36 residents—24 in private rooms, and 12 in semiprivate rooms. The total cost was $70,000 per bed, and the facility opened on July 1, 1991. The jury was attracted to the truly residential environment; the rural farmhouse style avoids the institutional character that so often marks this type of facility. The residential scale plan is set up as three independent houses for 12 residents, each with bedrooms, and living and dining areas. The typical nurse station was replaced by a kitchen and serving pantry, to which the residents have access and where they can practice their domestic skills. There are a variety of shared spaces, visible and accessible from the corridors, including country kitchens, guest rooms, music rooms, arts and crafts rooms, and an entertainment room.

The design reflects an understanding of changes resulting from Alzheimer's. Patients lose short-term memory and retain long-term memory. Environments with which people are familiar elicit appropriate behavior;

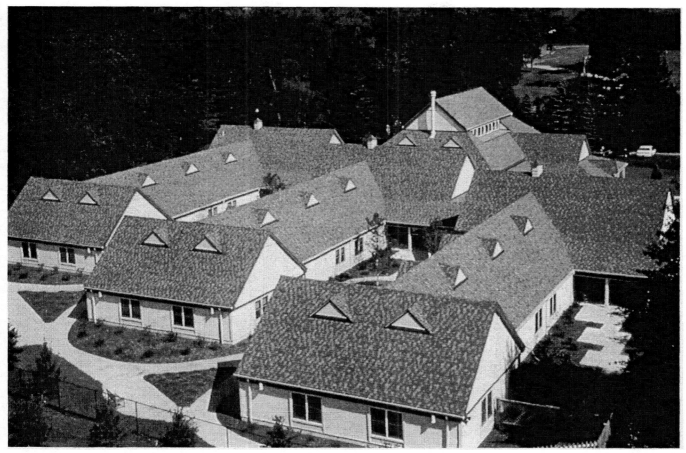

◆ **FIGURE 8–2** The rural farmhouse style of this residence in Oakmont, PA for 36 people with Alzheimer's disease is probably similar to the homes of many of its residents. A variety of porches open onto secure courtyards and a walking area. (*Project:* Woodside Place, Oakmont, PA. *Architecture/interior design:* Perkins Eastman Partners. *Photography:* Robert P. Ruschak.)

residents of typical nursing homes have no frame of reference for appropriate behavior. Residents can relate to the rural Pennsylvania residential design because many probably lived in similar homes. The resident rooms are truly homelike, with personal identification and a mailbox outside each room, Dutch doors, a Shaker pegboard and cup shelf, wall stenciling, and windows with pleasant views (see Figure C–28). The simple gabled roof and clapboard exterior are typical of the area and a variety of porches open onto secure courtyards customized for each house. The courtyards, in turn, open onto a larger secure walking area.

Open central facilities, including a library and a great room for large gatherings, are the focal point of each home. Quilt symbols in the great room combine the star, tree, and house, which are used in the decor of each of the three residential units.

The result is that family and staff, as well as residents, are likely to enjoy being in the facility. Since normative behavior is encouraged by the setting, families are more likely to visit and interact with residents through communication and participation in their activities. This will increase the quality of life for all parties, including the staff who will also be more efficient and satisfied.

Like the result, the process used to plan the project was unique. The state licensing agency was included as a member of the client's advisory board. It reviewed plans as they proceeded and this increased the flexibility of code interpretation. Not surprisingly, the facility is 100 percent occupied.

4. *Freeport Hospital Health Care Village,* designed by the NORR Partnership Limited, Architect & Engineers of Toronto, Canada, is a skilled nursing facility of 265 beds on an existing hospital campus in Ontario, Canada. The new campus employs a prominent courtyard on a town square concept, creating an urban space that is secure. The large scale of this project is broken down through strong architectural forms and the massing of buildings. The loop circulation that links buildings also allows clear orientation for residents.

Strong use of color and a rich palette of materials reduce the institutional feel of the complex. Each of the clusters has 15 beds arranged around living rooms and quiet rooms with lounge areas. Most of the rooms are semi's and quad's, but they employ a half wall, which is used in lieu of the traditional cubicle curtains and allows individual patient control. Semiprivate seating nooks in patient rooms are typical of the careful layering of private and public spaces and options for patients in this facility. The jury felt this project successfully resolved the major issues of a large-scale facility on an institutional campus through use of careful detailing and attention to individual patient needs.

5. *La Posada at Park Center* in Green Valley, AZ, was designed by Engelbrecht and Griffin of Des Moines, Iowa, and is operated by the Tucson Medical Center's "The Campus Group." This is a CCRC with 174 apartments; 128 are one-bedroom units and 46 are two-bedroom units. It also has a 20-bed healthcare facility. The facility is situated in the desert in the middle of a pecan tree grove. It maximizes its already spectacular site with a vista of the Arizona mountains. The architecture is indigenous to the Southwest and ties in beautifully with the region's natural beauty (see Figure C–29). The plan works well: A grand entrance plaza with covered parking on either side allows residents easy access to their apartments. Distances are minimal due to the spoke-type circulation from the commons facility in the center.

All apartment units face out toward the mountains and desert. This is probably a solution that is unique to this type of climate. The third floor has the most breathtaking views of the scenery. The second floor introduces some of the commons facilities, and the first floor is committed entirely to circulation and access for parking. Interior and exterior spaces are consistently strong in design and execution and continue to carry out the Southwest regional flavor. Adobe, exposed rafters, iron railings, and clay tile roofing identify the locale. The dining room is vivid and strong, providing a comforting feeling of home.

The desire to develop a project that was aesthetically pleasing and noninstitutional-looking appears to have been successfully carried out in all aspects of this community. The strong design tradition of the locale comes across without projecting a "cutesiness" or false feeling. It works. The overall impression is that of rich form and materials, yet La Posada was constructed for a very reasonable cost of $43 a square foot in 1989.

Juror Tim Johnson added a personal note. He said, "It's exciting to see a project such as this that is serious, yet playful, that appears to maximize independence and successfully deemphasize institutional feel. Everyone associated with the project has a right to be proud of it."

Goals and Objectives

It is hoped that the foregoing has provided a good overview of the product lines and facility types that are prevalent in today's design-for-aging marketplace. Environmental design can have an incredible impact on the lifestyles and well-being of the elderly. Perhaps no other population group is as severely affected by environmental insults and no other group seems to receive such dramatic benefits from knowledgeable designers working with well-informed clients. The principal goal of long-term care providers and design professionals is to create environments that maximize an individual's ability to enjoy a full life span with a minimum of dependence upon others. This is also the goal of the communities and governments that regulate long-term care facilities—indeed, of our entire society.

And yet, although independence is universally sought and treasured, what are we really talking about in facility terms when we talk about fostering and enabling independence? I believe we are searching for environments that enhance an individual's abilities to maintain his or her lifestyle—to retain family and friends and church, club, recreational, professional, social, and business affiliations. That means preserving neighborhood or community relationships to provide for daily needs: cooking, eating, sewing, cleaning; as well as travel, shopping, books, concerts, or sports. It also means being able to socialize and entertain or to be alone when one wants to be alone; being able to work, volunteer, dabble, or putter at whatever it is that one likes to do; and being able to preserve choice—to maintain control of the decisions of when to sleep, awaken, eat, dress, watch television, or talk on the telephone. In other words, we want to enhance the individual's ability to choose what to do and when to do it and make that choice because one wants to do it, not because the professional staff makes a decision. Residents want the freedom to choose either privacy or community, or both, and they want to be able to exercise the right and the ability to change that choice at will.

So, facilities have to be developed that do all those things. All these goals are most likely to be achieved in one's own home, which is a plus for so-called residential venues for healthcare. But, in fact, there is no way we will be able to afford or have the time or ability to build new residences and communities that will accommodate the entire burgeoning elderly population that has to be housed by the year 2030 (when the current baby boom generation is fully upon us). Thus, one's own home really does become the challenge for most people. Purpose-built residences and communities offer the next best solution for some; and residential environments in institutional settings are probably the least desired but are often the only reasonable alternative for many people.

In each case, residents are interested in security. Security in terms of physical safety, freedom from want or fear, from anxiety or stress. The Hebrew Rehabilitation Center for Aged in Roslindale, just outside Boston, maintains a group of 25 paid researchers with seven Ph.D.s and $5 million a year in funding for geriatric and gerontology studies. Before launching its first

CCRC, the center investigated CCRCs in 20 states and compared the lifestyles and responses to questionnaires. Some remarkable data was gathered. Questions like "Can you walk a mile?" were answered favorably by residents in CCRCs in their 90s. Many living outside the CCRC—but in the same communities—in their late 60s and early 70s could not answer the same. "Are you concerned about being a burden to anyone?" The answer from those inside CCRCs was almost always "no." Outside in the general community, it was almost always "yes."

While there's certainly no proof of linkage, the theory is that this data goes a long way to explain the incredible life expectancies that are being found in CCRCs. The average entering age today is 78 and the average life expectancy upon entrance is another 13 years. That means the average life expectancy inside these communities is 91 years of age, which is considerably better than the average life expectancy of the general population. But not everyone can afford a CCRC, and even some who can afford it are not interested in buying their way into a CCRC. This is why facility types such as assisted living, where people pay-as-they-go, are becoming popular. The brutal truth is that most of the population will not be able to afford either CCRCs or assisted living facilities, and therefore the issue is going to be how to make it possible for people to continue living in their own residences and communities with the services and support they need.

Jury Comments

The jury commented on the following categories of facility types:

- *Nursing Homes.* "Generally the jury was impressed with numerous projects exhibiting new design approaches to the nursing home concept. Designers developed unique responses to privacy issues in semiprivate rooms. Care was taken in these projects to give the resident a clear sense of place through better wayfinding and clearer definition of each person's territory. The jury rejected as inappropriate to residents' needs several medical models which were submitted with traditional approaches to nursing patterns and room layouts."
- *Continuing Care Retirement Communities.* "Rather than seeing strong new directions in CCRC design approaches, the jury noticed more subtle refinements. In several projects, the nursing component of the CCRC is more carefully layered into the overall complex rather than hidden in an obscure corner of the facility. Historical cliches such as bell towers, clock towers, town centers, and pedestrian malls still abound, but more attention is devoted to careful integration of parking and to site plans that are grander and more dramatic."
- *Assisted Living and Independent Apartments.* "The jury saw a great diversity of approaches to assisted living design solutions. Home care has been used successfully in some projects and several solutions incorporate assisted living units within the independent apartment areas. Independent apartments are generally larger and more traditionally homelike in layout than they have been in previous years with only a few projects exhibiting contrived, angular plans that would be hard to furnish or potentially alien to the residents' experience."
- *Codes and Regulations.* "Entrants were asked to comment on codes and

regulations that affected their designs. The most common variance from codes is the use of atrium and open activity spaces in the corridors. And the most frequent complaints relate to area and cost limitations that inhibit good design and force traditional operating patterns. Additionally, the zoning process and local interpretations of fire codes may stand in the way of innovative design. In light of the growing market for retirement facilities, the jury is encouraged by the interest in this Design for Aging Facilities Review program and pleased that established designs are being discarded in favor of new solutions that benefit architects, providers, and, most importantly, the residents."

AIA's Solution

I'd like to explain what AIA proposes to do about this problem. Back in 1982, AIA formed what was called the Task Force on Design for Aging. Based upon its work and in the ten years that have since passed, AIA has done a fairly decent job of making the architectural community aware of the problems of the aging and making design for aging a subject that most architects are at least conversant with, if not expert at. But there has been a lack of focus within AIA on aging issues, mostly because there are many standing committees in AIA—the Committee on Architecture for Health, Committee on Housing, Committee on Interiors, Committee on Building Performance and Regulations, and so on. These committees have some sense of ownership of this issue, but none wants to claim it. As far as the world outside of the AIA was concerned, there was no one to talk to about issues related to aging.

As a result, AIA formed another task force with representatives from each of those committees, which held a round table discussion in April 1991. The participants in this round table, which included representatives of caregivers, providers, physicians, advocates for the elderly, financing groups, manufacturers, and suppliers, urged AIA to get its act together and do something about the research required and the dissemination of information necessary to benefit the elderly. The task force wrote a white paper, recommending that the Aging Design Research Program be created, which it was! It is a program within the Council on Architectural Research, which is a group jointly administered by AIA and the Association of Collegiate Schools of Architecture (ACSA). Being outside of the AIA itself, the program is open to the membership and participation of anyone interested in elderly design issues.

The Council on Architectural Research approved the concept of the Aging Design Research Program as a membership organization that can reach out beyond architectural professionals and architectural schools, but can include them as well. Membership in the program will be solicited in 1992. Even though it's only embryonic, the program has already received its first grant from the Administration on Aging in Washington, DC.

In a joint program with the Association of Occupational Therapists of America (AOTA), AIA is organizing a demonstration program for occupational therapists (OTs) and architects on how to work together to better serve one another's needs and the needs of the elderly. The two professions have had very little contact. Yet, OTs are one of the groups of professionals who regularly visit the elderly in their own homes (along with such others as visiting nurses, physical therapists, and home care people). Since these therapists understand the needs of the elderly and are able to spot the physical barriers that exist within their homes, they can prescribe the corrections that are required. The demonstration project will put OTs together with architects to work with specific residents in homes, to develop responses and results. Those results will be published and disseminated through workshops all over the country sponsored by chapters of AIA and AOTA.

NAHB Demonstration House Video

I'd like to show a video borrowed from the National Association of Home Builders (NAHB). "It's All in the Planning" is about the demonstration house that NAHB has built for the dual purpose of convincing builders across the nation of the advantages of constructing fire-safe, as well as accessible, residences. First, I'll show the video and then discuss some of the issues it raised with my clients.

Person Number One: I've been in a wheelchair for more than 35 years. I've purchased three homes in my lifetime so far and each time has been almost a traumatic situation in trying to find homes that meet my needs.

Person Number Two: It is much more difficult to get around than it used to be. I find stairs a problem. I avoid them as much as possible. Another problem is reaching for things on high shelves. I can't manage it and it's very frustrating.

Person Number Three: I realize that, in the future, my condition is not going to get any better. It's probably going to get worse. Someday, I might be in a wheelchair or I might be restricted to using walkers or some other prosthetic aid. Planning a house anywhere today that is constructed to meet those future needs is almost impossible.

Person Number Four: If there were a fire in my house and if I were asleep, I wouldn't hear the alarm. If my wife weren't there, I would have a real problem getting out of the house.

Announcer: For 37 million people with disabilities and a growing number of our nation's elderly, suitable housing is a challenge that we're just beginning to meet. Here in the Washington, DC suburbs, the National Association of Home Builders Research Center has designed and built this demonstration house to show how a standard house plan can be easily modified to accommodate a wide variety of needs often at little or no expense. It's all in the planning.

From the very beginning, this house was designed to be easily accessible from the outside. The house is constructed on a two percent grade, sufficient to carry water away from the foundation, but not too steep for a wheelchair. And, by incorporating the wheelchair access ramp into the front porch, the house preserves its curb appeal without looking institutional.

Person Number Five: The most important feature for a house to have for me is enough room so I can maneuver my wheelchair.

Announcer: The entryway and all the doorways are just a little bit wider than typical door and entryways. The thresholds are nearly flat and the low pile carpets have been glued directly to the floor. Throughout the house, casement windows have been placed lower for a better view. This special mechanism makes it even easier to operate the window lock, and it costs less than $40. The fireplace hearth is flush with the floor and the fire box has been raised for easy reach. Wall outlet receptacles have been placed a foot higher than usual and wall switches four inches lower.

All the bathrooms in the house have reinforced walls to accommodate grab bars. The sink is hung lower on the wall and permits access by a wheelchair. A shroud protects legs from the hot water pipes below. The faucets have levers, not knobs, for easy grip. Even the mirror is hung lower for easy use. This barrier-free shower has a simple and inexpensive hand-held shower head that can be used by people with a wide range of special needs. This barrier-free bathroom costs only about $1,300 more than a comparable, standard bathroom.

The elevator is by far the most expensive option in this house. While it is convenient, it is not absolutely necessary. There's enough room at the base of the stairs to accommodate a less expensive platform lift or stair glide that rides along the banister. The upstairs shares many of the same design features as the rest of the house. The large closet in the master bedroom attracts a lot of attention with its motorized carousel. The master bath door has been hinged to swing both ways for ease in access. And for just a little bit more money than a standard unit, this state-of-the-art jetted bath has a door to help reduce falls while getting into and out of it. Again, these are subtle modifications that needn't cost much if they are planned from the start.

Person Number Six: The kitchen is lovely, but it's the small things that appeal mostly to me.

Announcer: This universal design kitchen shows how a little planning can keep the occupant from going a long way. Kitchen work can be done within a 22-foot triangle from refrigerator to stove to serving. These kitchen cabinets are mounted on brackets so they may be lowered to suit the occupants' needs. Lazy Susans help to utilize dead space in the corners. The sink has easier-to-grasp levers instead of turn-handle faucets to control the water. Similar quality levers add no extra cost. Control knobs have been placed on the front of the induction cook top stove. This design eliminates long reaches over open flames or hot coils and a potential for clothing or pot holders to catch fire. The oven door folds down so it may be used as a shelf when cooking. The oven controls are large and placed in front, making them easy to read and to reach. And the pass-through design cuts down on the distance the occupant has to walk or wheel in order to eat.

Person Number Seven: Right now I can move around fairly well. However, I realize because of my injuries that may not be the case in the future. When that happens, having an upstairs and a downstairs will mean more to my family than it does to me because I will be restricted to the use of the first floor of my home.

Announcer: This home's plans include adaptability as well as accessibility. The first floor plan includes a family room located conveniently next to the garage. The laundry facilities are located on the first floor, a convenience for some people but a necessity for someone with mobility limitations. The circuit box also is located on the main floor. And this room has been outfitted with an electric Murphy bed for a den or a study by day and a main-level bedroom at night to complete the potential for single-floor living.

Person Number Eight: I can't hear very well and I can't see very well. And also I have problems walking where it isn't light enough.

Announcer: Contrasting colors or shades are used to help the visually impaired distinguish the stairs or hallways. The fire safety control panel is located on the main floor. It connects the smoke detectors and sprinklers to the special fire alarm warning system. The main sleeping areas of the house are wired to activate special receptacles that operate in an emergency. A strobe light alerts a hearing-impaired person or a fan blowing onto the face alerts a hearing and visually impaired person of a fire emergency. And there are several means of escape from the main floor. Even the sliding glass doors have only a slight rise for easy wheelchair and walker access.

This house demonstrates many different features that help to meet the needs of people with disabilities. The important thing to remember is that accessibility and adaptability do not have to mean an institutional look. And as our country's population ages, many of these features we've just seen will come much more into demand to meet housing comfort and safety needs. In fact, the NAHB Research Center has compiled a catalog of adaptable products for builders to use as a reference for meeting their clients' special needs. But the most important thing to remember, whether it's modifications to help the sensory impaired, the elderly, or the infirm, is that for a total cost of as little as two percent over the home's base price almost any new house can be made adaptable for a wide range of special needs as long as it's all in the planning.

After seeing this video in Baltimore at a meeting of the Committee on Architecture for Health, I acquired it, along with the catalog of accessible products that NAHB puts out. I then said to the developers of Orchard Cove (Hebrew Rehab's new CCRC in Canton, MA), "Do you know we can get dishwashers that fit under a 34-inch counter? Why don't we lower all the counters to 34 inches to help these little old ladies?" Their response was, "We can't do that. The market will react negatively. They'll say it's not a 'real' kitchen. We won't be able to give them a 'real' stove."

One of the things I've been realizing, as a healthcare architect learning how to do residential design, is that there are fundamental differences in the housing and healthcare facilities markets. In both cases, the ultimate client is the same: the residents and the users of the facilities. But in health facilities design, there usually is a professional user group that advises design professionals. Even though we like to think we're designing universal environments that could be successfully used by any care provider, there usually is a sponsoring client who decides the details: what equipment and which materials, finishes, colors to use.

Housing, however, is much more speculative. Except in designing custom residences, specific occupants are rarely identified during the design phase of a project. Instead, one relies upon the experience of the developer, consultants, and focus groups of potential occupants to "psych out" what the marketplace really wants and needs.

Wants and needs may be two different things, however, because design professionals and developers are operating in a marketplace that's based on denial. They cannot impose their knowledge of what people need, unless people agree that they want the things design professionals and developers think they need. A perfectly designed accessible facility may stand empty, if the residents don't agree that it's a real house with a real kitchen and a real bathroom.

So, the decision was not to put in a unit with the grab bars already installed, but to make it possible to add them when they are needed later. It was not to put in the cabinets that can be lowered, but to bring some of the cupboards down to the counter-top levels so they're accessible. If changes have to be made later, the cabinet can be pulled out and a new one installed, because the unit with the visible gap telegraphs to the marketplace that this is accessible design. The home builders don't want accessible design. They want universal design, something that anybody will buy.

Marketing experts around the country know that the elderly typically think of themselves as 15 years younger than they really are, and they buy the products that were originally targeted for a younger generation. This is a philosophy that creates a lot of problems. How do design professionals convince a nursing home developer to do better than a plain vanilla, medical model, side-by-side two-bedded room, if nobody wants to see the nursing home when they check out a CCRC?

People want the comfort of knowing that, if they ever need it, the facility will be there. But, until then, they don't want to see or hear about it. Only a developer with experience (or advice that convinces him) is going to invest the money needed to build larger rooms with toe-to-toe arrangements, L-shaped arrangements, or whatever other configurations are required to give residents in a nursing home the kind of environments that are comparable to those they enjoyed in their independent living apartments.

Can a nursing home design be successfully marketed in a marketplace based on denial? Does every developer have to discover this on his own? Does every architect or design professional have to go through this set of issues with every client? Or is there some research that can be developed to provide proven directions that serve the needs of the residents, so that built facilities do not stand empty on their initial occupancy or become empty ten years later because better facilities have come on line since?

Predicting the future is something that operators of these care facilities are vitally interested in, because nonprofit developers like those in the AAHA group do not build and sell and walk away. They are developers who build and operate and expect to continue to operate for generations. How do they stay competitive in the next decade, the next time they have to fill up the CCRC? These are some of the challenges we hope to address in the new Aging Design Research Program of the AIA/ACSA Research Council. We invite anyone's interest, participation, and support.

Martin H. Cohen is an architect based in Armonk, New York, who assists owners, architects, and developers of healthcare facilities and senior living environments as a planning, design, design management, and project management consultant. With insights gained from 39 years of diverse experience, he serves as a resource, planner, advisor, and critic.

◆ ◆ ◆

THE CORINNE DOLAN ALZHEIMER CENTER

Fourth Symposium on Healthcare Design, Boston, MA, 1991

Margaret P. Calkins

I am going to talk about both process and product because they are integrally related. The process begins with setting goals. It is important to remember that the physical design of spaces should always follow the development of therapeutic goals.

Undoubtedly, building codes for any long-term care environment will ensure that biological needs and safety are addressed. The codes generally do not go much beyond that, but I believe that personal needs are very important. So, the goal at the Corinne Dolan Alzheimer Center was to go beyond safety and focus on love—the relationship between staff and residents, and residents and their families. We focused on self-esteem in terms of helping residents feel they still have dignity and control over their lives.

We also wanted to capture the spirit of a quote by Dr. Eisdorfer, who wrote that "one of the absolutely traumatic and debilitating processes in the human existence is the loss of mastery over your own life. The treatment objectives for the care of older persons with Alzheimer's disease, or a related disorder, are to maximize their functional effectiveness, freedom, and human dignity."

The literature suggests that there may be several different types of special care units. Ohta and Ohta conducted a study in 1988 and found three types or levels of care. A study conducted by Sloane and his colleagues found eight levels or types of care.

I would like to propose four levels of care:

- *Custodial Care* provides only those services necessary to maintain one's physical condition for as long as possible. In general, the individual needs of each patient are not considered—rather they are warehoused for the convenience of the staff.
- *Medical Care* is an advancement over custodial care because each patient is seen as an individual. However, care focuses on the medical condition, to the exclusion of the rest of the patient. It concentrates on keeping the patient alive and managing behavior as expeditiously as possible.
- *Functional Independence Care* views the resident (not patient) as an individual with social and psychological, as well as physical problems. The individual is assessed according to his or her ability to function rather than the extent of the pathology. This level of care encourages maintenance of remaining skills and includes individual care plans and activities.
- *Therapeutic Care* focuses on success, positive affect, social integration, and physical achievement. It goes beyond maintenance to provide a humanizing and existentially supportive context in which activities reaffirm the dignity, self-esteem, and happiness of the residents. A therapeutic milieu is based on a philosophy of humanism that attests to the dignity and worth of human beings and the right of the individual to self-realization and a sense of being accepted and valued.

Project Background

Heather Hill, a facility in Chardon, Ohio, had a one-year planning grant from the Robert Wood Johnson Foundation in 1985 to develop the program for the Corinne Dolan Alzheimer Center. We determined that there was a need for respite care, day care, and assisted living level care for people with dementia who did not need nursing level care. We also felt that there was a need for education and research. Heather Hill already had a special care unit for dementia that had been in existence since 1982, so we focused our efforts on these other needs.

Given the program that we wanted to run, we decided that the staff/resident ratio should be one-to-six. We were looking at two pods of 12 beds each. Keeping our goals and philosophy in mind, we then determined the program content.

- *Community Circle* is for the highest functioning level of residents who still have some social skills and the ability to work with others. The goals for this level of care are to maintain appropriate cognitive and social skills through activities, discussion, reminiscence, and outings to malls and parks.
- *Family Circle* is for moderately functioning residents who are more easily distracted and have fewer cognitive skills. The goal is to focus on activities that are familiar, through which the residents can succeed and feel productive: home chores, crafts, setting tables, and baking in the kitchen.
- *Men's Club* was developed because approximately one-quarter of our residents are male. The men's program is for a variety of levels and emphasizes activities that they would be more comfortable doing: gardening, woodworking, maintenance, and yard work.
- *Open Circle* is for residents with limited communication and social skills who are easily distracted. The goal is to meet individual needs primarily through one-on-one communication, music, reading, sensory stimulation, walks, and similar kinds of activities.

The next step was to identify the needs of the customers—residents, staff, families, social workers, and everyone else who comes in contact with the building. We developed a list of therapeutic goals that we used to judge and evaluate every design decision. Does this meet our philosophy; does it meet a specific goal? Does it meet the therapeutic goals that are primarily resident related? Does it serve the needs of other users?

We looked at existing facilities to help set up goals for how we wanted these areas to function. For the shared living spaces, we wanted to increase social interaction and decrease the institutional character. Increasing orientation was an important goal for the corridors—not just spatial orientation and wayfinding, but orientation to activity, to time of day. In the dining room, we also wanted to increase social interaction and decrease the institutional character. Bedroom issues were related to privacy and personalization.

We also looked at the normal aging deficits that this older population tends to experience. I won't go into any of them; but, we tried to relate any design decision back to what we know about aging—changes in vision, hearing, balance, and muscle tone—and how these might have implications for the physical environment.

I'm going to describe a variety of therapeutic goals that we set up, how we articulated them, and then how they were manifested in the built environment in the Corinne Dolan Alzheimer Center.

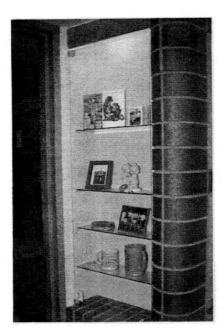

◆ **FIGURE 8–3** Each bedroom has a display case that is built into the wall with lockable glass doors. (*Project:* Corinne Dolan Alzheimer Center, Chardon, OH. *Architecture:* Stephen Nemtin. *Photo:* Margaret P. Calkins.)

Orientation

One of the first Alzheimer's facilities, the Weiss Pavilion at Philadelphia Geriatric Center, took an innovative approach and created a large open pavilion. When residents come out of their bedrooms, they can see the dining room, shared central spaces, and nurse station. It's all very clear—they don't have to make decisions as to which way to turn. We tried to utilize some of this openness, although we felt that one of the limitations of the Philadelphia Geriatric Center was its size. Forty residents in a single space is potentially overstimulating.

So we created two 12-bed pods that are virtually identical—because we were also conducting research in the building. As residents come out of their rooms, they can see the central space. There is a large kitchen and a dining room. We also wanted to increase opportunities for the residents to find their own bedrooms independently, so each bedroom has a display case that is built into the wall with lockable glass doors. If residents want to have access to the items in the case, they can ask the staff to help. Otherwise, the items are secure, so families can feel more comfortable in bringing in things that have sentimental, or even real, value; things that they don't want to be lost.

One of the first research projects we did in this building related to the display cases. There were two conditions: one having residents' own items in the display case and one having neutral items that did not have any significance. Over a four-week period, we asked the residents to take us to their rooms and we assessed whether or not personal versus nonpersonal items made a difference in their ability to find their rooms. In the analysis, we used CDR, the clinical dementia rating, for residents' levels of cognitive skills. CDR 1 means that a person is less confused and CDR 3 means they are more confused. We found that generally, people who were less confused were able to find their rooms better than people who were more confused, which makes sense.

But the difference was between the significant and the nonsignificant cues, particularly for people at CDR level 2. Residents at CDR level 2 with their own personal items in the case are twice as likely to be able to find their room than when there are neutral items. The residents were also very creative about finding other ways to identify their rooms when there were neutral items in the case. One woman put a poinsettia plant outside her door every day when she was in the condition of having neutral items in the case. We kept asking her if we could put the plant back in her room (because we didn't want her to use those kinds of cues). But, she clearly knew that without her own items in the display case, she couldn't find her room and had to do something else.

Orientation is more than just finding the bedroom. It relates to other levels of functioning. In our existing nursing home unit, we noticed that a number of residents seemed to be incontinent because they couldn't find the bathroom. So we specifically designed the bathroom area of the bedroom to be open and visible. We had to answer a lot of questions before the building opened as to whether or not it was ethical and appropriate to do this. But we had discussed what was more important: maintaining continence, or the potential loss of some privacy. There is a privacy curtain, and residents tend to close their doors when they are in their rooms. We did not feel that the privacy issue was as significant.

We also wanted to make sure that the toilet was very visible and stood out

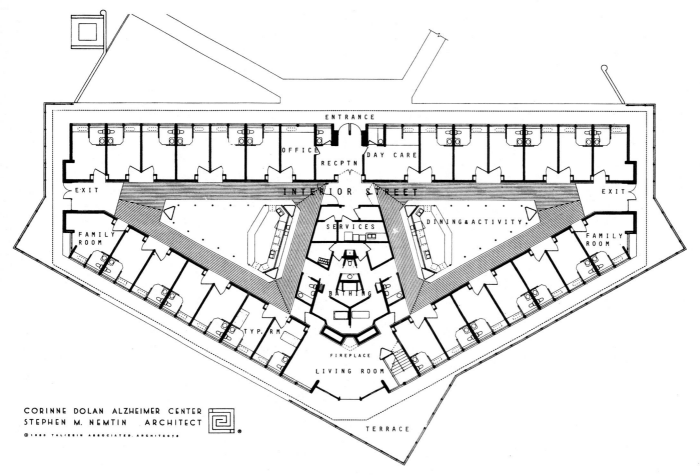

ENTRANCE

OFFICE   DAY CARE

RECPTN

EXIT

INTERIOR STREET

EXIT

FAMILY ROOM

SERVICES

DINING & ACTIVITY

FAMILY ROOM

BATHING

TYP. RM

FIREPLACE

LIVING ROOM

TERRACE

CORINNE DOLAN ALZHEIMER CENTER
STEPHEN M. NEMTIN ARCHITECT
© 1988 TALIESIN ASSOCIATED ARCHITECTS

◆ **FIGURE 8–4**   Floor plan shows the identical 12-bed pods in the Corinne Dolan Alzheimer Center. (*Architecture:* Stephen Nemtin. *Drawing:* Stephen Nemtin.)

from the wall space, so we installed white fixtures that contrast with the brick-colored wall and floor. Having a white ceramic toilet with white walls and a white floor is more likely to cause accidents because some will miss the toilet.

Our research investigated toilet use when the toilets were visible versus when the privacy curtain was closed. Unfortunately, in the research, the residents whom we had hypothesized would be most likely to be influenced by the visibility or the nonvisibility of the toilet were in the nonvisible condition first. They became so incontinent that within three days, they and/or the staff and/or families requested that they be removed from the study. Even without their participation, however, the difference in toilet use was substantial. Therefore, making the toilet very visible can significantly increase the residents' ability to maintain continence independently.

We also conducted a study on signage. We looked at different nomenclature and graphics, and we tested a number of different signs with various colors and patterns. When none of these were as effective as we wanted them to be, we put signs on the floor. And in fact, this was most effective.

Residents would come out, look at the arrow, and although they might not know what it meant or where it led to, they were intrigued by it, and followed it to the bathroom. This signage might not be right for every situation, but in our building it was what was most effective.

Wandering

The first thing that has to be done with wandering is to find out the residents' agenda. Why are they wandering? Do they want to go home? Do they want to go to work? If it's an 8 A.M. exit-seeking behavior, it may mean that the person feels as if he or she should be going to work. If that is the case, what needs to be done is to give these wanderers something productive to do so that they feel as though they are going to work.

For some people, wandering may be a manifestation of boredom or anxiety. Wandering is not inherently negative. There are times when wandering is very therapeutic. There are also times when it's not therapeutic. Wandering in the traditional double-loaded nursing home corridor does not provide any positive reinforcement. There are often lots of carts and equipment stored in the corridor that residents can trip over if they are not careful.

We looked at creating opportunities for residents to wander and examined what happens along that wandering path. Each 12-bed unit has a triangular wandering path because we wanted to avoid dead ends. We know that people can have a hard time turning around if they are in a narrow space. We also looked at what happens at the ends of the paths and located seating areas, family rooms, program activity spaces, and access to a living room there. We encourage tactile experiences and put quilts on the wall so that residents will reach out and touch and explore their environment. There is also a brick and a concrete block wall for tactile variety.

Art work by Mardel Sanzotta has a teddy bear with real fur, real lace curtains, a real ball and blocks that stick out, and real flowers. So again, not just the quilts, but all of the art work in the building encourages residents to reach out and explore their environment. We want it to be a rich environment, but one that doesn't overstimulate; residents have control over how much stimulation they want to get.

In talking about wandering, we know that some people seem to get into a pattern and never stop. So we created spaces at the end of the hallway to encourage them to sit down and rest. They can look outside and see the park, or look inside toward the dining area and watch any ongoing activity.

We also created places for them to "rummage." We were somewhat concerned about potential rummaging through other people's bedrooms, so we created positive opportunities for rummaging. Drawers on the back side of the kitchen contain magazines, pieces of fabric, or whatever the residents seem to be most attracted to.

We also looked at how wandering can be appropriately manifested outside. There is a fence that encloses a two-acre park that is adjacent to the building (Figure 8–6). Residents have free access to this park. It took us a while to teach the staff to let the residents outside on their own. There are a few residents whom we feel are not safe and appropriate outside by themselves, so they are accompanied by staff or volunteers. But we give most of the residents the ability to control their actions. If they want to go wandering outside on these paths, that is part of their right and part of our philosophy. The

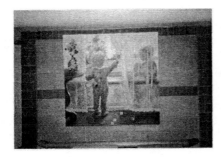

◆ **FIGURE 8–5** Tactile experiences are encouraged by putting quilts and art work on the wall so that residents will reach out and touch and explore their environment. (*Project:* Corinne Dolan Alzheimer Center, Chardon, OH. *Architecture:* Stephen Nemtin. *Art work:* Mardel Sanzotta. *Photo:* Margaret P. Calkins.)

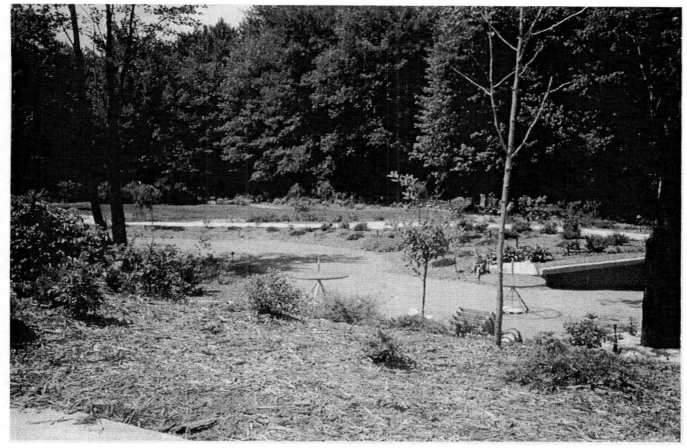

◆ **FIGURE 8–6**   A fence encloses a two-acre park adjacent to the building, to which residents have free access. (*Project:* Corinne Dolan Alzheimer Center, Chardon, OH. *Architecture:* Stephen Nemtin. *Photo:* Margaret P. Calkins.)

residents also go with each other on a regular basis, because they feel that they are helping each other.

Privacy and Social Interaction

Privacy and social interaction are linked together, because in a sense, they are on a continuum. We need to look at how people can manage and control opportunities for both privacy and social interaction. There is enough data on behavior patterns in humans to suggest that both are necessary for high quality of life.

In some of the places we had seen when we were doing the research for our building, the chairs were lined up around the outside of a room. This makes it much more difficult to have a conversation because it is harder to turn one's head 90 degrees to talk to someone. There were a few positive attempts to make conversation easier—such as a table with some chairs.

We created a variety of different spaces for different-sized groups. There is the dining room, which is used only as a dining room. This practice reinforces for the residents what types of behavior are appropriate in this space. There is the living room—used as a living room, not as a program activity space. Each 12-bed unit has a family room at the end of the building that is used for more structured activities. There is also a craft room, where some of the messier activities take place.

We decided to provide private bedrooms. There is some controversy about private versus semiprivate bedrooms. Generally, I feel that a mix is most appropriate. There are some residents who do benefit from the positive aspects of having a roommate. But in general, unless the rooms are designed in such a way that each person has clear territory and opportunity for privacy, private rooms allow more personal control.

The family room furniture gets moved around a lot because it's a changing space. The residents themselves will come in and change the space around—they feel that they have control over their space.

Homelike Environment

We are located 22 miles outside of Cleveland in a very rural area where there are many farmers and people from working classes who did not experience "high-style architecture." We also get people from downtown Cleveland, Shaker Heights, and the eastern suburbs who are used to a higher style of finishes and furniture.

Finding one style of furniture to meet everyone's expectation of what is "homelike" did not seem the appropriate way to go. So we looked at other aspects of what is "home," and decided one of the things that is fundamental about home is control. When people are at home, they decorate it the way they want. They can get up in the middle of the night and get cookies and milk. They can control the temperature. They can control whether or not their windows are open.

Those are the kinds of directions that we went in to make this a homelike environment. While the building is noninstitutional, it is not "residential" in its appearance.

We looked at things like group sizes. I've already mentioned that we were looking at a one-to-six staff ratio. Most of the activities happen with six or fewer residents. The staffing is consistent so that the residents get to know their staff member—the person who is ultimately responsible for their partnership and care.

We looked at dining. Trays are one of the most institutional ways of serving food. The fact that these people may be eating in the same dining room with the same furniture, china, and often the same food for several years made us question whether they should have to eat off a tray as in a cafeteria. So we designed the food service system to be very residential—family style.

Is the schedule rigid or flexible? Again, that relates to the residents having control. Our residents get up when they want to get up. They go to bed when they want to go to bed. We try to meet their own needs for when they bathe—whether they want a shower or a bath.

Terminology also makes a difference. How many of us have a day room in our house? Does anyone know what one does in a day room? If a nurse says to a resident, "Go down to the day room and be good," what is the definition of "good" in a day room? By making the spaces look familiar, giving them terms that are familiar, and have them function in familiar ways, we are more likely to encourage appropriate behavior.

One of the things that is most institutional is the nurse station. In a recently constructed facility, the nurse station is 36 feet long. How can there be a "residential" program with a 36-foot-long nurse station that encourages separation between the staff and the residents? It doesn't allow the staff to function like a family.

Our staff do not wear uniforms—they are part of the family. We do wear big yellow name tags. One of the residents once asked us, "Why do you all wear name tags? I want one." So we started making name tags for the residents. There is much less differentiation between who is a resident and who is staff; who is helping whom.

We did have to have something like a nurse station in order to get the plans approved. It's in the kitchen—and is noninstitutional, since it is fairly common to have a desk in the kitchen. It's where the telephone is located. There are two file drawers that are lockable, where the staff keep their records. But the staff can sit there and watch the residents throughout the rest of the space—and residents know somebody is often working at the desk in the kitchen. It breaks down that institutional feeling of who is in control.

We also wanted residents to be able to relate to familiar activities. Since we recognized that a majority of the residents would be women, and the residents who were likely to be coming into our building were not ones who had a lot of outside support, they were likely to have spent considerable time in a kitchen. So having a kitchen that was readily accessible to the residents was a fundamental component of the program.

Access to a washer and dryer is also something that is very important from a family point of view, because families can do that activity with the resident and it is productive. It relates to familiar things that they may have done at home. It provides positive reinforcement for ways of interacting.

The home is different from other places we spend time in because we have the ability to personalize it, to control what is put in it, and where things are put. We continued this pattern—all the residents bring in their own furniture. For those who may be coming from another care facility and may not have their own furniture anymore, we encourage families to bring in things that were familiar or look similar to the furniture the person had lived with.

I talked about the ability to have control, which even relates to lights and thermostats. Each room has its own thermostat and the residents have the opportunity to control it. Sometimes it means that the controls are set on 85 degrees. There are a couple of residents who no longer know how to use the thermostat appropriately. But we didn't want to start with the assumption that this was something that the residents couldn't do anymore. We start with the assumption that this is something that they can do: they can state a preference for how warm or cool they want their room. And then we work from there to make sure that the thermostat works with the resident's level of comfort.

A variety of different kinds of outside spaces is important. In a private backyard, there might be a large lawn, a small patio, and some deck furniture. There are different kinds of spaces—private backyards are not as uniform as many of our institutional environments are. So, we wanted to create different spaces. A retaining wall is used for gardening, so people can pull up a chair and garden while seated. It isn't one of those wooden structures that begins to look like "handicap-accessible" gardening. We wanted an environment that doesn't have the stigma of serving people who need support or help reinforce an image of health as opposed to sickness.

Excess Disabilities and Functional Independence

Excess disabilities are a common problem with this population, often related to functional independence. Having high contrast on the tables and contrast between the chair and the floor is important. The arms of the dining room chairs are rounded and very easy on the hands, so that if people are going to push up, they can do it without getting indentations in their hands.

Light switches in bedrooms contrast with the wallpaper. The set of lights for the front hall, central dining room, and kitchen space is also accessible to residents. However, we anticipated that there might be someone walking around the wandering path who would go along and flip all of the lights on and off all day long. So we painted these switches the same color as the wall. Again, we didn't want to prevent access to the switches, but we wanted to discourage their inappropriate use. It has been very effective. It wouldn't work in every situation—some people would go along and flip them all of the time. But, most of our residents don't see the switches, and therefore don't play with them.

We did one study on what constitutes a distraction. We had three conditions: One was with no barriers, and two were with two different-height barriers to see whether or not residents would concentrate on an activity longer in the different barrier conditions. What we found was that the presence of any barrier, high or low, was enough to keep the residents focused significantly longer on their activity. This study is applicable to a facility with a large day room that might effectively be subdivided. We're beginning to explore what level of separation is necessary. Should it be acoustic? Should it be visual? How high does it have to be? Most of these studies are just pilot studies and the results are not meant to provide the final answer. But they begin to suggest patterns that we can use in future research studies.

We also looked at functioning in terms of dressing. We wanted to encourage the residents to have their own clothes and more of a choice of what to wear. We looked at the closets in our existing nursing home. The staff told us that some residents didn't have enough hanging space; some didn't have enough shelf space; some needed more drawers; and some needed long hanging for dresses. They wanted to be able to customize the closets for each person.

So we created an open space into which we can put wire shelf systems. If someone needs a lot of hanging space and doesn't need the baskets, we take the baskets out. If someone has long dresses and a lot of blouses and still needs some baskets, we can use the bottom half of the basket system. It's very flexible and we work with the families before the resident comes in to make sure that the closet will meet the storage needs of that resident.

We then went beyond that to look at how we could design a closet that would enable the residents to dress themselves independently. We designed a modification with bars; clothes are laid out the night before with a staff member so that residents have a choice of what they will wear. The clothes they put on first in the morning are in front, so the decision-making process is taken out of the dressing activity. Each item is presented in the relative location to where it goes on the body so that pants, socks, underwear are down below; and blouses, sweat shirts, and other similar items are on top. Again, results are preliminary, but for some residents, this system did seem to make a difference.

Safety and Security

Safety and security is not what we call one of our primary, therapeutic goals, but it is something that we are responsible for. The kitchen area presents the potential for many hazardous situations. There is a stove to which residents have access, and there is also a microwave. We wanted the staff to be able to turn off the power to the stove but in a way that was not obvious. So we hid the switch for the stove inside a cabinet; when the cabinet is closed it looks like any of the other kitchen cabinets. We also put a separate fire suppression system that is on a heat-sensitive lock above the stove. Thus if there is a fire on the stove, it doesn't set the sprinklers off throughout the whole building.

We also wanted to, at times, discourage residents from going into the kitchen. So there is a section of the counter that flips up and latches onto the adjacent counter. It's not foolproof—there are some people who crawl underneath but, for the most part, it's enough to tell the residents that this is a space they should not be using right now. It's very effective at suggesting security without making it so absolutely fundamental.

One of the other concerns about security in environments for people with dementia is limiting access in and out of buildings and the units. The only entrance that the residents do not have free access to is the front door. There is a gate system so that residents are not right up against the door. We tried to limit their visual access to areas we were not giving them physical access to. We don't want them to be focused on the front of the building where people are coming and going, so the main entrance has solid-core doors with no windows. Instead, we encouraged increased visual access to spaces that we were giving them physical access to by using glass in doors that lead to the park.

There are a couple of different kinds of locks. We use a mechanical lock on the storage room, housekeeping closet, and the door that goes down to the lower level where the offices are. Because these mechanical locks are all on solid doors, none of the residents play with them. Whereas, at exits, where there are views to the park to entice residents outside, we installed a keypad. Therefore when it is very cold in the winter, we can secure the doors and make sure that residents are properly dressed before they go outside. Sometimes residents will stand at the keypad, which is by these glass exit doors, and play with it until they figure out the combination. We have had to change the combination a number of times.

In general, keypads can be very effective. However, I visited a facility in Wisconsin that had put in a system where operators didn't have the opportunity to change the code and they hadn't really assessed their residents very well. Within three days, the residents were helping the families leave the unit because the families couldn't remember the code but the residents all knew it. The system should have the ability to be reprogrammed and the numbers recoded.

In general, I don't like securing doors if there are other alternatives. Securing a door has both advantages and disadvantages compared with some other patient monitoring systems. I'm also not very fond of tagging residents, for ethical reasons. I have a real problem with putting a tag on a resident who locks or unlocks a door. There are certain situations where there is no alternative but to tag the patient. Nonetheless I look for other alternatives first.

Security also relates to how residents are "told" that they are in a secure or nonsecure environment. Creating barriers that are very obvious is more likely to increase frustration. Our outside space has a fence that secures the area, but which "fades into the background" and becomes very unobtrusive. Thus residents aren't constantly reminded that they are in an enclosed, secured space.

Conclusion

Where do we go from here? This has been a brief introduction to the Corinne Dolan Alzheimer Center at Heather Hill, designed by Stephen Nemitin of Taliesin Associated Architects. We have found that it is very successful. We conducted eight research projects under the direction of Dr. Kevan Namazi, which have been published in *The American Journal of Alzheimer Care and Research* (Vol. 6, 1991 and Vol. 1, 1992). We also went back and assessed our nursing care unit; while the staffing and the programs are pretty good, the environment was not ideal. So Heather Hill has just broken ground on a new nursing care facility. We tried to incorporate many of the lessons that we learned in the Dolan center in the new unit.

In summary, design and healthcare professionals should not look at environments in isolation. Programs, activities, administrative policies, and the environment all need to work together in order to produce a facility that is successful for everyone.

Margaret P. Calkins is president of I.D.E.A.S.: Innovative Designs in Environments for an Aging Society, in Milwaukee, Wisconsin. She is also a senior fellow of the Insitute on Aging and Environment at the University of Wisconsin–Milwaukee. Calkins integrates the disciplines of psychology and architecture in her research on environments for people with Alzheimer's disease and related dementias. A member of several national organizations and panels that focus on issues of care for cognitively impaired older Americans, she also is a frequent speaker at conferences in the United States and abroad. Her book, Design for Dementia: Planning Environments for the Elderly and the Confused, *was the first comprehensive design guide for special care units.*

◆

◆

◆

◆

◆

P   O   S   T   S   C   R   I   P   T

Wayne Ruga, AIA, IIDA,
Allied Member ASID

The National Symposium on Healthcare Design, the organization that produced the First through Fifth Symposia (the proceedings from which all the presentations in this book were excerpted from) had its origin in two concepts. Both concepts are based on the observation that there is substantially underutilized potential to use physical design to improve the quality of healthcare.

The first concept was to convene a forum of healthcare executives, design professionals, and manufacturers. Prior to the First Symposium, there was little, if no integration of the *design* and *healthcare* industries. Now, as a result of the Symposium, there is a thriving *healthcare design industry* with almost 20,000 active individuals worldwide and many more who serve in a supportive role.

The forum concept has served as a place for people of different needs, interests, and professional backgrounds to come together to learn, network, and share ideas. Through this forum, many new strategies have been formulated and new technologies created to meet the current needs of those who participate in the Symposia.

The second concept was to generate an inquiry to explore the variety of ways that design of the physical environment can be used to improve the quality of healthcare. Although this inquiry has brought a substantial volume of vital material into everyday use, its nature is ongoing and without an end. The richness and vitality of this inquiry is fueling the growth of a new industry that has the opportunity for continued development and expansion far into the foreseeable future.

Fundamental to those who participate in the Symposia is a collective desire to create a future that would not have happened otherwise. The very essence of the Symposia as an event is that it is a progressive, future-oriented undertaking that endeavors to bring viable, new ideas, strategies, and technologies into current application. Each Symposium has gently nudged the status quo of both the design and healthcare industries to the degree that the cumulative effect of the almost 5000 individuals who have attended six Symposia has been to transform the "healthscape." As I look back to when the Symposium first began in 1988, I can see that the healthscape is clearly different. This certainly represents a future that would not have happened otherwise.

As I look further into the future, I am proud of what we have accomplished as an industry and am inspired by the possibility of transformation that is still available.

Next Steps

As we prepare to challenge continually the status quo, deepen our inquiry, and expand the participation in our forum and its influence, let us consider the following activities, or "next steps," as a road map for sustained progress. The nature of the progress that we have collectively produced can be characterized as evolution. For us to sustain this evolution, each one of us must continue actively to apply ourselves.

It is important to recognize and keep in mind that the original observation about the mediocre design of the healthcare facilities that created the Symposium is still true today. This is unfortunate, as a reflection of the slow rate of change, yet encouraging, because of the amount of work that still needs to be done. The near future holds the realization that healthcare design is just as essential to healthcare as is medical technology, pharmaceutical interventions, and lifestyle management. Once this realization takes place, and the power of design to contribute to the quality of healthcare is universally acknowledged, we will enter what healthcare futurist Leland Kaiser refers to as "the decade of design."

Most of us are familiar with physical design's ability to improve how things look and to organize elements and people for enhanced efficiency. Yet, in the specific field of healthcare design, there is little application of design as a means to influence positively therapeutic outcomes, support enhanced staff performance, improve visitor participation, or encourage community support. It is in these areas that the breakthroughs of the next design decade will occur. It is here that the designers of the future will realize the potential for physical design to influence positively levels of performance. It is in this dimension of design that a future will be created that would not have happened otherwise.

To create this new future, I believe the following steps are critical:

1. *Continue to grow as an industry.* At its most basic level, expansion of the healthcare design industry provides recognition of design's ability to improve the quality of healthcare, and it enhances the credibility of the industry. Crucial to the growth of the industry is the need for its members to become organized and to communicate with one another.

Design competitions and award programs provide a platform for high quality, life-enhancing design to be recognized, both within the industry and by the general public. At all times, it must be kept in the forefront of awareness that the general public is the recipient of the benefits of design's contributions.

Growth as an industry means much more than numbers of people. Growth is a natural reflection of an industry that invests in itself. Areas in which this investment may be seen is in the creation of *new research*, development of *new technologies*, and realization of *new strategic opportunities*.

Particularly in the area of healthcare design, in which the background of facility decision makers is deeply rooted in science and business, the need for quality *research* is critical to demonstrate design's ability to influence positively desired levels of performance. Investment by the healthcare design industry is required for industry growth to occur. This necessary research will take time and financial resources. For useful, accessible, quality research to become available as an industry resource, the industry will have to be sufficiently well organized to manage the creation and dissemination of the material.

The development of new *technologies* also requires research and development investment. This is clearly true for product manufacturers, but equally true for healthcare providers and design professionals as well. For providers, this investment might be in program development, while for design professionals it might be in the utilization of computer applications. In all three of these cases, progress cannot occur without the investment of time and money.

Investment for the realization of new *strategic opportunities* is also crucial for the growth of the industry. Recent examples of strategic investment include the development of the LDRP concept or the Planetree unit. In each example, innovative program strategies were integrated with sophisticated design applications to produce a new departure in healthcare. Without an investment in strategy, neither would have been possible.

2. *Approach each project as an opportunity to experiment and demonstrate.* The industry can benefit from developing progressive benchmarks. To sustain the advancement of progress, it is necessary for new projects to be influenced by those that have been previously executed and evaluated. Scientific rigor is essential for developing progressive benchmarks. Project programming must include quantifiable measures of desired performance characteristics, as well as the investigation and inclusion of pertinent research. Design professionals must become accountable for project performance, which is measured in a series of follow-up, postoccupancy evaluations. Since most design professionals are not trained in the scientific methods required for this type of rigor, it will be necessary to engage the consulting services of additional project team members, such as environmental psychologists, social scientists, statisticians, and researchers.

The basis for publication of projects in magazines should be the measure that it advances the benchmark of the industry. If this were the case, each published project would serve as a demonstration of what design is capable of contributing to the quality of healthcare.

3. *Remember that design is simply and only a reflection of values.* The organization that commissions design articulates its values by establishing the design direction, setting priorities, and creating an expression of its culture. Equally so, the design professional is responsible for collecting the necessary data, interpreting it, and translating it into the design of an environment that outwardly states what the organization believes in. An organization with strong beliefs and deep values will have these clearly expressed in the environment.

Organizations that value patients' lives, staff well-being, visitor participation, and community health guide the expression of their environment's design so that these core values are clearly stated and understood. Good design, in this sense, is a measure of the designer's ability to assist the organization in articulating its values and creating a design that positively influences the desired performance outcomes.

In the contemporary environments of our technologically sophisticated age, one frequently finds basic human needs compromised. True progress, in the sense of realizing the contribution that design can make to the quality of healthcare, will only be made when environments provide direct access to both daylight and fresh air.

Furthermore, giving inhabitants the ability personally to control aspects of their environment is an important step in recognizing the very nature of human beings. What each person needs is different and the ideal environment—particularly a healthcare environment—should be able to respond to an individual's preference for air quantity, quality, temperature, humidity, and movement; quality and quantity of light; color; acoustical privacy and control; odor and fragrance; art; dietary selection; decoration; privacy; room size and shape; audiovisual media; bed adjustment; and room layout. Although this degree of choice may seem extreme, it is only a brief matter of time before the patient in a progressive setting will be able to make these selections.

4. *Be a lifelong learner.* The final suggested "next step" to create a future that would not have happened otherwise is for each of us to continue learning. As the healthscape evolves and our industry continues to make progress, new opportunities will continually present themselves. For the industry to grow, the individuals within the industry must grow. They must read, tour projects, attend symposia, and network. They must welcome opportunities to stretch their capabilities.

The very nature of work related to healthcare requires a big heart. We must create opportunities to enlarge our hearts and express this in the design of caring, compassionate, joyful environments. When our growth and learning stops, our industry will lose its responsiveness and vitality.

One thing that is certain about the future is that it just keeps happening. As human beings, we can choose to be observers or active participants in the crafting of our personal and global future. Each life situation presents us with a fresh choice. We are fortunate to be living at a time in history in which the choices we are currently making will benefit the world population for generations to come. Collectively, we can create a desired future that would not have happened otherwise.

Wayne Ruga, AIA, IIDA, Allied Member ASID, is an architect, as well as the president and CEO of The Center for Health Design, a nonprofit organization in Martinez, California that was formed in 1993 to promote the widespread development of health-enhancing environments through research and education. The center oversees the activities of the National Symposium on Healthcare Design, which has, since 1988, been dedicated to producing educational programs and publications that explore how the design of the physical environment can positively affect the quality of healthcare.

INDEX